MEDICAL RADIOLOGY

Radiation Oncology

Editors:
L. W. Brady, Philadelphia
H.-P. Heilmann, Hamburg
M. Molls, Munich

Springer-Verlag Berlin Heidelberg GmbH

V. Grégoire · P. Scalliet · K. K. Ang (Eds.)

Clinical Target Volumes in Conformal and Intensity Modulated Radiation Therapy

A Clinical Guide to Cancer Treatment

With Contributions by

A. Bosly · R. Bristow · M. Cengiz · K. S. C. Chao · E. E. Coche · G. Cosnard · T. Duprez
P. A. Gervaz · M. Gospodarowicz · V. Grégoire · L. L. Gunderson · M. G. Haddock · M. Hamoir
K. Haustermans · T. Haycocks · T. Herzog · M. Jewett · I. C. Kiricuta · B. G. Lengelé
A. Lerut · M. Lonneux · P. Loubeyre · M. Milosevic · F. Mornex · H. Nelson · B. O'Sullivan
P. W. T. Pisters · L. Renard · H. Reychler · P. Rocmans · P. Scalliet · B. Tombal · P. van Houtte
F. Vaylet · J. Wunder

Foreword by

L. W. Brady, H.-P. Heilmann and M. Molls

Preface by

H. Suit

With 92 Figures in 222 Separate Illustrations, 129 in Color and 73 Tables

Springer

Vincent Grégoire, MD, PhD
Pierre Scalliet, MD, PhD
Department of Radiation Oncology
Université Catholique de Louvain
Cliniques Universitaires Saint-Luc
Avenue Hippocrate 10, UCL 10/4752
1200 Bruxelles
Belgium

K. Kian Ang, MD, PhD
Department of Radiation Oncology
UT MD Anderson Cancer Center
Houston, TX 77030
USA

Medical Radiology · Diagnostic Imaging and Radiation Oncology
Series Editors: A. L. Baert · L. W. Brady · H.-P. Heilmann · M. Molls · K. Sartor

Continuation of
Handbuch der medizinischen Radiologie
Encyclopedia of Medical Radiology

ISBN 978-3-642-07463-9

Library of Congress Cataloging-in-Publication Data

Clinical target volumes in conformal and intensity modulated radiation therapy: a
clinical guide to cancer treatment / V. Grégoire, P. Scalliet, K. K. Ang (eds.); with
contributions by K. K. Ang ... [et al.]; foreword by L. W. Brady, H.-P. Heilmann, and M. Molls.
p. ; cm. -- (Medical radiology)
Includes bibliographical references and index.
ISBN 978-3-642-07463-9 ISBN 978-3-662-06270-8 (eBook)
DOI 10.1007/978-3-662-06270-8

1. Cancer--Radiotherapy. I. Grégoire, V. (Vincent), 1962- II. Scalliet, P. (Pierre),
1953- III. Ang, K. K. (K. Kian) IV. Series.
[DNLM: 1. Neoplasms--radiotherapy. 2. Radiotherapy Dosage. 3. Radiotherapy,
Conformal--methods. QZ 269 C6416 2002]
RC271.R3 C58 2002
616.99'40642--dc21 2002075846

springeronline.com

Originally published by Springer-Verlag Berlin Heidelberg New York in 2004
Softcover reprint of the hardcover 1st edition 2004

Cover-Design and Typesetting: Verlagsservice Teichmann, 69256 Mauer

21/3111 - 5 4 3 2 1 - Printed on acid-free paper SPIN 11502388

Foreword

The advances in radiation oncology in the past 50 years are probably more dramatic than those that occurred in the first half of the 20th century. There have been major technical achievements associated with increased overall cure rates for cancer from 20% at 5 years 50 years ago to now nearly 60% at 5 years. The cure rates in selected tumor sites at 5 years in 1950 and in 2000 respectively were as follows: breast, 50% and 80%; colon and rectum, 40% and 85%; lung, 5% and 15–20%; prostate, 40% and 80%; Hodgkin's disease, 50% and more than 90%; cervix, 40% and 70–80%; uterus (endometrium), 80% and more than 90%; bladder, 30% and 50%; head and neck, 30% and 60%; esophagus, 2% and 15%. A significant proportion of these advancements have been due to a broader array of techniques available in radiation oncology for treatment, as well as emphasis on combined integrated multimodal treatment with surgery, radiation therapy, and chemotherapy.

The volume by Grégoire, Scalliet and Ang identifies a new technique with regard to conformal radiation therapy that allows for appropriate selection and delineation of clinical target volumes for different tumor sites. Included within that definition is the knowledge of lymph node areas with potential microscopic involvement, addressing the issues of those areas that must be included in the target volumes.

The volume makes significant and important data available relative to clinical, radiological, and pathological examiniation for surgical specimens as well as the patterns of local regional relapse to influence the recommendations for the selection of clinical target volumes. Three-dimensional reconstructed treatment planning and three-dimensional reconstructed treatment delivery to the identified primary tumor as well as the potentially involved regional lymph node involvement would be associated with improvement in the ultimate outcome. These basic data allow for decisions that are important in selection and delineation of the target volume, emphasizing the appropriate radiation therapy techniques. This information is crucial with regard to the maximization of tumor control and the minimization of complications from the treatment regimen.

Without question, these data are important in making more appropriate and proper use of the radiation therapy technology. These advances, based on major clinical information from surgical and pathologic studies along with clever and careful biologic research, form the foundation for conformal treatment and its ultimate contribution to the care of the cancer patient.

Philadelphia
Hamburg
Munich

Luther W. Brady
Hans-Peter Heilmann
Michael Molls

Preface

This book deals comprehensively with the critically important requirement for radiation oncologists to integrate knowledge of the anatomy and the new imaging techniques for planning and delivery of radiation treatment. The remarkable and rapid gains in the technical ability of the physicists and engineers to deliver radiation dose to any defined target volumes in patients with an uncertainty of only a few millimeters has resulted in much more intense emphasis on defining the target and the secure knowledge of the position of the entirety of the target relative to the beam throughout each treatment session.

Currently, high-technology radiation treatments include three-dimensional conformal, intensity-modulated radiation treatment planning/delivery and high-resolution online portal imaging. Thus, there is the requirement for accurate knowledge in the individual patient of the exact position of the primary and secondary targets. This book places heavy and appropriate emphasis on defining the location of lymph node chains in each patient. That is, the treatment volume should not be based on the volumes of tissues in which a particular nodal chain is found in a patient population, but rather on the location of the node chain of concern in the particular patient whose treatment is being planned. In parallel, it is necessary to define the extent and pattern of subclinical tumor. Further, the distinction between edema and inflammatory changes owing to tumor infiltration is essential. These considerations apply similarly to radiation therapy and surgery, as the target volumes are, of course, exactly the same for the two modalities. These imaging techniques include very thin section CT, MRI, MRS, ultrasound and PET. Advances in both the precision and the accuracy of these techniques are in development for specific sites, e.g., paramagnetic iron oxide as the contrast agent for visualization of lymph nodes.

A central theme in this book is the detailed presentation of the anatomy of the lymph node chains and the likelihood of nodal involvement for tumors at different body sites. The opening chapter is an extensive and scholarly description of the anatomy of the lymph vessels and nodes at various parts of the human body. This is followed by analysis of imaging of lymph nodes using CT, MRI and PET.

The ensuing chapters are valuable contributions on the anatomy and treatment planning at specific sites: head and neck, lung, esophagus, breast, prostate, bladder, gynecologic tumors, rectum/anus, sarcoma of soft tissues and lymphomas. In most of these, there is consideration of identification of the number, size and anatomic distribution of lymph nodes and the probability of their involvement by metastatic tumor.

The authors are well recognized for their expertise in their respective fields. The information contained in this book will serve as a valuable resource for daily practice for both the clinician and the physicist. Significantly, this book constitutes a highly useful aid in the education of young doctors.

Herman Suit
Andres Sorian Distinguished Professor of Radiation Oncology,
Harvard Medical School / Radiation Oncologist,
Massachusetts General Hospital, Boston, Massachusetts, USA

Introduction

Radiation oncology is a relatively young medical speciality that focuses on the treatment of neoplastic diseases using ionizing radiation. The fascination for using ionizing radiation in medical treatment started right after the discovery of X-rays by Wilhelm Conrad Röntgen in 1895 and isolation of radium by Marie and Pierre Curie in 1898. Among the first documented medical uses of radiation was that in 1896, when a Viennese dermatologist, Leopold Freund, treated the hairy nevus utilizing the very low dose rate X-rate tube available at that time. However, without rudimentary understanding of how radiation affected living tissues, radiation was mostly used by dermatologists and surgeons during the first two decades of the twentieth century as a form of cautery. High single radiation doses were generally administered that caused tissue sloughing, which led to morbid sequelae. Such casual applications of radiation resulted in a general skepticism about its usefulness as a therapeutic modality during the first two decades of the twentieth century, but the specialty has come a long way since then.

More systematic applications and investigations of radiation for medical treatments began around 1920. This was characterized by a swing toward fractionated treatment in Paris, Zurich, and Vienna, based on the pioneering clinical work of Regaud, Coutard, Schwarz, Holzknecht and others complemented by experimental findings on the sterilization of testicles in the grasshopper and rabbit. The field of radiation oncology then evolved gradually, starting in Europe, at first in combination with diagnostic radiology but subsequently growing to a separate speciality at varying speeds in different countries. "Fractionation in Radiotherapy", edited by Thames and Hendry and published by Taylor and Francis in 1987, is an excellent reference for readers interested in the history of the specialty.

Radiation oncology has experienced a number of "quantum leaps" brought about by combinations of advances in equipment engineering and better insight into biological processes governing cellular and tissue responses to ionizing radiation. The advent of telecobalt units followed by invention of accelerators producing both high-energy photons and electrons, for instance, made it possible to deliver potentially tumoricidal radiation doses even to deep-seated neoplasms without exceeding the tolerance of the skin and subcutaneous tissues. The development of technology for portal shaping (e.g., lead collimation or Cerrobend block) and beam intensity modulation (e.g., wedges and missing tissue compensator) along with computerized treatment-planning systems gradually improved the flexibility and precision of radiation dose delivery.

Simultaneous with gradual refinement of radiotherapy techniques, conceptions of basic biological principles had an important impact on radiation therapy. The idea of decreasing "density of clonogenic infestation" with increasing distance from the tumor epicenter, for example, led to the conception and validation of the "shrinking field" technique and laid the foundation for combining surgery and radiotherapy. More recently critical scrutiny of clinical and experimental data on the effects of radiation dose fractionation resulted in the design of biologically rational altered fractionation regimes, i.e., hyperfractionation and accelerated fractionation. The collective data of many phase III trials designed to test these biologically sound regimes indeed validated the superiority of some of the altered frationation regimens in yielding local-regional tumor control.

Advances in the knowledge of drug-radiation interaction have also generated enthusiasm for combining radiation with cytotoxic agents to improve therapy outcome. Numerous radiation-chemotherapy regimens, particularly when given concurrently, have been found in phase III studies to be better than radiation alone in obtaining local-regional control and survival of patients with a variety of cancers, but, unfortunately, too often at the cost of increased late normal tissues toxicity. Roaring progress in molecular and tumor biology is beginning, forming the foundation for development of a new generation of therapies targeting specific molecules or signaling pathways to selectively enhance the response of tumors with distinct molecular make-up.

Finally, the explosive growth in computer hardware and software along with improved design of medical linear accelerators has begun to revolutionize radiotherapy. The availability of computer-operated multi-leaf collimators offers the flexibility not only to dynamically shape the radiation portal but also to vary the beam intensity across the portal. This capacity, along with improvements in the accuracy of tumor delineation through progress in diagnostic imaging methodology, has introduced an unprecedented era of high-precision radiation therapy. This relatively new technology will improve physical targeting of tumors, i.e., deliver high radiation doses to three-dimensional volumes that conform to the shapes of tumors and involved nodes, thereby reducing the dose administered to normal tissues. In general terms, such high-precision radiation delivery is, therefore, referred to as three-dimensional conformal radiotherapy (3-D CRT) or simply conformal radiotherapy.

Proper application of conformal radiotherapy, however, demands greater familiarity with tumor and normal tissue anatomy and better knowledge of the patterns of contiguous and lymphatic spread to minimize the risk of geographically missing tumors or their potential microscopic extension. Therefore, this volume attempts to provide general introductory guidelines for delineation of the gross target volume and clinical target volume for a number of common neoplasms as a practical day-to-day reference for novices in the field. We are grateful that many radiation oncologists who pioneered the clinical use of conformal radiotherapy have contributed to this project. It is important to keep in mind in using this handbook that general guidelines cannot address all possible clinical permutations, so that it may be prudent to apply rational clinical judgement or consult more experienced colleagues in unusual cases. We also anticipate that these general guidelines will require further refinement based on emerging clinical experience. Therefore, we will appreciate feedback, remarks, and advice.

Bruxelles
Houston
Bruxelles

Vincent Grégoire
K. Kian Ang
Pierre Scalliet

Contents

1 The Lymphatic System

Anatomical Bases for Radiological Delineation of Lymph Node Areas

B. G. Lengelé

CONTENTS

B. G. Lengelé, MD, PhD, FCCP
Professor and Head of the Human Anatomy Department, Université Catholique de Louvain, Avenue E. Mounier 52.40, 1200 Brussels, Belgium

1.1 Introduction

The lymphatic system is constituted of numerous fine vessels which traverse several groups of nodes and transport the lymph into the venous system. The capillaries of origin have closed extremities which are disseminated within the connective tissues beyond the epithelial lining, and which through several interconnecting anastomoses form primary networks which drain the lymphatic fluid into the first collecting ducts. Passing through the successive groups of lymph nodes, these ducts again divide into capillaries and then finally give rise to the larger collecting vessels which are usually two in number: the thoracic duct and right lymphatic duct, which join the left and right brachiocephalic veins respectively.

The lymphatic vessels have very thin endothelial walls, are filled with a clear colourless fluid, and are usually not visible in living tissue so that various staining or radio-opaque substances have to be injected before their distribution and general pathways can be studied. In the small intestine, however, they have a milk-white appearance during the immediate postprandial period, which explains their original name of *lacteal veins*. They possess numerous valves which result in a characteristic moniliform appearance and are present in all tissues of the human body except for avascular structures such as the epidermis, the cornea and the cartilage. They are also absent in the brain, spinal cord, and bone marrow.

According to their location, the lymphatic vessels branch into two networks located respectively above and below the deep fasciae. The superficial lymph vessels drain the skin and the subcutaneous tissue and tend to run alongside the superficial veins, though some may be independently situated. Vessels of the deep subfascial network similarly course alongside the arteries and veins. They are connected to the nodes and unite to form deep main lymphatic channels which are usually located at the outer surface of the large veins. In rare cases, however, some of them may pass behind the venous blood vessels. Such an arrangement, which was already emphasised by Poirier two centuries ago, appears to be of major clinical importance not only for surgical dissection of the lymphatic chains, but also for the radiological delineation of the main lymph node areas which are invariably located on the superficial aspect of the large deep veins.

A relative separation exists between the lymph vessels of the epi- and subfascial plexuses. Nevertheless, anastomoses occur between both networks which as a rule lead the superficial channels to drain into the deeper channels. On the other hand, a large number of connecting channels unite neighbouring ducts so that most of the lymphatic areas of the body communicate freely with the adjacent regions. Major drainage pathways are thus constituted from the proximal capillary networks originating in the peripheral organs through collecting ducts which penetrate the lymph nodes and finally rejoin the main ducts. Some of these pathways cross the midline, while others directly reach the thoracic duct without traversing any node. From one region, several distinct pedicles also extend that reach the same distal destination but take different routes with various intermediate nodal relays. When considering these anatomical aspects, for each organ or topographical area it is possible to define a preferential pathway of lymphatic drainage which is also the principal means of lymphatic spread for neoplastic or inflammatory cells in pathological situations. On this main axis, the first targeted lymph node is called the *sentinel node*. Nevertheless, the large number of alternative connecting channels, combined with the plasticity of the lymph vessels which have a marked capacity for regeneration after obstruction or damage, provide the lymphatic system with a dynamic functional structure in which all the areas described below have a constant anatomical location, but display variable circulating relationships and a relative independence from the neighbouring regions.

1.2 Major Collecting Ducts

1.2.1 The Thoracic Duct

The *thoracic duct* (Fig. 1.1) drains the lymph from the subdiaphragmatic part of the body and from the left chest, left upper limb and left part of the head and neck, back into the blood circulation. Originating from the cisterna chyli located in front of the first and second lumbar vertebrae, it enters the thorax through the aortic hiatus of the diaphragm and then follows the anterior aspect of the vertebral column to reach the posterior mediastinum. Usually not visible on computed tomography (CT) or magnetic resonance (MR) images, it occupies a narrow space between the azygos vein on its right, the hemi-azygos vein on its left, the thoracic vertebrae located posteriorly, and the aorta and oesophagus on its anterior surface (Fig. 1.1). At the level of the fourth thoracic vertebra the duct then inclines to the left, running along the posterior aspect of the aortic arch and then along the left side of the oesophagus behind the origin of the subclavian artery. Reaching the lower part of the neck through the left side of the thoracic inlet, it finally arches laterally near the transverse process of the seventh cervical vertebra, crosses over the prescalenic portion of the subclavian artery and finally ends by opening into the area between the left internal jugular and subclavian veins. At this point, a valvular bicuspid system prevents the blood from being sent back into the terminal part of the duct, but sometimes inducing blockage of the latter by metastatic cellular thrombi.

During its course, tributaries from the intercostal and posterior mediastinal nodes flow into the thoracic duct. At its origin in the cisterna chyli, it drains both lumbar trunks that collect lymph from the lower limbs, the pelvis and the posterior abdominal walls, together with large intestinal trunks originating from all parts of the intra-abdominal digestive system. In the neck, the thoracic duct is joined by the left jugular trunk from the left side of the head and neck, the left subclavian trunk from the left upper limb, and the left bronchomediastinal trunk which usually collects the ascending lymph from the left chest viscera together with the parietal lymphatic channel from the parasternal nodes.

1.2.2 The Right Lymphatic Duct

Described by Poirier and Charpy as the great lymphatic vein, the *right lymphatic duct* (Fig. 1.1) is formed by the union of the right jugular, subclavian and bronchomediastinal trunks which collect the lymph from the right half of the head and neck, the right upper limb, the right side of the thorax and right lung, and part of the convex surface of the

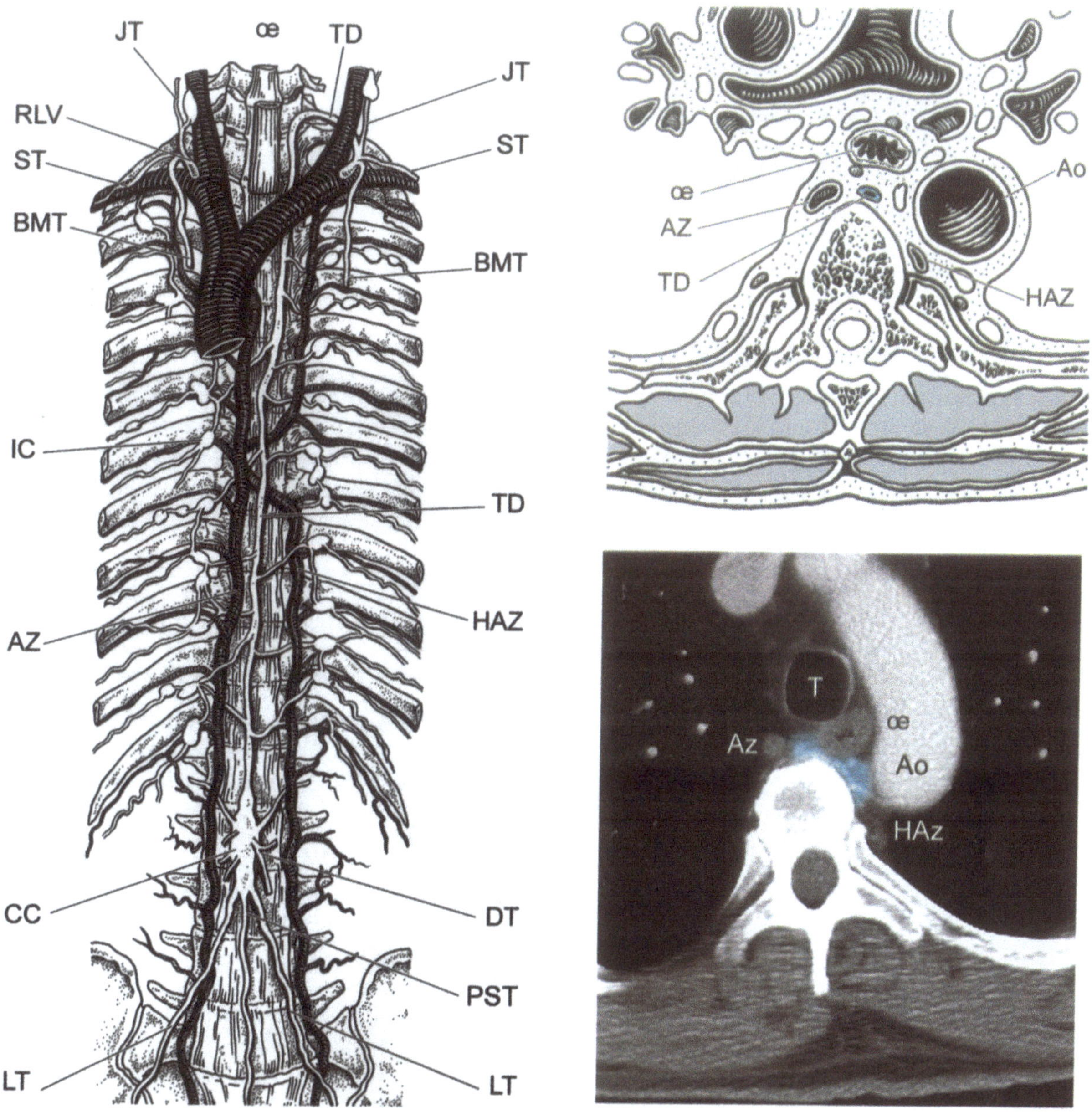

Fig. 1.1. Major collecting ducts of the lymphatic system. Anterior anatomical view of the main ducts and trunks, with the corresponding anatomical and CT sections at the thoracic level. The key structures for the delineation of the thoracic duct area (*green frame*) are as follows: the azygos (*AZ*) and hemiazygos veins (*HAZ*), thoracic aorta (*Ao*) and the oesophagus (*Oe*). *TD* thoracic duct, *RLV* right lymphatic duct, *ST* subclavian trunks, *JT* jugular trunks, *BMT* bronchomediastinal trunks, *CC* cisterna chyli, *LT* lumbar trunks, *PST* presacral trunk, *DT* digestive trunks, *IC* intercostal nodes

liver, respectively. The duct measures about 1 cm in length and runs along the medial side of the scalenus anterior, displays a large number of variations in the confluence pattern of its tributaries and finally enters the venous system at Pirogoff's angle, located at the junction of the right subclavian and internal jugular veins.

1.3 Lymphatics of the Head and Neck

Following the general arrangement of the lymphatic system in the various parts of the body, the lymph nodes of the head and neck area (Fig. 1.2) consist of superficial and deep groups of nodes which form a

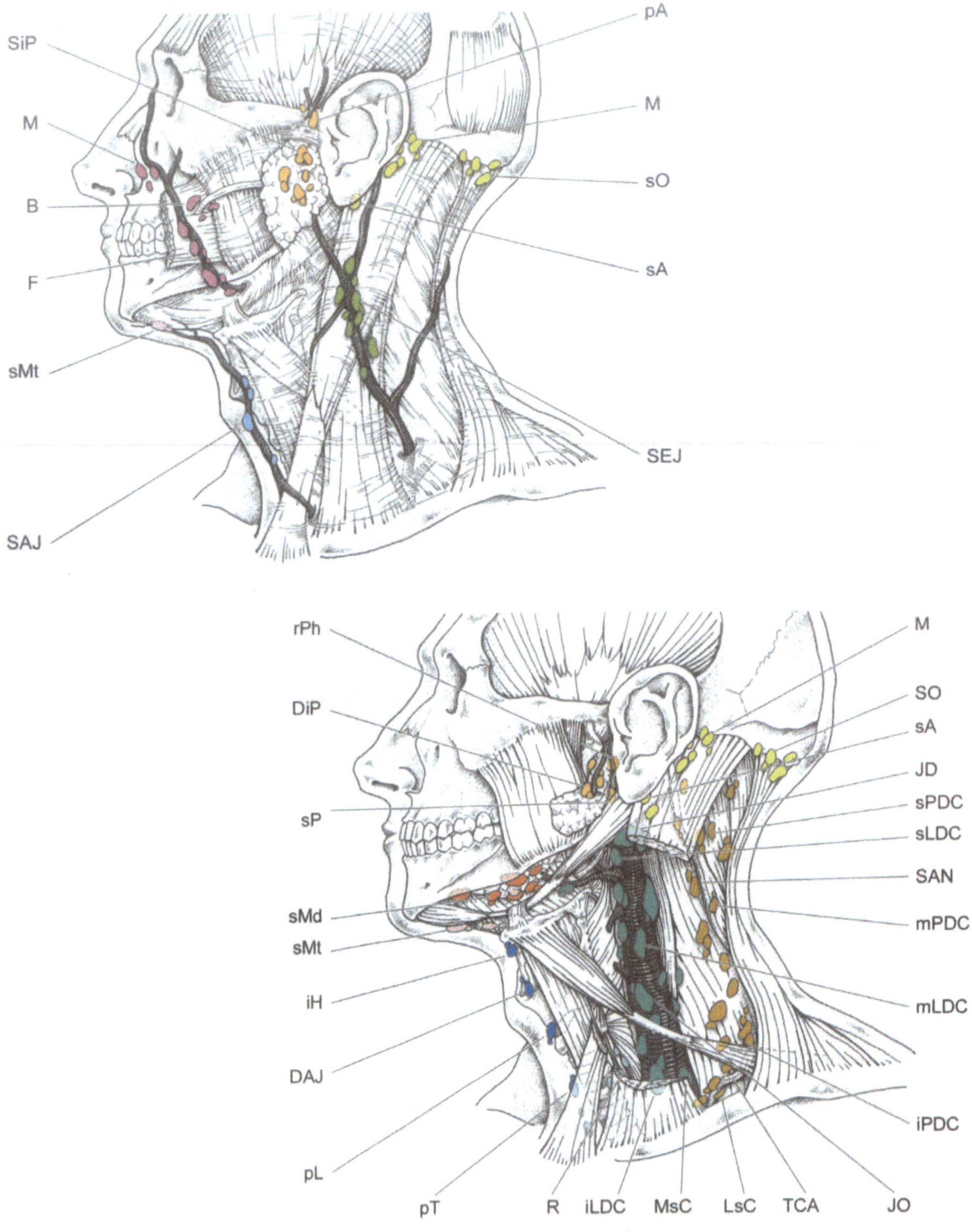

Fig. 1.2. Lymphatic nodes of the head and neck. Lateral view of the superficial and deep node groups of the cervicocephalic region. Node groups are identified by different *colours* corresponding to the surgical and radiological classification given in Fig. 1.3. *B* buccal n.; *DAJ* deep anterior jugular n.; *DiP* deep intraparotid n.; *F* facial n.; *iH* infrahyoid n.; *JD* jugulodigastric n. (Kütner's); *JO* jugulo-omohyoid n. (Poirier's); *LDC* superior (*s*), middle (*m*) and inferior (*i*) lateral deep cervical n.; *LsC* lateral supraclavicular n.; *M* malar n.; *MsC* medial supraclavicular n.; *PDC* superior (*s*), middle (*m*) and inferior (*i*) posterior deep cervical n.; *M* mastoid n.; *pA* preauricular n.; *pL* prelaryngeal n.; *pT* pretracheal n.; *R* recurrent n.; *SAJ* superficial anterior jugular n.; *sA* subauricular n.; *SEJ* superficial external jugular n.; *SiP* superficial intraparotid n.; *sMd* submandibular n.; *sMt* submental n.; *sO* suboccipital n.; *sP* subparotid n.; *rPh* retropharyngeal n.

transverse collar along the cervicocephalic junction and then a vertical chain which lies under the sternocleidomastoid muscle, along the large vessels of the neck and the last cranial nerves, from the base of the skull downwards to the supraclavicular area. All these nodes are connected by numerous small vessels within the loose adipose tissue between the superficial, pretracheal and prevertebral laminae of the cervical fascia. These vessels give rise to a complex subcutaneous and subfascial lymphatic network, and, with the interposed node groups, constitute major and accessory chains which following a specific pattern drain all the visceral and cutaneous parts of the face and neck regions. In each area there is an ipsilateral drainage pathway into the main jugular or accessory chains. However, some median skin areas and organs located posteriorly in the facial region have bilateral pathways of lymphatic drainage with significant clinical implications in the treatment of head and neck cancers.

1.3.1 Lymph Node Groups of the Pericervical Circle

The *pericervical circle* (Fig. 1.2) is divided into five nodal groups which are named according to their specific location. They can be distinguished according to where they are situated, i.e. their position from posterior to anterior: the occipital, mastoid, parotid, submandibular and submental groups. Additional often isolated nodes are classified as the facial and retropharyngeal groups.

The *occipital nodes* are usually from one to three in number. Lying near the lateral insertions of the trapezius muscle, they always occupy a subfascial plane and receive their afferent vessels from the posterior part of the hairy scalp. Their efferent vessels run downwards in the posterior cervical triangle and join the upper part of the posterior cervical accessory chain.

The *mastoid nodes* are located in the retro-auricular area, lie superficially to the attachments of the sternocleidomastoid muscle and are covered by the fascial extension of the auricularis posterior. Draining the temporal region of the hairy scalp, the posterior surface of the auricle and the posterior wall of the external acoustic meatus, they have efferent vessels which traverse the upper insertions of the sternocleidomastoid muscle to join the superior deep lateral cervical lymph nodes.

The *parotid nodes* are divided into four subgroups according to their specific relationship with the parotid gland and its fascial sheath. The most superficial of these nodes is situated in the subcutaneous tissue, immediately in front of the tragus. Usually characterised as the *subcutaneous pre-auricular node*, it drains lymph from the frontal skin, the eyelids and the conjunctiva into the intraparotid nodes which lie within the parotid space. Among these, the *superficial intraparotid nodes* are usually two to three in number, and are situated on the external surface of the gland beneath the parotid fascia. On the contrary, the *deep intraparotid nodes* are scattered throughout the glandular tissue and are mainly grouped along the external carotid artery and the intraparotid part of the external jugular vein. One of these nodes is invariably situated in the lower extremity of the gland near the mandibular angle. All these intraparotid nodes mainly receive their afferent vessels from the anterior surface of the auricle, the anterior wall of the external acoustic meatus, the tympanum, the frontal and temporal areas, and the root of the nose. Nevertheless, some of the deep intraglandular nodes are also connected to the *subparotid nodes* which are located between the parotid gland and the pharynx near the retrostylian space. In close contact with the internal carotid artery and internal jugular vein, these nodes receive afferent lymph vessels from the nasal cavities, the nasopharynx and the eustachian tube. Also linked to the retropharyngeal nodes, they share the caudal drainage of the intraparotid nodes into the superior nodes of the deep lateral cervical chains.

The *submandibular nodes* are located beneath the cervical fascia in the submandibular triangle. The latter is bounded medially by the lateral border of the anterior belly of the digastric muscle, cranially by the mylohyoid muscle and laterally by the medial surface of the mandible, from the mylohyoid line downwards to its basilar border. The submandibular nodes are usually from three to ten in number and are located on the bony and cutaneous surfaces of the submandibular gland, although some may be found on its deep surface facing the muscles of the floor of the oral cavity. One node is always present at the anterior end of the gland, while the others are located between the gland and the mandible, in front of and behind the facial artery where the latter curves around the bone. Additional nodes in this group also surround the course of the facial vein on the cutaneous surface of the gland, or are embedded in the glandular tissue itself. Their afferent vessels arise in the following areas: the alae, dorsum and tip of the nose, the cheek, the mandibular and maxillar alveolar ridges, the upper lip and lateral part of the lower lip, and finally the anterior third of the lateral borders of the tongue. Their efferent vessels cross the hyoid bone and terminate in the upper deep lateral cervical nodes.

Some of the afferent lymphatic vessels to the submandibular nodes make an additional relay in small *facial nodes*, also described as genian or *buccal nodes*. Located under the superficial musculo-aponeurotic layer of the face, these small nodes are distributed throughout the oblique course of the facial vessels in the infra-orbital area (*malar node*), within the nasogenian groove (*nasolabial nodes*), on the outer surface of the buccinator muscle near Stenon's duct (*buccinator node*), or between the anterior border of the masseter and the posterior border of the depressor anguli oris, beneath the platysma (*mandibular node*).

The *submental nodes* are located within the median suprahyoid triangle bounded posteriorly by the body of the hyoid bone and laterally by the medial borders of both anterior bellies of the digastric muscles. Lying in a subfascial plane, the submental nodes rest on the outer surface of the mylohyoid muscles and display a variable arrangement between the mandibular symphysis anteriorly and hyoid bone dorsally. Their afferent vessels drain the integuments of the chin, the central part of the lower lip, the floor of the oral cavity, and finally the tip of the tongue. Often decussating over the midline, their efferents join the nodes of the submandibular group or pass directly in the middle deep cervical lymph nodes.

Located behind the cephalic part of the pharynx, the *retropharyngeal nodes* can be considered the deepest-seated part of the peri-cervical circle. Facing the longus capitis that covers the lateral mass of the atlas, these nodes are usually two in number and occupy the narrow space between the prevertebral and peri-pharyngeal fasciae. They are laterally located, are highly inconstant on the midline and are in close relation with the pharyngeal constrictors anteriorly and the internal carotid artery laterally. They receive afferent vessels from the nasopharynx, the eustachian tube and the soft palate. Their efferent vessels pass behind the internal carotid artery to mainly reach the upper deep cervical lymph nodes. Nevertheless, some of them drain into the nodes of the subparotid group.

1.3.2 Descending Cervical Chains

The cervical chain nodes are distributed within the anterior and lateral areas of the neck, mainly alongside the various jugular veins (Fig. 1.2). Most of them form part of the deep lateral cervical chain which runs along the lateral side of the internal jugular vein located deep within the sternocleidomastoid muscle, and which drains directly into the jugular lymphatic trunk. Other nodes, however, join to form alternative pathways, i.e. the posterior cervical accessory chain, the superficial external jugular chain, and two anterior cervical chains known as the superficial anterior jugular chain and the deep prelaryngo-tracheal chain. In the lower part of the neck, a paratracheal recurrent chain is also present.

1.3.2.1 The Deep Lateral Cervical Chain

The *deep lateral cervical chain* is variably described as the carotid, internal jugular or substernomastoid chain. Extending from the tip of the mastoid process downwards to the clavicle, it contains three groups of large lymph nodes which are always arranged in a chain parallel to the antero-lateral side of the internal jugular vein medially and located beneath the sternocleidomastoid muscle laterally. According to their respective locations, these nodes are termed superior (upper), middle or inferior (lower) deep lateral cervical nodes.

The lymph nodes of the *superior deep lateral cervical group* lie in the triangular area delineated by the posterior belly of the digastric muscle cranially, the upper third of the internal jugular vein dorsally and the thyrolinguofacial venous trunk caudally. Also known as Kütner's jugulodigastric nodes, they receive afferent vessels from the parotid, submandibular and submental groups but are also directly connected to lymphatic vessels that drain the tongue and the oropharynx. Their efferents extend to the nodes of the middle and lower groups of the lateral cervical chain, or directly join the jugular trunk.

The *middle deep lateral cervical nodes* are related to the middle third of the internal jugular vein. Usually less numerous and smaller in size than those of the upper group, they are located between the hyoid bone and cricoid cartilage, above the point where the intermediate tendon of the omohyoid muscle crosses the internal jugular vein. Usually one of these nodes displays greater development than the others. It lies directly on the intermediate tendon of the omohyoid and is known as Poirier's jugulo-omohyoid node. Most of the afferent vessels in this group arise from the upper deep lateral cervical nodes, while the efferents descend into the lower nodes. However, Poirier's main node is also connected to the efferent vessels from the submandibular and submental nodes. Furthermore, the latter receives direct pathways that drain the tongue and the floor of the oral cavity.

The *inferior deep lateral cervical nodes* lie between the distal part of the sternocleidomastoid muscle and the lower third of the internal jugular vein. Their area is limited cranially by the omohyoid muscle and caudally by the sternal end of the clavicle. They receive afferent vessels from the upper and middle node groups of the chain, and also drain the lymph vessels from the supraclavicular nodes. Their efferent vessels drain into the jugular trunk or directly into the right or left collecting ducts.

1.3.2.2 The Deep Posterior Cervical Chain

The *deep posterior cervical nodes* are distributed within the posterior cervical triangle, bounded anteriorly by the posterior border of the sternocleidomastoid, posteriorly by the anterior border of the trapezius and inferiorly by the clavicle. They are usually small in size and round, and are situated on the dorsal aspect of the internal jugular vein, on the muscular bellies of the splenius, levator scapulae and scaleni muscles. Embedded in the cellulo-adipose tissue that occupies the space between the superficial and deep laminae of the cervical fascia, they show close relationships with the branches of the cervical plexus cranially, and with those of the brachial plexus in the subclavian area. Depending on their location in the upper, middle and lower parts of the posterior cervical triangle, they can be classified into three successive groups:

- The *superior posterior cervical nodes* are located in the narrow apex of the triangle, above the point where the spinal accessory nerve exits the posterior border of the deep surface of the sternocleidomastoid muscle. They are connected to the occipital nodes and drain the lymph from the posterior hairy scalp.
- The *middle posterior cervical nodes* surround the subcutaneous course of the accessory nerve. Occupying the middle part of the posterior cervical triangle, they are linked proximally to the submandibular and retropharyngeal nodes and thus collect the lymph from the naso- and oro-pharyngeal regions in addition to the nuchal region. Distally, their efferents terminate in the nodes of the supraclavicular group.
- The *inferior posterior cervical nodes* occupy the supraclavicular or subclavian area, and are situated distally to the posterior belly of the omohyoid muscle. They are connected to one another, and form a slightly oblique chain directed anteriorly and located around their accompanying anatomical structure, i.e. the cervical transverse artery. Their main afferent vessels originate from the upper (supraspinal) and middle (perispinal) groups of the posterior cervical chain. However, these infraspinal supraclavicular nodes also drain additional lymphatic vessels from the integuments of the arm and pectoral regions, and sometimes efferent vessels from the axillary nodes.

1.3.2.3 The Superficial Lateral Cervical Chain

The *superficial external jugular chain* extends along the external jugular vein and includes three to five superficial cervical nodes situated on the outer surface of the sternocleidomastoid muscle. Collecting the lymph from the lobule of the auricle, the floor of the acoustic meatus and the skin over the angle of the mandible, the highest node of the group is usually located near the point where the external jugular vein leaves the lower extremity of the parotid gland. Distally, the efferent vessels of this subcutaneous chain pass around the borders of the sternocleidomastoid muscle to enter the middle or lower deep lateral cervical nodes.

1.3.2.4 The Anterior Cervical Chains

The *superficial anterior jugular chain* runs parallel to the anterior jugular vein and comprises two to three small inconstant nodes located between the superficial and pretracheal lamina of the cervical fascia at the surface of the infrahyoid muscles. Draining the lymph from the anterior cervical skin regions, these nodes are connected proximally to those of the submental group and their efferent vessels extend into the nodes of the deep lateral cervical chain. Distally, the lower node occupies the suprasternal space and can sometimes use the bronchomediastinal trunk as an efferent pathway.

The *deep anterior cervical chain* contains several small lymph nodes which are situated beneath the lamina pretrachealis of the cervical fascia and usually below the infrahyoid muscles, immediately in front of the larynx and trachea. Depending on their specific location, they are referred to as the infrahyoid, prelaryngeal and pretracheal nodes, and are usually represented by a single inconstant node at each level. If present, the infrahyoid node is located in front of the thyrohyoid membrane. The prelaryngeal node, known as the 'delphian' node, is present on the cricothyroid membrane, in the narrow V-shaped space between the two cricothyroid muscles. Finally, the pretracheal nodes are spread along the anterior aspect of the trachea in close relation with the isthmus of the thyroid gland cranially and caudally with the inferior thyroid veins. All these nodes receive their afferent vessels from the glottic and subglottic parts of the larynx, the hypopharynx and the thyroid gland. Their efferent vessels run downwards into the inferior nodes of the main internal jugular chain.

The *recurrent chain* is associated with the recurrent laryngeal nerve. Deeply located in the visceral spaces of the neck, these nodes are very small and usually remain unrecognised during a cervical surgical procedure. Scattered within the areolar adipose tissue between the trachea and the oesophagus, they form a chain which continues caudally without any clear demarcation with the tracheobronchial group. As afferents, these nodes receive the lymphatic vessels from the inferior laryngeal pedicle, the lateral lobes of the thyroid gland and the cervical parts of the trachea and oesophagus. Their efferent vessels usually terminate in the lower deep lateral cervical or supraclavicular nodes. They never seem to drain into the neighbouring upper mediastinal node groups.

1.3.3 Functional Drainage Pathways

Arising from the various superficial or visceral parts of the cephalic region, the lymphatics of the head and neck follow several drainage pathways depending on their origin (Fig. 1.3). Taking into consideration the usual metastatic nodal extensions that can develop in malignant tumours from various sites, these preferential pathways can be classified as follows:

- The main lymphatic pathway starts from the submental nodes (level Ia) and passes through the submandibular (level Ib) and anterior jugulodigastric (level IIa) groups. So reaching the upper part of the internal jugular chain, the lymph then descends along the middle (level III) and lower (level IV) deep lateral cervical nodes and finally reaches the jugular collecting trunk. Connected proximally to the parotid and buccal groups of nodes, this central pathway basically drains the superficial areas of the face and the anterior segments of the oral and nasal cavities.
- The posterior accessory pathway originates from the posterior part of the jugulodigastric group (level IIb) and thereafter traverses the middle (level Va) and lower (level Vb) deep posterior cervical groups. So running successively alongside the accessory nerve and alongside the transverse cervical vessels, this additional lymphatic pathway offers an alternative means of drainage to the deep dorsal parts of the visceral cavities of the face including the nasopharynx, the oropharynx, the velum and the root of the tongue.
- The anterior lymphatic pathway is connected with the drainage of the median part of the lower lip, the anterior oral floor and the apex of the tongue. It follows direct connecting channels spread between the submental (level Ia) and the jugulo-omohyoid (level III) nodes or, more rarely, reaching the lower internal jugular (level IV) nodes. This alternative anterior pathway of nodal dissemination explains the routine clinical observation of inferior cervical skip metastases developing in the course of anterior tumours of the oral cavity. In cases of superficial or deep tumours located in the anterior cervical triangle (level VI), these may also extend along the superficial or deep anterior cervical chains respectively, before reaching the distal part of the main lymphatic pathway (level IV).
- Finally, the superficial lateral pathway is associated with the external jugular chain. Connected to the occipital and the mastoid node groups, it terminates in the deep main pathway. Functionally speaking, it is solely linked with the lymphatic drainage of the integuments of the posterior scalp and retro-auricular area.

In this complex lymphatic network consisting of numerous vessels and nodes, each tumour has a preferential pattern of dissemination whereby metastases enter the main chain, often invading a first group of nodes depending on where the primary tumour is located. From that point however, further spread may also follow several different routes, for instance via the anterior or posterior additional pathways. The more anterior the primary site, the greater the likelihood of

Fig. 1.3a–c. Surgical and radiological delineation of head and neck lymph nodes areas. Node groups (a) are currently classified into six levels (I–VI) to which should be added the parotid (*P*), retropharyngeal (*rp*) and buccal (*B*) areas. An additional external jugular level (VII) should also be considered. The corresponding volumes are delineated on anatomical sections and corresponding CT images of the head and successive neck regions respectively. The key structures for the delineation of the various target volumes are as follows: the sternocleidomastoid (*SCM*), infrahyoid (*IH*), digastric (*D*), pterygoid (*Pt*), longus capitis (*LC*), scaleni (*S*), splenius (*Sp*), levator scapulae (*LS*) and trapezius (*T*) muscles. Other landmarks are the internal (*IJV*), external (*EJV*), anterior (*AJV*) and posterior (*PJV*) jugular veins, the facial vein (*FV*), the submandibular (*SMG*) and thyroid glands (*TG*), cervical transverse artery (*CTA*) and the facial (*FN*), lingual (*LN*), vagus (*VN*) and spinal accessory (*SAN*) nerves. Legend and *colours* used to indicate the node groups are identical to those in Fig. 1.2

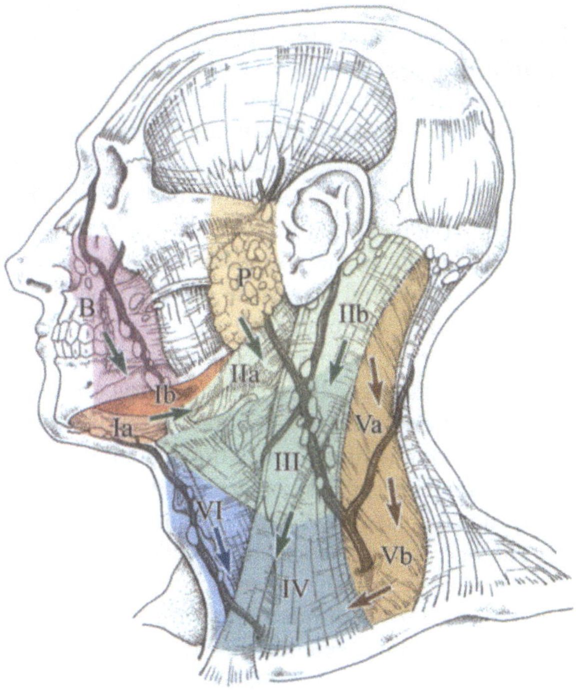
B
P
IIa
IIb
Ib
Ia
III
Va
VI
IV
Vb

a

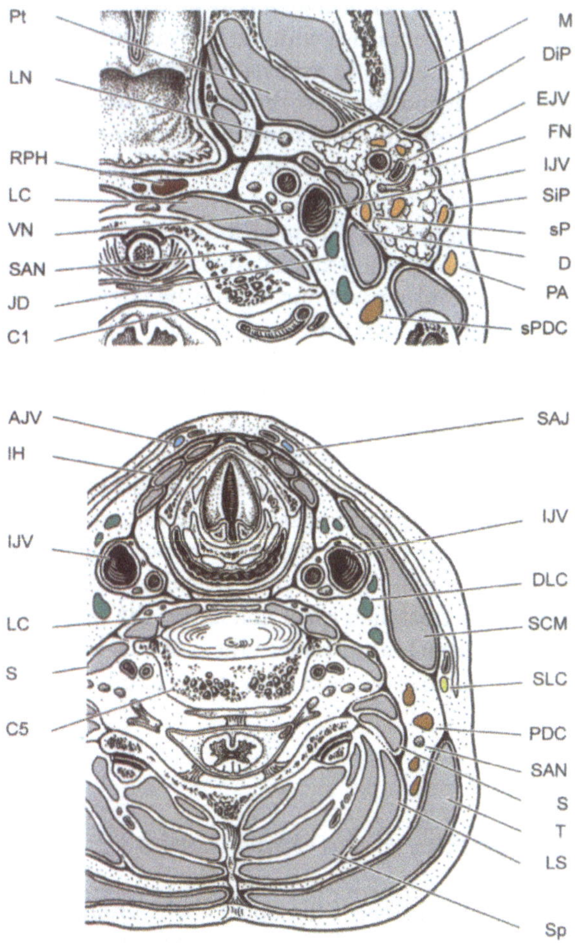
Pt
LN
RPH
LC
VN
SAN
JD
C1
M
DiP
EJV
FN
IJV
SiP
sP
D
PA
sPDC
AJV
IH
IJV
LC
S
C5
SAJ
IJV
DLC
SCM
SLC
PDC
SAN
S
T
LS
Sp

b

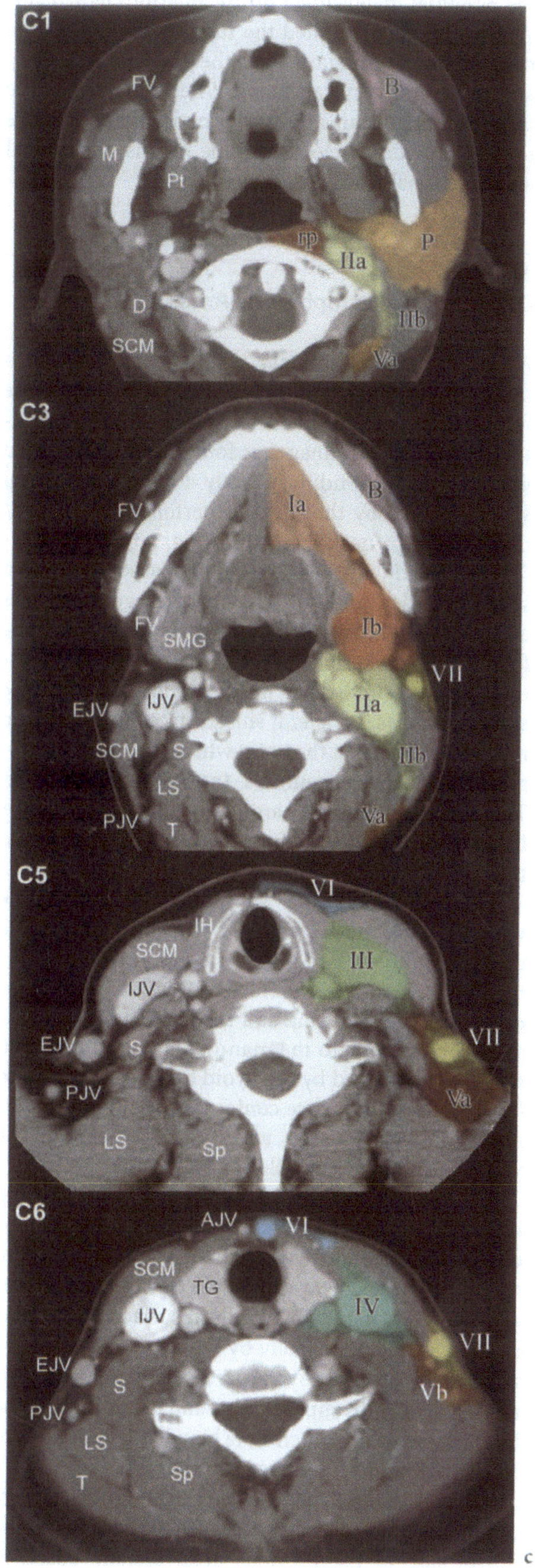
C1
FV
B
M
Pt
rp
P
IIa
D
IIb
SCM
Va
C3
FV
Ia
B
FV
SMG
Ib
VII
EJV
IJV
IIa
SCM
S
IIb
LS
PJV
T
Va
C5
VI
IH
SCM
III
IJV
EJV
S
VII
PJV
Va
LS
Sp
C6
AJV
VI
SCM
TG
IV
IJV
VII
EJV
S
Vb
PJV
LS
T
Sp

c

the potential involvement of the anterior chain. Conversely, the deeper seated the tumour, the higher the risk of lymphatic metastases in the posterior accessory and transverse cervical chains. When considering the three potential chains of dissemination, cancer of the tongue provides a clear example of this anatomical and functional reality.

1.3.4 Delineation of Lymph Node Areas

As an immediate corollary of the anatomical landmarks mentioned in the previous description, the lymph node areas of the head and neck can be identified on CT or MR images as four pyramidal-shaped volumes corresponding exactly to the anatomical spaces cleared by the surgeon performing a parotidectomy and a neck dissection (Fig. 1.3).

The *parotid area* is a cranially-based pyramidal space bounded anteriorly by the pterygoid muscles and the mandibular ramus, and posteriorly by a plane following the anterior border of the sternocleidomastoid, the posterior belly of the digastric muscle and the stylian muscles. Its lateral surface faces the skin, and its apex is located at the point where the sternocleidomastoid muscle encounters the mandibular angle. This space contains the parotid gland, the facial nerve, the external carotid and jugular vessels, in addition to the pre-auricular, superficial and deep parotid nodes.

The submental and submandibular nodes lie within the pyramidal volume between the inner side of the mandible laterally and the suprahyoid muscles medially. The inferior surface of this *submandibular area* faces the platysma at a sub-cutaneous level. Its apex corresponds to the mandibular symphysis and its base is bounded by the hyoid bone. In addition to level I nodes, this space contains the submandibular gland, the facial vessels, and on its medial wall, the vascular and nerve bundles of the tongue.

The *jugulocarotid area* (Fig. 1.3c) forms a long inverted pyramid which comprises the three groups of the deep lateral cervical chain and extends from the cranial base downwards to the clavicle. Its surfaces are bounded laterally by the deep surface of the sternocleidomastoid, medially by the large vessels of the neck, and posteriorly by the prevertebral muscles. This area is filled with adipose tissue and in addition to the blood vessels also contains the lymphatic structures of levels II, III and IV and the vagus nerve.

The *posterior cervical area* (Fig. 1.3c) is the last pyramidal-shaped volume located adjacent to the dorsal side of the previous area. Distally based in the supraclavicular zone, it has a narrow apical part located in the suboccipital plane. The volume then enlarges progressively in a caudal direction, and its lateral subcutaneous face follows the posterior border of the sternocleidomastoid and the anterior border of the trapezius. Responding anteriorly to the posterior face of the carotid artery and internal jugular vein, it is bounded dorsally by the bellies of the deep cervical muscles. Including the lymphatic vessels and nodes of the posterior and transverse cervical chains (level V), this dorsal cellulo-adipose area also contains the accessory nerve, the nerve roots of the cervical and brachial plexuses and the transverse cervical vessels.

In addition to these four main lymphatic areas, there are four laminar zones that circumscribe the buccal, anterior cervical, external jugular and retropharyngeal areas (Fig. 1.3c).

The *buccal area* is located between the nasolabial fold anteriorly and the anterior border of the masseter posteriorly. Bounded superiorly by the infraorbital foramen, it extends downwards to the lower mandibular edge and contains the satellite lymph nodes of the facial vessels.

The *anterior cervical area* is located in front of the larynx and the trachea with the lateral borders of the infrahyoid muscles as external boundary. Extending from the hyoid bone to the suprasternal notch, it crosses the midline and contains the superficial and deep anterior cervical chains (level VI), connected to the anterior jugular veins.

The *external jugular area* forms a narrow plane extending over the external surface of the sternocleidomastoid muscle and should be considered as an additional cervical level (level VII). Covered superficially by the thin layer of the platysma, it includes the superficial lateral cervical lymph nodes and the external jugular vein.

The *retropharyngeal area* is located at the level of the first two cervical vertebrae between the lateral half of the posterior pharyngeal wall and the prevertebral muscles. More laterally this space, which contains the retropharyngeal nodes, then becomes continuous with the retrostylian space containing the subparotid nodes, internal carotid artery, the proximal part of the internal jugular vein and the last four cranial nerves.

1.4 Lymphatics of the Upper Limbs

All the lymphatics of the upper limbs drain into the large nodes of the axilla, either directly or after passing through an intermediate group of small nodes. They are arranged in two layers, and either run superficially in the subcutaneous tissue converging towards the superficial veins, or course under the deep fasciae as close satellites of the main neurovascular bundles.

1.4.1 Axillary Lymph Nodes

The axillary nodes collect the lymph not only from the entire upper limb, but also from the cutaneous tissue of the upper part of the trunk and from the subjacent muscles (Fig. 1.4). Very large in size, they vary from 12 to 30 in number, and are scattered in the cellulo-adipose tissue within the axilla. According to their afferent vessels and respective relationships with the vascular structures of the axilla, they are divided into five groups which, however, are not clearly delineated:

- The *lateral* or *brachial group* includes four to six nodes situated on the infero-medial side of the axillary vein. Their afferent vessels drain the lymph from the superficial and deep compartments of upper limb, except for the superficial vessels of the arm that run alongside the cephalic vein. Their efferents have a threefold termination: most of them terminate in the central or apical groups, while others pass into the supraclavicular nodes.
- The *anterior* or *pectoral group* is composed of four to five nodes located behind the pectoralis major muscle and along the lower border of the pectoralis minor. Forming a chain along and behind the lateral thoracic vessels, these nodes receive afferent vessels from the skin and muscles of the anterior and lateral walls of the trunk above the umbilicus. They also drain the lateral parts of the breast, and their efferent vessels extend to the central and apical groups of axillary nodes.
- The *posterior* or *subscapular group* comprises six to seven nodes arranged above one another in a chain that follows the subscapular vessels, in the groove which separates, on the posterior wall of the axilla, the teres major and subscapularis muscles. The afferent vessels of this group collect the lymph arising from the muscles and skin of the back and from the scapular area downwards to the iliac crest. Their efferent vessels drain into the central and apical lymph nodes.
- The *central group* of axillary nodes usually contains three to five extremely large nodes, located in the central part of the adipose tissue of the axilla between the preceding chains which progressively converge towards them. Their efferent vessels then extend to the apical group.
- The *apical group* contains six to 12 large lenticular nodes which occupy the apex of the axilla, behind the upper portion of the pectoralis minor and partly above this muscle. The majority of these nodes rest on the infero-medial side of the proximal part of the axillary vein, in close contact with the upper digitations of the serratus anterior. Receiving afferent vessels from all the other axillary nodes, they also drain some superficial vessels running along the cephalic vein. The efferent vessels of this group unite to form the subclavian trunk which finally opens into the right lymphatic duct on the right side, or into the thoracic duct on the left side.

1.4.2 Superficial Lymph Nodes

Located on the surface of the deep fasciae, the superficial lymph nodes of the upper limbs are few in number and are invariably located in the subcutaneous tissue. Interposed on the superficial lymphatic pathways, they are known as the *supratrochlear* and *infraclavicular* groups (Fig. 1.5).

The *supratrochlear node* is usually isolated and deeply embedded in the subcutaneous fat, just over the deep fascia about 4–5 cm above the medial epicondyle of the humerus. Draining the superficial lymphatic pathways ascending from the ulnar side of the forearm, it sends efferent vessels which accompany the basilic vein to join the deep subfascial vessels.

The *infraclavicular nodes* are one to two in number, and consist of small interrupting nodes located near the cephalic vein in the deltopectoral groove. They are traversed by the superficial lymphatic vessels which drain the lateral skin of the arm and shoulder. Their efferent vessels pierce the clavipectoral fascia immediately below the clavicle and terminate in the apical group of axillary nodes. Nevertheless, some other vessels cross the anterior border of the clavicle and finally reach the deep cervical nodes of the supraclavicular group.

1.4.3 Functional Drainage Pathways

On a functional level, the superficial and deep lymphatic pathways of the upper limbs are almost completely segregated by the deep fasciae. Nevertheless, they finally converge towards the axilla and communicate with each other at both locations where the

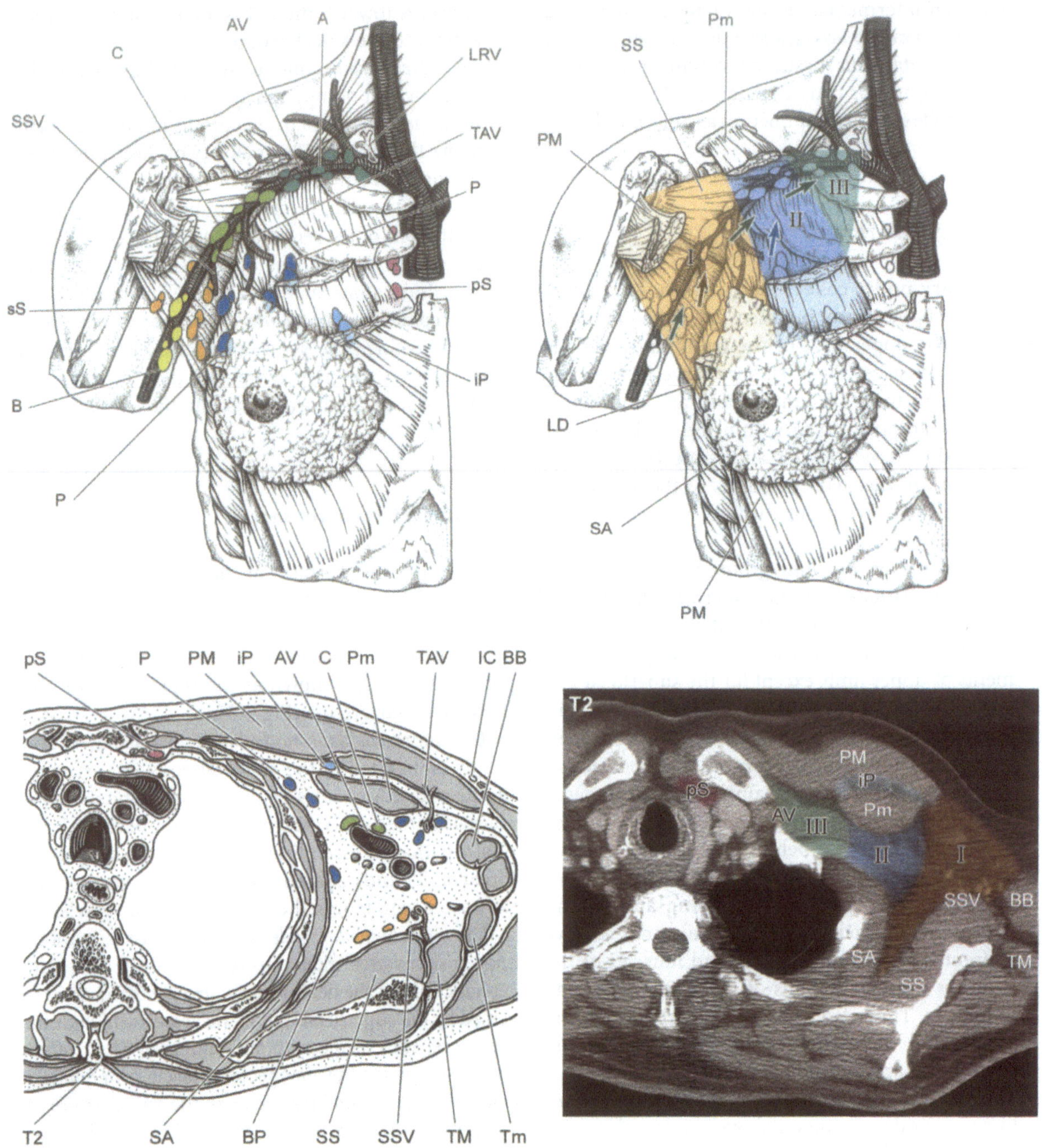

Fig. 1.4. Anatomical, surgical and radiological delineation of axillary lymph node areas. Anterior view of the axilla and chest after partial removal of the pectoral muscles with the corresponding levels (I–III) indicated on anatomical and CT sections. Lymph nodes are identified as follows: the brachial (*B*), pectoral (*P*), interpectoral (*iP*), subscapular (*sS*), central (*C*), apical (*A*) and the parasternal (*pS*) groups. The anatomical key structures to delineate the target volumes are: the pectoralis major (*PM*), pectoralis minor (*Pm*), serratus anterior (*SA*), latissimus dorsi (*LD*), teres minor (*Tm*), teres major (*TM*) and the subscapular (*SS*) and biceps brachii (*BB*) muscles. Other landmarks are given by the axillary vessels (*AV*), surrounded by the nerves of the brachial plexus (*BP*), and by the subscapular (*SSV*) and thoraco-acromial (*TAV*) arteries and veins. Levels (I–III) are bounded by the successive borders of the PM and Pm muscles, respectively, and do not match the limits of the anatomical node groups

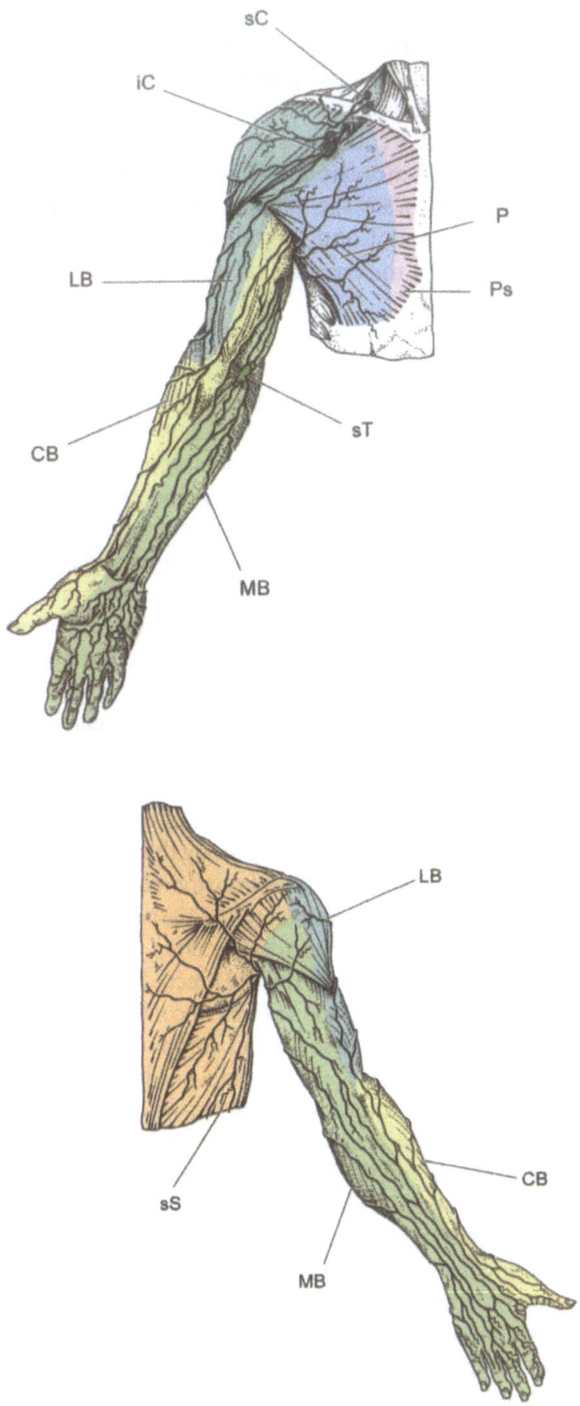

Fig. 1.5. Superficial lymphatic pathways of the upper limbs. Anterior and posterior anatomical views showing the distribution of vessels and nodes of the upper limbs. Nodes are identified as follows: the supratrochlear (*sT*), infraclavicular (*iC*) and supraclavicular (*sC*) nodes. Collecting vessels form three ascending drainage pathways classified as the medial brachial (*MB*), central brachial (*CB*) and lateral brachial (*LB*) pathways. Parietal vessels of the anterior and posterior chest walls run into the pectoral (*P*), parasternal (*pS*) and subscapular (*sS*) groups of nodes, respectively

superficial vessels, running alongside the basilic and cephalic veins accompany them through Morestin's and Cruveilhier's fascial foramina and then join the deep perivascular lymphatic channels.

The *superficial lymphatic pathways* (Fig. 1.5) issue from all parts of the cutaneous layers of the upper limb and originate in the hand from an extremely dense network with maximal development on the palmar surface of the fingers. These digital plexuses are drained by small collecting vessels which first follow the corresponding collateral artery but then incline backwards and pass into the dorsal aspect of the hand. The remainder of the palm is drained by vessels which course in front of the wrist and divide into medial, lateral and central small trunklets which then ascend towards the forearm along its ulnar, radial and palmar aspects. On the posterior surface of the forearm, the dorsal antebrachial channels pass progressively around the medial and lateral borders of the limb to join the vessels that course in front of the elbow. As they run upwards, these channels gradually decrease in number, and finally separate into three distinct superficial brachial pathways:

- The *medial brachial collecting vessels* follow the basilic vein, and some of them pass through the supratrochlear nodes above the elbow. Thereafter they perforate the fascia with the vein, join the deep collectors, and end in the brachial group of axillary nodes.
- The *central brachial collecting vessels* run longitudinally over the fascial sheath of the biceps brachii, pierce the axillary fascia along the anterior axillary fold, and terminate in the brachial nodes.
- The *lateral brachial collecting vessels* are associated with the cephalic vein and continue their course on the lateral side of the biceps brachii until they reach the deltopectoral groove. At this point most of them empty into the brachial group of axillary nodes. A few transit by the infraclavicular nodes which also receive lateral afferents from the deltoid area. Efferents from these nodes end, as previously stated, in the apical axillary nodes and sometimes in the cervical supraclavicular nodes.

During their course, the longitudinal superficial vessels undergo many divisions which sometimes diverge and sometimes converge, thereby creating several connections between the dorsal, central, lateral and medial pathways organised around the arm and forearm. Because of the large number of randomly distributed anastomosing channels, the pattern of lymphatic spread of a cutaneous tumour such as a melanoma is difficult to predict: for instance, the dissemination of a dorsomedial melanoma of the hand can first involve the palmar supratrochlear node, then the brachial group of the axilla. The potential however exists that if the dorsal collecting trunklets incline more likely around the lateral border of the forearm, there is a possibility of primary metastatic nodes being present in the infraclavicular group and then immediately in the apex of the axilla.

The *deep lymphatic pathways* of the upper limb comprise large collectors which are few in number and relatively less anastomosing than the superficial channels. Running around the axial vessels, they form radial, ulnar, interosseous and brachial ascending pathways which drain into the lateral brachial nodes of the axilla. Along their course small nodes can be found. Within the axilla, the main lymphatic channels arising from the lateral, anterior and posterior nodes successively pass through the central and apical groups of nodes. During their course along the axillary vein, they sequentially cross three topographical segments located respectively behind the lower part of the pectoralis major (level I), behind the pectoralis minor (level II), and finally above the upper border of the pectoralis minor in the subclavicular triangle (level III).

Closely linked to the lymphatic pathways of the upper limb, the *lymphatic vessels of the breast* are mainly directed toward the axilla (Fig. 1.4). Originating from a dense plexus in the interlobular connective tissue of the breast they communicate with the overlying subcutaneous network, especially around the nipple, giving rise to a subareolar circular plexus. The latter is drained by two or three main collectors which turn around the inferior border of the pectoralis major and which become satellites of the lateral thoracic vessels. Behind the muscle the *principal lymphatic pathway of the breast* thus reaches the anterior pectoral group of axillary nodes. Nevertheless, three *alternative drainage pathways* also exist, explaining the other primary locations of metastatic lymph nodes observed in breast cancer:

- The first accessory route is constituted by direct lymphatic vessels of the inferolateral part of the breast which adopt a more dorsal route and join the posterior subscapular nodes of the axilla.
- The second route involves lymphatic channels which arise from the upper parts of the gland and tend to follow the cutaneous branches of the thoraco-acromial artery. Most of these vessels pass through the fascicles of the pectoralis major and drain immediately into the apical axillary nodes. Between the pectoralis major and minor muscles, some of these vessels are interrupted by a large inconstant interpectoral node, usually known as Rotter's node. Others encounter the infraclavicular and supraclavicular nodes.
- The third alternative pathway is directed medially and comprises several channels running alongside the cutaneous perforating branches of the internal thoracic artery. Like the latter, these vessels perforate the medial attachments of the pectoralis major and the intercostal muscles and terminate in the parasternal lymph nodes.

1.4.4 Delineation of Lymph Node Areas

Except for the infraclavicular nodes which are located in the subcutaneous tissue facing the deltopectoral groove, all the main lymphatic groups of the upper limb are scattered within the quadrangular pyramidal space of the axilla. Filled with adipose tissue, the latter is easily delineated on CT and MR images as follows (Fig. 1.4): its anterior wall is constituted by the deep surfaces of the pectoralis major and minor muscles. Posteriorly, it is bounded by the subscapularis, teres major and latissimus dorsi muscles while the serratus anterior, covering the chest, delineates its medial boundary. Its lateral surface is usually narrowed and corresponds to the muscles of the arm running along the anteromedial surface of the humerus. The almost virtual base of the axillary volume corresponds to the tissue between the inferior borders of the pectoralis major anteriorly and the latissimus dorsi posteriorly. Directed upwards and medially, the apex of this volume is confined between the clavicle and the first rib and communicates in the manner of the constricted part of a sandglass, with the enlarged base of the supraclavicular area.

Within this volume, the inferior border of the pectoralis major and the inferolateral and superomedial edges of the pectoralis minor can be used as anatomical landmarks to separate the inferior (I), middle (II) and superior (III) levels of the axillary space. Narrowing progressively, these levels contain the anterior (pectoral), lateral (brachial), posterior (subscapular) and central groups of nodes (level I), then the central and apical groups of nodes (levels II and III), contiguous with their satellite vessels and nerves.

1.5 Lymphatics of the Thorax

The lymphatic system of the chest is clearly divided into two different functional groups of vessels and nodes. The first comprises the parietal lymphatics which drain the diaphragmatic and sternocostal walls of the thorax. The second concerns the visceral lymphatic system, associated with the various organs within the thoracic cavity.

1.5.1 Parietal Vessels and Nodes

Linked to the anterior, lateral and posterior integuments of the chest, the *superficial lymphatic vessels* of the thoracic walls ramify subcutaneously and converge towards the subscapular or pectoral axillary lymph nodes (Fig. 1.5). Those running along the anterior surface of the sternum may cross the midline and usually drain into the parasternal nodes, as previously described for the medial breast collectors.

The lymph vessels of the *deep parietal system* drain the muscles of the chest wall and, depending on their origin, join three groups of nodes, i.e. the parasternal, intercostal and superior diaphragmatic nodes (Fig. 1.6).

There are four to five *parasternal* or *internal thoracic nodes* on each side. Located behind the anterior ends of the intercostal spaces alongside the internal thoracic vessels, these nodes are separated from the anterior aspect of the pleura by the transversus thoracis muscle and the endothoracic fascia. Collecting vessels from the breast, they also receive afferents from the deepest parts of the anterior thoracic and abdominal walls above the umbilicus. Through a small group of nodes concealed behind the xiphoid process, they also drain the lymph from the superior part of the diaphragmatic surface of the liver. Their efferent vessels usually unite with those of the visceral nodes to form a single channel, the bronchomediastinal trunk, which terminates in the right or left large collectors, but which may also open directly into the internal jugular or subclavian veins.

The *intercostal nodes* are located dorsally and occupy the posterior extremities of the intercostal spaces in front of the head and neck of the ribs. They receive afferent vessels that are satellites of the posterior intercostal arteries. Their efferents drain into the thoracic duct on the left, or into the right lymphatic duct on the right side.

Scattered over the upper surface of the diaphragm, the superior *diaphragmatic nodes* are distributed into three separate groups on the anterior, lateral and posterior fleshy fascicles of the muscle. The anterior nodes are connected by their afferents to the liver and drain into the parasternal nodes. Arranged around the point where the phrenic nerve enters the diaphragm, the lateral diaphragmatic nodes are located close to the pericardium, and on the lateral aspect of the inferior vena cava on the right side; they collect the lymph from the costal part of the diaphragm and their efferents empty into the brachiocephalic or the posterior mediastinal nodes. Finally, the posterior diaphragmatic group consists of a few nodes on the back of the diaphragm, associated on the one hand with the abdominal aortic nodes, and on the other with the posterior mediastinal nodes.

1.5.2 Visceral Vessels and Nodes

The lymphatic nodes which drain the vessels originating from the thoracic viscera are all spread in the anterior, middle and posterior compartments of the mediastinum (Fig. 1.6). Depending on their location, they are classified as brachiocephalic, tracheobronchial and posterior mediastinal nodes.

The *brachiocephalic nodes* occupy the anterior part of the mediastinum around the brachiocephalic vein (level I), in front of the aortic arch (level V), and the pulmonary trunk (level VI) or between the large arterial vessels arising from the heart. Usually, enlarged lenticular nodes are found on the lateral side of the superior vena cava (Barthels' azygocaval node), between the latter and the ascending part of the aorta (interaorticocaval node) and between the aortic arch and the pulmonary trunk (Engels' aorticopulmonary node, also known as the ligamentum arteriosum node). Receiving their afferents from the thymus, the thyroid gland, the pericardium and the lateral diaphragmatic nodes, these anterior mediastinal nodes give rise to efferent ducts which unite with those from the tracheobronchial nodes to form the bronchomediastinal trunk.

The *tracheobronchial nodes* are concentrated around the tracheal bifurcation and include five different groups which frequently contain the largest nodes of the body: the *paratracheal nodes* (levels II and III) on the lateral sides of the trachea; the *superior (latero)tracheobronchial nodes* (level IV), situated in the angles between the trachea and the right and left main bronchi; the *inferior (inter)tracheobronchial nodes* (level VII), located below the carina between the two main bronchial stems, the *bronchopulmonary nodes* (level X), in the hilum of each lung, and the *intrapulmonary nodes* (levels XI–XV), scattered within the central

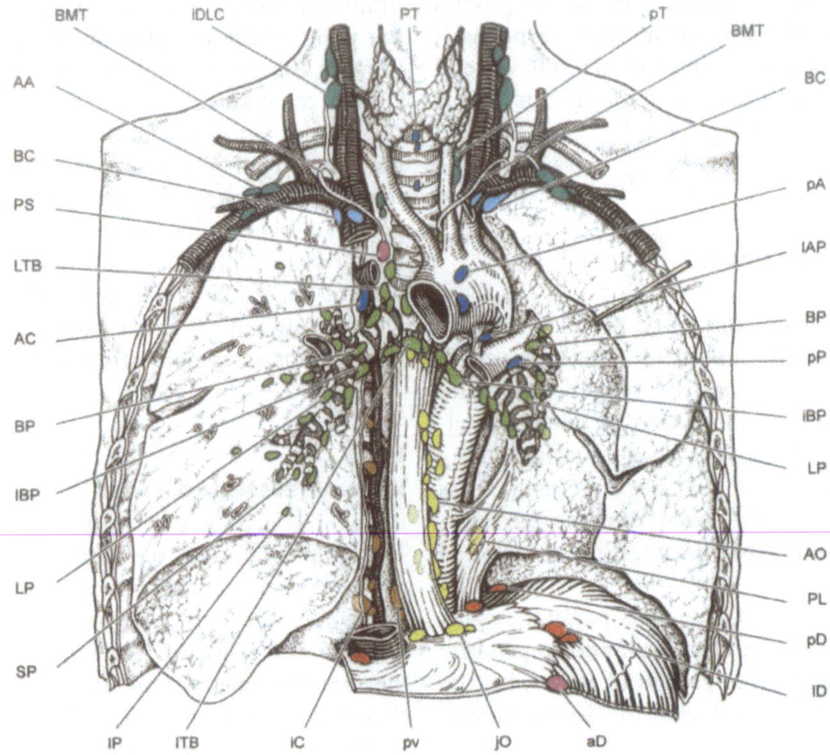
BMT
iDLC
PT
pT
BMT
AA
BC
BC
PS
pA
LTB
lAP
AC
BP
pP
BP
iBP
IBP
LP
AO
LP
PL
pD
SP
lD
IP
ITB
iC
pv
jO
aD

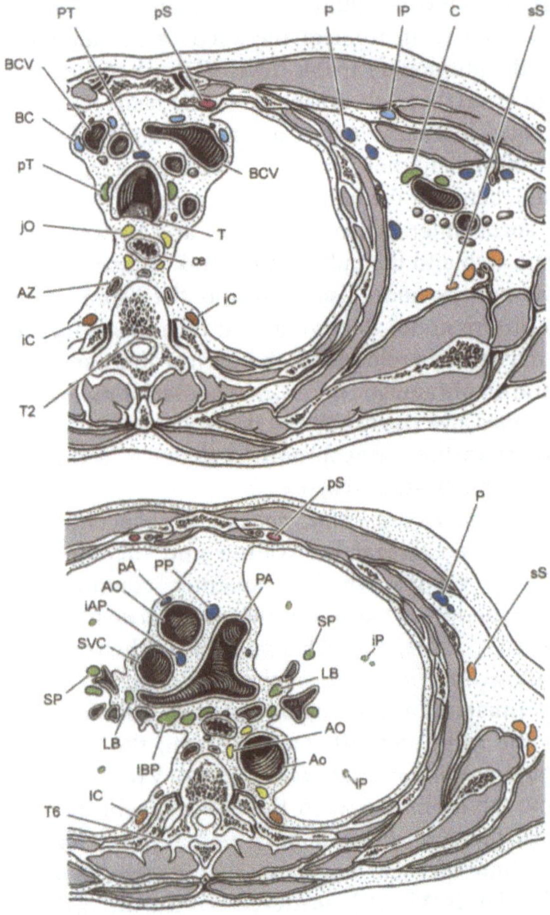
PT
pS
P
IP
C
sS
BCV
BC
BCV
pT
jO
T
œ
AZ
iC
iC
T2
pS
P
pA
PP
AO
PA
sS
iAP
SP
iP
SVC
LB
SP
LB
AO
Ao
IBP
iP
IC
T6

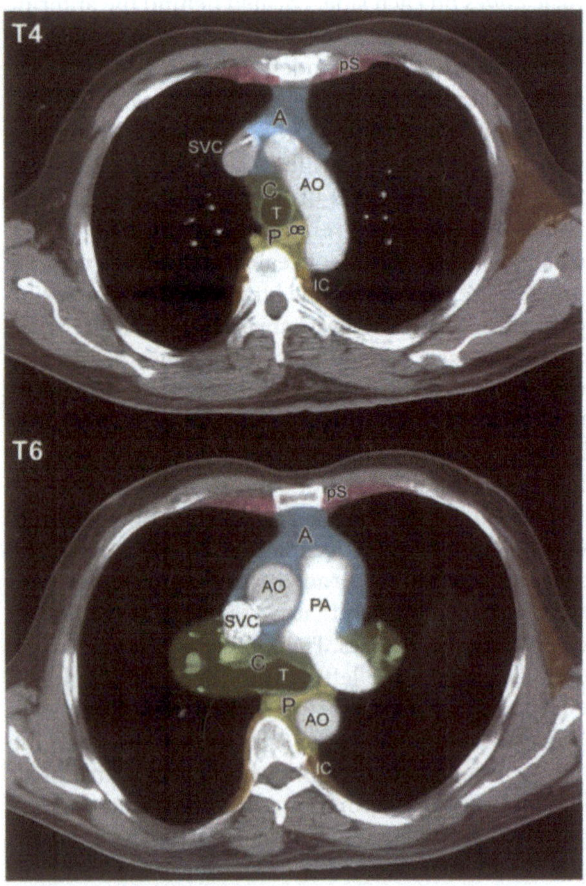
T4
pS
A
SVC
AO
C
T
P
œ
IC
T6
pS
A
AO
PA
SVC
C
T
P
AO
IC

lung substance inside the divisions of the lobar and segmentar branches of the bronchial tree. The afferent vessels of the tracheobronchial nodes drain the lymph from the superficial (subpleural) and deep (peribronchial) networks of the lung, and also from the thoracic part of the trachea and the heart. Together with those of the brachiocephalic group their efferents constitute the right and left bronchomediastinal trunks.

The *posterior mediastinal nodes* are spread within the posterior mediastinal fat, behind the pericardium, along the pulmonary ligament (level IX), and around the aorta and the oesophagus (level VIII). Receiving afferent vessels from the posterior part of the pericardium, the oesophagus and the posterior diaphragmatic nodes, they send efferents which mostly terminate in the thoracic duct, although some may end in the tracheobronchial chain.

1.5.3 Functional Drainage Pathways

Of immediate interest in understanding the way in which intrathoracic tumours are disseminated, the lymph nodes of the chest and their connecting vessels are arranged in three main ascending streams:

- The anterior stream (A) is located in the anterior mediastinum. Including the xiphoid, parasternal and brachiocephalic nodes, it may become invaded as a result of the dissemination of breast, thyroid, or thymic tumours.
- The central stream (C) occupies the middle part of the mediastinum. Linked inferiorly to the lateral diaphragmatic nodes, it is formed by the successive subgroups of tracheobronchial nodes. Immediately adjacent to the respiratory tree, this main drainage pathway of the thoracic viscera represents the usual route of dissemination for lung cancers, but also for malignant tumours of the oesophagus.
- The posterior stream (P) runs behind the heart, in the narrow fatty space of the posterior mediastinum. Grouping the posterior diaphragmatic nodes and the posterior mediastinal nodes arranged in a continuous chain around the aorta and the oesophagus, it mostly ends in the thoracic duct. Its metastatic involvement is usually observed in cases of oesophageal cancer.

Although each represents an individual preferential pathway of lymphatic dispersion, the anterior, central and posterior mediastinal chains described herein are not completely separated from one another. In the superior mediastinum, the terminal ducts of the anterior and central chains unite to give rise to a common bronchomediastinal trunk, while the posterior chain remains isolated, mainly connected to the thoracic duct. On the contrary, the posterior and central pathways may encounter one another inferiorly since the lower peri-oesophageal nodes send divergent efferent vessels that end either in the inferior tracheobronchial nodes or in the thoracic duct. Finally, it should be noted that both anterior and posterior pathways are connected by transdiaphragmatic channels with the parietal lymphatics of the peritoneal cavity: they may thus become involved in the spread of intra-abdominal tumours.

1.5.4 Delineation of Lymph Node Areas

On transverse sections of the chest, the lymphatic target volumes can be delineated according to the following anatomical landmarks (Fig. 1.6):

◄

Fig. 1.6. Lymphatic nodes of the thorax. Anterior view of the chest showing the distribution of the thoracic node groups and levels. Corresponding target volumes are indicated on anatomical and CT sections through the upper and lower parts of the thorax. Node groups of the parietal system and of the anterior, central and posterior visceral pathways are indicated by different *colours*, matching those of the corresponding target areas: *AA* apical axillary n., *AC* azygo-caval n. (Barthels'), *aD* anterior diaphragmatic n., *AO* aortico-oesophageal n., *BC* brachiocephalic n., *BMT* bronchomediastinal trunk, *BP* bronchial pulmonary n., *iAP* interaortopulmonary n. (Engels'), *iBP* interbronchial pulmonary n., *iC* intercostal n., *iDLC* inferior deep lateral cervical n., *iP* intrapulmonary n., *TB* intertracheobronchial n., *jO* juxtaoesophageal n., *lD* lateral diaphragmatic n., *LP* lobar pulmonary n., *LTB* superior laterotracheobronchial n., *P* pectoral n., *pA* preaortic n., *pD* posterior diaphragmatic n., *PL* pulmonary ligament n., *pP* prepulmonary n., *pS* parasternal n., *pT* paratracheal n., *pv* prevertebral n., *SP* segmental pulmonary n., *sS* subscapular n. Key anatomical structures used to delineate the target volumes are as follows: the aorta (*Ao*), pulmonary arteries (*PA*), superior vena cava (*SVC*), brachiocephalic veins (*BCV*), tracheobronchial tree (*T*) and the oesophagus (*Oe*). The target volumes are indicated as follows: the parasternal (*PS*), anterior brachiocephalic (*A*), central intertracheobronchial (*C*), posterior mediastinal (*P*) and intercostal (*IC*) areas

- The *parasternal lymphatic area* is a lenticular laminar plane bounded anteriorly by the deep surface of the sternum and anterior intercostal spaces and dorsally by the transversus thoracis muscle. It extends from the xiphoid process upwards to the sternoclavicular joints with the internal thoracic artery as a central anatomical landmark.
- The *brachiocephalic lymphatic area* occupies the anterior mediastinal fat, in front of the large supracardiac vessels. Anteriorly facing the posterior aspect of the sternum, this volume is bounded laterally by the anterior parts of the right and left mediastinal pleurae. Caudally it disappears nearly below the level of the sixth thoracic vertebra and cranially it communicates through the thoracic inlet, alongside the carotid arteries and internal jugular veins, with the lower part of the cervical jugulocarotid areas. Conventionally, the inferior edge of clavicle can be used as landmark to trace the limit between these intrathoracic and deep cervical areas. Taking the brachiocephalic vein, the aortic arch and the pulmonary trunk as successive anatomical landmarks, this volume can be divided into supra-aortic, pre-aortic and subaortic stages which respectively contain the upper (level I), middle (level V) and lower (level VI) anterior mediastinal lymph node groups.
- The *intertracheobronchial area* is centred around the thoracic trachea and the main bronchi. Its anterior and posterior limits can be defined as running respectively along the posterior aspect of the superior vena cava and aortic arch anteriorly and along the ventral aspect of the oesophagus posteriorly. Delineated by the middle parts of the mediastinal pleurae, its lateral boundaries include the right and left pulmonary hilia which enter into both lungs. Inferiorly, this area does not extend below the level of the sixth thoracic vertebra, but includes all the node groups associated with the trachea (levels II, III and IV) and the bronchial tree (levels VIII–XV).
- The *posterior mediastinal area* is a narrow fatty channel located behind a plane running along the posterior aspect of the heart caudally and along the anterior surface of the oesophagus cranially. It is bounded by the ventral aspect of the vertebral column posteriorly, and laterally by the dorsal part of the mediastinal pleurae. This volume contains the thoracic oesophagus, the descending aorta, both azygos and hemi-azygos veins and between these landmarks, the posterior mediastinal nodes (levels IX and XIII) and the thoracic duct. Posterolateral extensions on both sides of the vertebrae up to the costal angles allow it to also include the posterior intercostal node groups.

1.6 Lymphatics of the Abdomen

Following the same arrangement as that in the thorax, the lymphatics of the abdomen are divided into parietal and visceral vessels and nodes, and respectively drain the walls and contents of the abdominal cavity. As a general rule, they all follow the course of the parietal and visceral branches of the abdominal aorta and they all return – except for some lymphatics arising from the liver – into the venous bloodstream via the thoracic duct. Before reaching the latter, most of them are interrupted by very large retroperitoneal nodes scattered around the inferior vena cava and the aorta, commonly described as the terminal lumbo-aortic nodes.

1.6.1 Parietal Vessels and Nodes

The *superficial parietal lymphatic vessels* of the abdominal wall drain the lymph from the anterior and posterior abdominal skin and subcutaneous tissue upwards into the pectoral and subscapular axillary nodes, respectively (Fig. 1.5). Nevertheless, the low abdominal integuments located below the umbilicus are supplied by descending lymph vessels which terminate in the superficial inguinal nodes.

The *deep parietal vessels* originate from the muscles and fasciae of the abdominal wall. Running in the subperitoneal adipose tissue, they converge superiorly in a few small inferior diaphragmatic nodes and inferiorly they follow the deep inferior epigastric vessels to join the external iliac nodes. Posteriorly, they cross the quadratus lumborum and the psoas to end in the lateral or posterior lumbo-aortic nodes.

1.6.2 Visceral Vessels and Nodes

Arising from the various abdominal organs, the visceral lymphatic vessels pass through several outlying nodes firstly located close to the viscera, then occupy an intermediate position in the peritoneal ligaments and mesos. Finally, they reach larger groups of nodes associated with the major paired or uneven branches of the abdominal aorta, and terminate in the lumbar peri-aortic nodes (Fig. 1.7).

The *lumbar peri-aortic nodes* include four groups of nodes which are not clearly differentiated from each other topographically, although functionally each of them possesses a specific lymphatic territory. These four groups are divided into pre-aortic nodes, right and left lateral aortic nodes, and postaortic nodes.

The *median pre-aortic nodes* drain the lymphatics of the digestive tract running along the ventral branches of the abdominal aorta. Their efferents form the intestinal trunks which open into the cisterna chyli.

On both sides the *lateral aortic nodes* receive efferent vessels arising from the common iliac nodes as well as terminal lymphatic collectors originating along the lateral branches of the aorta, from the kidneys, the suprarenal glands and the male or female gonadic glands. Therefore they constitute the main terminal group of nodes of all the abdominal or pelvic viscera of the urogenital system. They give rise to several large efferent vessels which constitute the right and left lumbar trunks, ending on both sides in the inferolateral corners of the cisterna chyli.

The *post-aortic nodes* do not possess a specific lymphatic territory. Initially described as mostly collecting the posterior deep parietal lymph vessels, they are now more accurately regarded as functionally linked to the lateral aortic nodes and share the same drainage area. Obviously, they never receive direct visceral afferents and have to be considered as additional relays of the previous groups of nodes before they reach the thoracic duct.

1.6.2.1 The Pre-aortic Group of Nodes and Their Digestive Affluents

The pre-aortic nodes are located immediately on the anterior surface of the abdominal aorta, forming a discontinuous chain divided into three distinct masses respectively grouping the coeliac, superior mesenteric and inferior mesenteric nodes, closely associated with the origin of the corresponding arteries.

The *coeliac nodes* are usually two or three in number and surround the coeliac trunk at the level of the 12th thoracic vertebra. They collect the lymphatics from the stomach, duodenum, the major part of the liver, the gallbladder, pancreas and spleen. Their outlying intermediate nodes, located close to these organs and around their supplying blood vessels, are arranged in three main sets: the gastric, hepatic and pancreaticosplenic node groups.

The *gastric nodes* are situated along the arterial vessels running along the lesser and greater curvatures of the stomach. Therefore, they are distinguished as *right* and *left gastric nodes* which are located in the lesser omentum on the lesser curvature of the stomach, or as *right* and *left gastro-epiploic nodes*, which lie between the two sheaths of the greater omentum in the lower part of the great curvature of the stomach. The upper nodes of the left gastric chain rest against the cardia and collect the lymph from the abdominal part of the oesophagus. Although they drain mainly into the coeliac group of aortic nodes, these *paracardial nodes* may also have some efferent vessels which extend to the lower posterior mediastinal lymph nodes. Below the central part of the stomach, the right gastro-epiploic nodes are relayed by a group of four to five *pyloric nodes* which lie close to the division of the gastroduodenal artery and receive afferent vessels originating from the pylorus but also from the first part of the duodenum and from the head of the pancreas. The efferent vessels of these pyloric nodes usually follow the course of the gastroduodenal artery, crossing the first part of the duodenum posteriorly to join the coeliac group of pre-aortic nodes. Alternatively however, they may pass in front of the horizontal part of the duodenum to join the superior mesenteric nodes.

The *hepatic nodes* form a chain of three to six nodes which are situated along the course of the hepatic artery. The first nodes are located at the origin of the artery and consequently correspond to the superior border of the pancreas. The following nodes are distributed on the anterior surface of the portal vein, on the anterior border of Winslow's epiploic foramen. The upper nodes finally occupy the hilum of the liver, randomly distributed around the right and left divisions of the hepatic artery. One of these nodes, however, has a fairly constant location at the junction of the cystic and common bile ducts near the neck of the gallbladder: it is known as Quenu's *cystic node*. Commonly, the hepatic nodes receive afferents from the liver, bile ducts and gallbladder, but also from the stomach, duodenum and pancreas; their efferents all pass through the pre-aortic nodes.

The *pancreaticosplenic nodes* are associated with the splenic artery and are consequently related to the upper border and posterior aspect of the pancreas. The largest of these nodes, described by Cunéo, is located medially behind the body of the pancreas. Laterally, one or two smaller nodes are located in the pancreaticosplenic ligament, near the hilum of the spleen. Collecting afferent vessels running alongside the branches of the splenic artery, these nodes drain the spleen, the tail and the body of the pancreas and the fundus of the stomach. Their efferents end in the coeliac group of pre-aortic nodes.

The *superior mesenteric nodes* form a large mass of lymphatic tissue surrounding the origin of the

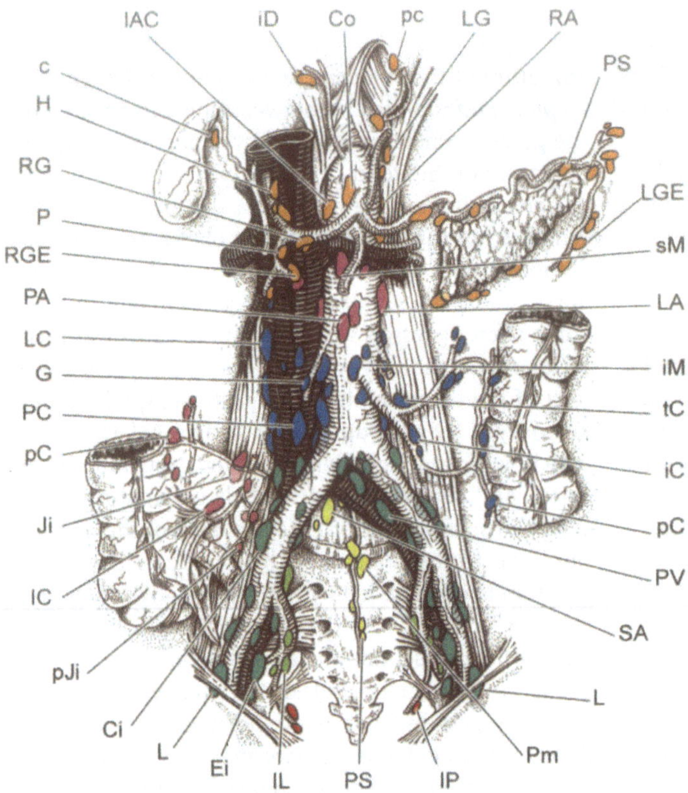
IAC
iD
Co
pc
LG
RA
PS
c
H
RG
P
RGE
PA
LC
G
PC
pC
Ji
IC
pJi
Ci
L
Ei
IL
PS
IP
Pm
L
SA
PV
pC
iC
tC
iM
LA
sM
LGE

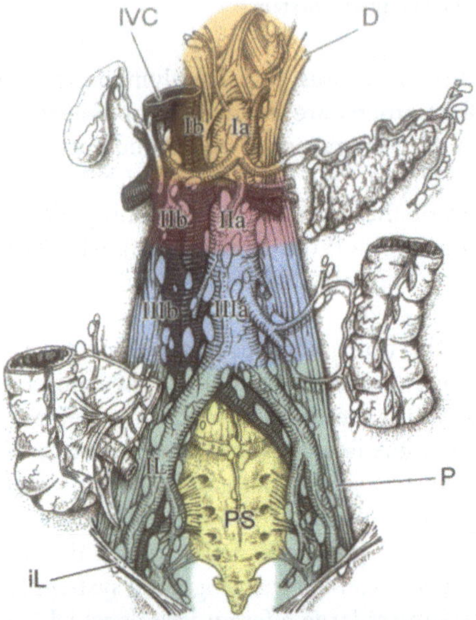
IVC
D
Ib
Ia
IIb
IIa
IIIb
IIIa
IL
PS
P
iL

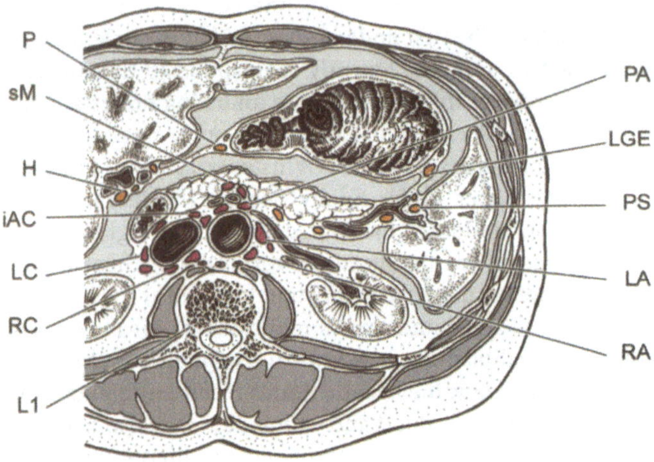
P
sM
H
iAC
LC
RC
L1
PA
LGE
PS
LA
RA

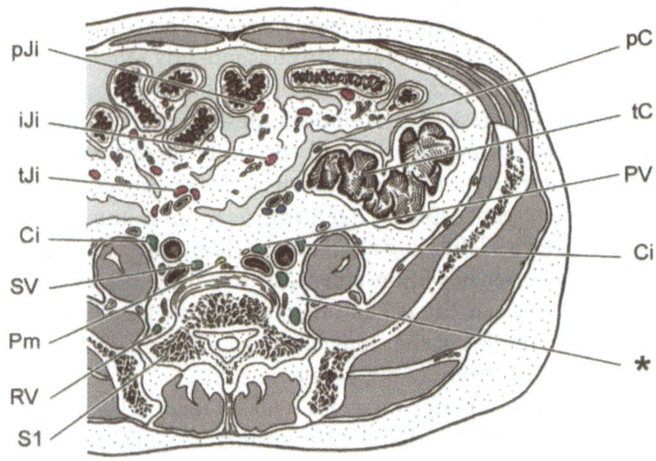
pJi
iJi
tJi
Ci
SV
Pm
RV
S1
pC
tC
PV
Ci
*

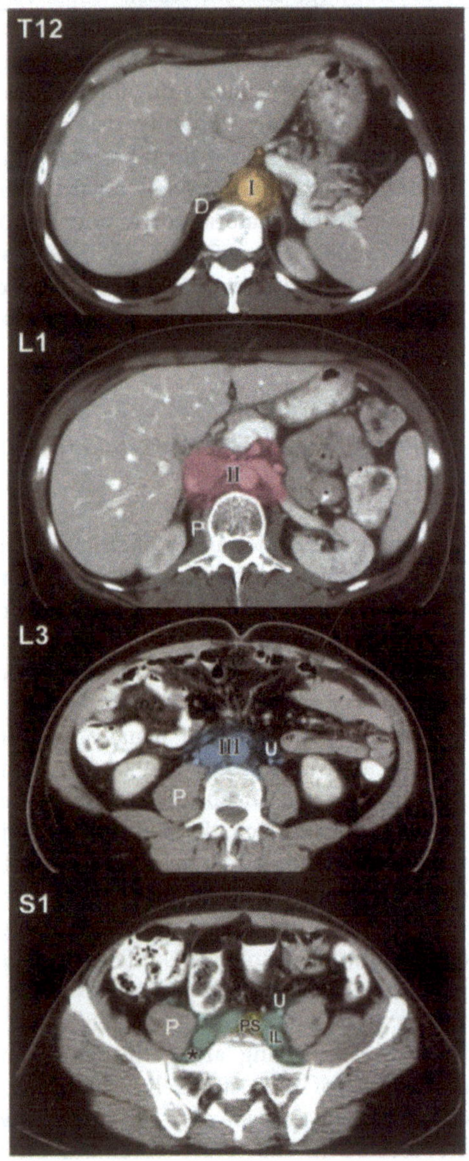
T12
D
I
L1
II
P
L3
III
U
P
S1
P
PS
IL
U
*

superior mesenteric artery on the anterior aspect of the aorta. Located behind the pancreas at the level of the first lumbar vertebra, they are almost continuous, without a clear line of demarcation, with the large mesenteric lymph nodes situated at the root of the mesentery. Their numerous afferent vessels drain the mesenteric and ileocolic lymph nodes, and in this manner the last parts of the duodenum, the small intestine and the right part of the colon.

The *mesenteric lymph nodes* are approximately 100 to 150 in number. They are usually distributed within the mesenteric fat and constitute three successive relays: the most peripheral nodes are known as the *juxta-intestinal mesenteric nodes* and lie close to the intestinal walls between the terminal jejunal and ileal arteries; the second group of nodes occupies an intermediate position within the mesentery between the primary or secondary loops of the superior mesenteric artery; the last nodes, which are less numerous but larger, are located along the main stem of this vessel, near the mesenteric root, and constitute the *central mesenteric nodes.*

The *ileocolic nodes* constitute a continuous chain of about 20 nodes around the ileocolic artery, and are sometimes artificially differentiated into upper and lower ileocolic nodes. At the point where the vessel divides into its terminal branches, the lower nodes form three subgroups known as the *recurrent ileal* and *anterior* or *posterior ileocolic nodes,* which occupy the corresponding ileocaecal folds. A single node is usually found in the meso-appendix.

The *inferior mesenteric nodes* usually consist of two large elongated nodes symmetrically located on each side of the origin of the inferior mesenteric artery. In these lymph nodes situated at the level of the third lumbar vertebra terminate the lymphatic trunks originating from the upper part of the rectum and from the left half of the colon. Moreover, these vessels have already passed through three or four successive relays which are very similar to those of the small intestine: among these are the *epicolic nodes,* which are small nodules embedded in the walls of the colon itself. They are connected to the *paracolic nodes* which are located along the mesenteric borders of the colon and followed by the *intermediate colic nodes,* located along the middle and left colic arteries. Their efferents finally drain into the *terminal colic nodes,* along the main stem of the inferior mesenteric artery. An identical nodal arrangement is observed in the ascending and transverse parts of the colon, although the terminal collectors end in the ileocolic group of superior mesenteric nodes.

1.6.2.2
The Lateral Aortic Lymph Nodes and Their Urogenital Affluents

The *left lateral aortic nodes* form an almost continuous vertical chain on the left side of the abdominal aorta. Dorsally, this chain lies on the vertebral attachments of the psoas muscle and on the left pillar of the diaphragm. Laterally facing the sympathetic nervous trunks, it is crossed on its anterior aspect by the left renal vessels.

The *right lateral aortic nodes* are located either in front of the inferior vena cava or behind it. A few of them lie on the lateral side of the vein or seem to be interposed between the latter and the aorta. According to their various locations, the right latero-aortic nodes can be characterised as *precaval, laterocaval* or *postcaval nodes.* However, they have the same topographical relationships as those of the left lateral aortic nodes.

On both sides, the lateral aortic nodes receive afferent vessels from all the structures supplied by the posterior and lateral paired branches of the abdominal aorta and also collect the ascending lymphatic trunks arising from the pelvis through the common iliac nodes. In addition to the posterior parietal vessels, their major affluents are the following:

Fig. 1.7. Lymphatic nodes of the abdomen. Anterior view of the abdominal blood vessels and satellite lymph node groups. The corresponding target volumes are indicated on anatomical and CT sections through the upper, middle and lower parts of the abdominal cavity. Median and lateral groups of the lumbar periaortic nodes and related juxtavisceral nodes of the successive abdominal levels (I–III) are indicated by different *colours,* matching those of the corresponding target areas. *c* cystic n. (Quenu's), *Co* coeliac n., *G* gonadic n., *H* hepatic n., *IAC* interaorticocaval n., *IC* ileocolic n., *iC* intermediate colic n., *iD* inferior diaphragmatic n., *iM* inferior mesenteric n., *Ji* jejunoileal n., subclassified as para-intestinal (*p*), intermediate (*i*) and terminal (*t*), *LA* lateroaortic n., *LC* laterocaval n., *LG* left gastric n., *LGE* left gastroepiploic n., *p* pyloric n., *PA* preaortic n., *PC* precaval n., *pC* paracolic n., *pc* paracardial n., *RA* retroaortic n., *RC* retrocaval n., *RG* right gastric n., *RGE* right gastroepiploic n., *sM* superior mesenteric n., *tC* terminal colic n. Key anatomical structures to delineate the target volumes are as follows: the aorta (*Ao*), inferior vena cava (*IVC*), iliac vessels (*IV*), ureters (*U*), diaphragmatic pillars (*D*) and the psoas muscles (*P*). The *asterisks* indicate Cuneo's and Marcille's fossae. Inferiorly, the lymphatics of the abdomen are continuous with those of the lateral and central chains of the pelvis, emphasised with the same *colours* and legend as in Fig. 1.8

- The *lymphatics from the suprarenal glands* running along the renal, suprarenal and inferior diaphragmatic vessels
- The *lymphatics from the kidneys*, also draining the perirenal fat capsule and the abdominal part of the ureter, which enter the nodes located near the first lumbar vertebra
- The *gonadic lymphatics* arising from the testes in the male, or from the ovaries and lateral part of the uterine tubes in the female

All these afferent vessels form tortuous networks around the suprarenal, renal and gonadic vessels. Furthermore, they issue directly from their respective organs without making any relay in the intermediate nodes. Finally, among the efferent vessels leaving the lateral aortic nodes, some send multiple connections to the pre- and postaortic nodes, thereby giving rise to a rich peri-aortocaval lymphatic plexus, partially bypassing the main lumbar collecting trunks.

1.6.3 Functional Drainage Pathways

Because of the complex three-dimensional organisation of the abdominal lymphatic network, the major drainage pathways are difficult to delineate for the different visceral groups (Fig. 1.7).

Widely distributed between the immediate vicinity of the various derivatives of the alimentary tract and the origin of their successive supplying vessels, the *digestive lymphatic pathways* occupy the multiplanar spaces of their mesos and peritoneal ligaments. Running between the complex arrangement of organs, these pathways cannot be easily confined in a simple volume with well-defined boundaries. Distally however, they all converge towards a *central ascending axis*, giving rise to a median pre-aortic pathway. The latter longitudinal chain can be divided into three successive functional levels:

- The *coeliac level (IA)* is located in front of the T12 vertebra. It receives the terminal lymphatic pathways of all the viscera located in the supramesocolic part of the peritoneal cavity. Consequently, its metastatic involvement is thus usually observed in tumours of the liver, bile ducts, stomach, abdominal oesophagus or pancreas.
- The height of the *superior mesenteric level (IIA)* corresponds to that of the L1 vertebra. Receiving the lymphatic pathways from the small intestine and right hemicolon, it may also be invaded in cases of pancreaticoduodenal cancer.
- The height of the *inferior mesenteric level (IIIA)* is situated in front of the L3 vertebra and may show enlarged metastatic nodes as a result of the lymphatic spread of malignant tumours of the left hemicolon or upper part of the rectum.

More precisely located in the retroperitoneal space, the *genito-urinary lymphatic pathways* on both sides of the abdominal aorta form two *lateral ascending chains* facing the psoas muscles posteriorly and the right and left diaphragmatic pillars. As in the case of the central digestive axis, the anatomical landmarks of the T12, L1 and L3 vertebrae can be used to define the three functional levels (IB, IIB, IIIB) where primary metastatic nodes of suprarenal, renal and gonadic tumours may be respectively found.

1.6.4 Delineation of Lymph Node Areas

As an extension of the previous considerations, it is difficult to include all the juxtavisceral or intermediate groups of abdominal nodes and interposed lymph vessels within simple geometric compartments with well defined anatomical boundaries. However, the possibility exists of more accurately delineating the three-dimensional space that contains the terminal lumbar peri-aortic nodes, their efferent trunks, the cisterna chyli and the abdominal part of the thoracic duct (Fig. 1.7).

On radiological CT or MR sections, the so obtained *lumbar peri-aortic lymphatic area* is bounded dorsally by the anterior aspect of the vertebral column and extends laterally towards the lateral borders of the psoas muscles and, more superiorly to the edges of both pillars of the diaphragm. Ventrally, its anterior limit corresponds to the posterior peritoneal lining of the omental bursa, then to the posterior surface of the pancreas, and finally to the root of the mesentery. This longitudinal volume extends from the 12th thoracic vertebra downwards to the fourth lumbar vertebra, and in addition to the various lumbar groups of nodes includes the abdominal aorta, the inferior vena cava, the ureters, the gonadic, renal and suprarenal vessels and the sympathetic nerves of the coeliac plexus, all embedded within the retroperitoneal fat.

1.7 Lymphatics of the Pelvis

Divided into parietal and visceral networks of lymph vessels and nodes, the lymphatics of the pelvis all drain into successive groups of nodes located at the level of the pelvic inlet, along the arcuate line of the coxal bone and in front of the fifth lumbar vertebra. Mostly associated with the iliac vessels and their branches, they form several ascending chains which include the external iliac, internal iliac, common iliac and sacral groups of nodes. Finally, their collecting ducts terminate in the inferior part of the lateral aortic chain on the corresponding side (Figs. 1.7, 1.8).

1.7.1 Parietal Lymph Vessels and Nodes

The parietal lymphatics collect the lymph from the anterior, lateral, posterior and inferior walls of the pelvis and include superficial and deep networks that drain the integuments of the perineum and the muscles covering the pelvic girdle respectively (Fig. 1.8).

The *superficial parietal vessels* are only present on the pelvic floor. Running under the perineal skin from the coccygeal area towards the pubis, they cross anteriorly the medial side of the root of the thigh around the outer surface of the adductor muscles, and then join the superomedial group of superficial inguinal nodes. Their functional territory comprises all the soft tissues of the perineum below the outer fascial sheath of the urogenital diaphragm, but also the distal part of the vagina below the hymen and the inferior part of the anal canal below the ano-cutaneous line.

The *deep parietal vessels* follow the parietal branches of the external and internal iliac vessels and thereby make their first relay into the inferior epigastric, circumflex iliac and sacral groups of nodes:

- The *deep inferior epigastric nodes* consist of three to six small nodes situated over the lower third of the course of the corresponding artery, behind and along the lateral border of the rectus abdominis muscle. These nodes may sometimes be absent, but when present mostly drain the lower part of the anterior abdominal wall but also the retropubic part of the anterior pelvic wall. Their efferent vessels terminate in the lateral chains of external iliac nodes.
- The *deep circumflex iliac nodes* are from two to four in number but are frequently absent. Located around the artery which bears the same name, they receive afferent vessels arising from the iliac muscle and the parietal peritoneal lining of the iliac fossa. Their efferent vessels then extend to the external iliac nodes.
- The *sacral groups of nodes* are located around the lateral and median sacral arteries, and constitute three ascending chains running respectively along the lateral borders of the sacrum and in front of its anterior aspect on the midline. Draining the presacral space between the fascia recti anteriorly and the sacrum posteriorly, they send their efferent vessels towards the internal iliac nodes laterally and towards the subaortic nodes in the median area. The largest of these median sacral nodes is usually resting on the anterior aspect of the L5–S1 intervertebral disc and because of this location is known as the *promontorial node.*

On the lateral pelvic walls, the lymph vessels run along the surface of the endopelvic fascia and join the external and internal chains of iliac nodes above the plane of the levator ani and coccygeal muscles. Below the plane of the levator ani, the muscles and fasciae are drained by the lymphatic vessels that follow the internal pudendal artery at the surface of the obturatorius internus, in Alcock's pudendal canal. These deep lymphatics originate in the prevesical space, bounded anteriorly by the pubic symphysis and posteriorly by the umbilicoprevesical fascia. They also collect the lymph from the ischiorectal fossa, then pass around the posterior aspect of the ischial spine and finally join the lower part of the internal iliac chain.

1.7.2 Visceral Vessels and Nodes

Like those of the abdomen, the visceral lymphatic vessels of the pelvis usually include several successive relays first located close to the viscera, then around the different vascular pedicles of each organ and finally along the large iliac vessels. At this level, they form rich plexuses which are much more developed than in the upper part of the abdominal cavity and give rise to multiple ascending drainage pathways, all converging towards the lateral groups of lumbar aortic nodes (Fig. 1.8).

1.7.2.1 Juxtavisceral Nodes

According to their respective locations, the *juxtavisceral nodes* are distinguished as follows:

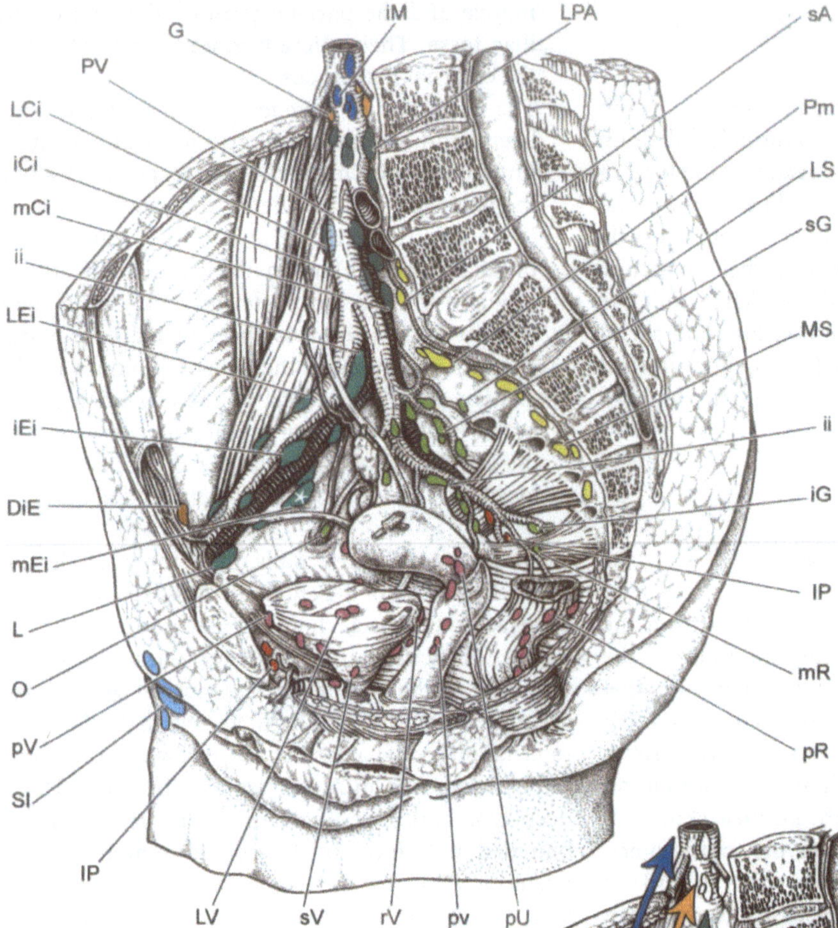
iM
LPA
sA
G
PV
LCi
iCi
mCi
ii
LEi
iEi
DiE
mEi
L
O
pV
Sl
IP
LV
sV
rV
pv
pU
Pm
LS
sG
MS
ii
iG
IP
mR
pR

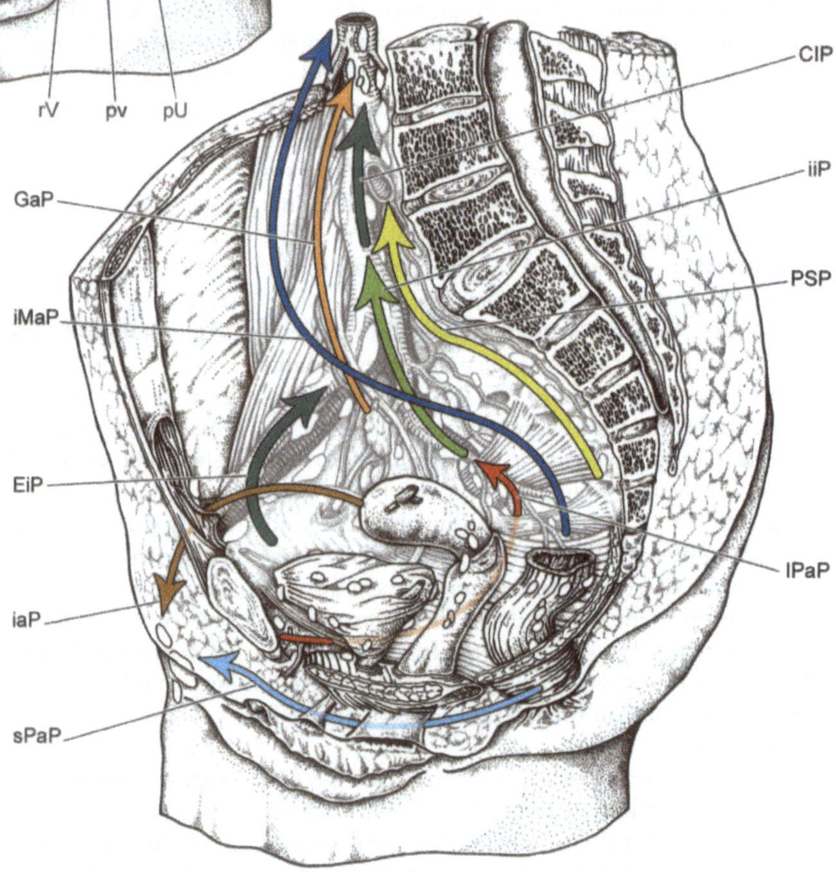
CIP
iiP
GaP
PSP
iMaP
EiP
IPaP
iaP
sPaP

- *Pre-, lateral-, post-* and *subvesical lymph nodes* are located on the corresponding surfaces of the bladder, in the urinary compartment of the pelvis.
- *Paravaginal* and *parauterine lymph nodes* are found respectively on the lateral edges of the vagina and the cervix, in the genital compartment of the female pelvis.
- *Pararectal lymph nodes* are ranged around the right and left aspects of the rectum, in the posterior digestive pelvic compartment.

Afferent vessels to these nodes arise directly from the neighbouring viscera, while the respective routes of the efferent vessels extend to the external iliac, internal iliac or presacral chains.

1.7.2.2 External Iliac Nodes

Grouped around the external iliac vessels, the external iliac nodes are usually from nine to ten in number and have a constant arrangement, forming three distinct chains each consisting of about three nodes: the lateral, middle and medial groups of external iliac nodes (Fig. 1.8).

The *lateral chain* comprises three nodes which are interposed between the medial border of the psoas and the lateral side of the external iliac artery. The lower node is located under the inguinal ligament, frequently passes through the femoral septum, and is known as the lateral lacunar lymph node. Closely related to the origin of the deep inferior epigastric and deep circumflex iliac arteries, it receives the efferent vessels from the corresponding groups of nodes.

The *middle* or *intermediate chain* usually comprises two or three nodes which lie on the anterior aspect of the external iliac vein, along the medial side of the artery. The lower node is termed the intermediate lacunar node, but is frequently absent. The middle node, however, is always well developed and rests in front of the vein, midway between the inguinal ligament and the bifurcation of the common iliac artery. The upper node is located in the angle between the origins of the external and internal iliac arteries. Known as the *interiliac lymph node*, the latter is usually covered by the iliac segment of the ureter.

The *medial chain* includes three to four nodes and is placed on the medial side of the external iliac vein, against the lateral wall of the pelvic cavity above the obturator nerve. The lower node of this group is located immediately behind the femoral septum in contact with Cloquet's deep inguinal lymph node, and is commonly termed the medial lacunar lymph node. The suprajacent node, which is often very large, elongated and lenticular, tends to separate itself from the vein and descend downwards into the pelvic cavity. Through this prolapse into the pelvis, a number of authors regard the medial chain as belonging to the internal iliac groups of nodes. Nevertheless, its pelvic affluents are relatively few in comparison to the majority of its afferent vessels originating from the lower limb. Therefore it has to be considered functionally linked to the external iliac chain. Furthermore, from the surgeon's point of view, this group of nodes, located in a quadrangular area bounded superiorly by the external iliac vein, posteriorly by the internal iliac artery followed by the pelvic part of the ureter, and inferiorly by the obturator nerve, corresponds to the so-called *obturator nodes*. As previously noted by Cruveilhier and Sappey, this surgical terminology should not lead to these nodes becoming confused with the isolated small *obturator node* which occupies the internal foramen of the obturator canal in the lower part of the obturator fossa. The latter indeed drains satellite lymph vessels running along the obturator artery, and through its efferents is functionally linked to the internal iliac chain.

As regards their afferent vessels, the lateral, intermediate and medial chains of the external iliac

Fig. 1.8. Lymphatic node groups and drainage pathways of the pelvis. Medial view of the right female hemipelvis showing the distribution of the pelvic lymph node groups and their eight connecting pathways, identified by different *colours*. *DiE* deep inferior epigastric n., *G* gonadic n., *iCi* intermediate common iliac n., *iEi* intermediate lateral iliac n., *iG* inferior gluteal n., *iI* interiliac n., *ii* internal iliac n., *iM* inferior mesenteric n., *IP* internal pudendal n., *L* lacunar n., *LCI* lateral common iliac n., *LEI* lateroexternal iliac n., *LPA* lumbar periaortic n., *LS* lateral sacral n., *LV* laterovesical n., *mCi* medial common iliac n., *mEi* medial external iliac n., *mR* middle rectal n., *MS* median sacral n., *O* obturator n. (Cruveilhier's), *Pm* promontory n., *pR* pararectal n., *pU* parauterine n., *pv* paravaginal n., *PV* prevenous n., *pV* prevesical n., *RV* retrovenous n., *rV* retrovesical n., *sA* suboartic n., *sG* superior gluteal n., *SI* superficial inguinal n., *SV* subvenous n., *sV* subvesical n. Note that the surgical obturator node (*) differs from the true anatomical obturator node. The major lymphatic pathways of the pelvis are identified as the external iliac (*EiP*), internal iliac (*iiP*) and presacral (*PSP*) pathways and converge in a common iliac pathway (*CIP*), ending in the lateral lumbar periaortic nodes. Alternative routes follow the internal pudendal (*IPAP*) gonadic (*GaP*), inferior mesenteric (*iMaP*) and superficial perineal accessory pathways (*sPaP*). The existence of an inguinal accessory pathway (*iaP*) seems possible

nodes mostly receive collectors from the lower limb through the superficial and deep inguinal nodes. Furthermore, all of these also drain deep lymphatic vessels arising from the subumbilical part of the abdominal wall and deep collecting trunks from the glans, penis or clitoris which pass through the inguinal canal, coursing along the vas deferens in the male and the round ligament of the uterus in the female. In addition, the medial chain and to a lesser degree the intermediate chain receive lymphatic satellites of the obturator vessels originating from the muscles of the medial compartment of the thigh and some visceral vessels ascending from the lateral lobes of the prostate, the fundus of the urinary bladder, the cervix uteri or the upper part of the vagina. The latter originate from the laterouterine and laterovaginal juxtavisceral nodes which, as first described by Lucas Championnière, are located near the corresponding organs in the base of the broad ligament of the uterus alongside the terminal arch of the uterine artery and close to the origin of its upper vaginal branches in the parametrium. The fact that these vessels have a long course along the levator ani and obturatorius internus muscles before reaching the pelvic inlet and the fact that they end in the intermediate and medial chains of external iliac nodes may appear somewhat odd, since their route would be much shorter if they joined the internal iliac nodes, over which they are compelled to cross. According to Cunéo and Poirier, this arrangement is in fact explained by their specific development. In the fetus indeed, the prostate, vagina and cervix uteri are positioned much higher than in the infant or the adult, and are situated at the level of the pelvic inlet. At this stage, their developing lymph vessels thus create their primary connections with the medial nodes of the external iliac chain and later on, when the organs occupy a lower position within the pelvic cavity, their route then becomes more elongated and complicated. The same phenomenon occurs with the lymphatics of the ovary and testis.

The efferent vessels of each external chain iliac drain into the lower nodes of the corresponding common iliac chains. Several anastomosing channels run from the medial to the intermediate and from the intermediate to the lateral chains in such a manner that the medial pelvic lymphatic flow mixes progressively with the lateral flow mostly originating from the lower limb. The perivascular network thus constituted is mostly located on the anterior surface of the blood vessels, though some connecting vessels also cross their posterior aspect.

1.7.2.3
Internal Iliac Lymph Nodes

Often described as *hypogastric nodes*, the *internal iliac nodes* surround the internal iliac vessels and are placed near the origin of their different branches or in the angles formed by their separation (Fig. 1.8). Most of them combine to form a crescent-shaped chain, facing anteriorly and running in front of the sacro-iliac joint downwards to the lower part of the greater sciatic foramen. Inferiorly, the most anterior node of the chain is located between the umbilical and obturator arteries below the point where the obturator nerve enters its canal. Posteriorly the most superior node lies against the origin of the superior gluteal artery. Intermediate nodes are distributed along the initial course of the uterine, internal pudendal, inferior gluteal and middle rectal arteries. All of these nodes have the same name as the vessel they accompany.

Afferent vessels of the internal lymph nodes originate from all the pelvic viscera including those from the posterior part of the prostate, the lateral and lower parts of the urinary bladder, the membranous and prostatic segments of the urethra, the seminal vesicles, the middle and lower parts of the vagina, the body of the uterus, and the middle part of the rectum.

In addition, the *superior gluteal nodes* drain the deep regions of the buttock, including the gluteal muscles, while the *inferior gluteal nodes* similarly collect lymph from the lower part of the gluteal region, in continuity with the posterior compartment of the thigh and the dorsal part of the posterior perineum. The previously mentioned *internal pudendal lymphatic vessels* join the nodes of the internal iliac chain in front of the origin of the sciatic nerve just above the ischial spine, and drain the lymph from the deepest parts of the perineum, the ischio-anal fossa and the lower parts of the prostate, vagina and rectum.

The efferent vessels of the internal iliac nodes are directed upwards and outwards, course within the hypogastric lamina, then pass underneath the common iliac vein and terminate in the intermediate group of common iliac lymph nodes.

1.7.2.4
Common Iliac Lymph Nodes

Usually ranging from four to seven in number, the *common iliac nodes* are grouped around the common iliac vessels and, according to their topographical distribution and afferent vessels, can be differentiated into the lateral, intermediate and medial groups of nodes:

- The *lateral chain* usually consists of two large nodes interposed between the lateral side of the common iliac artery and the medial border of the psoas. This group forms an extension of the lateral chain of external iliac nodes, and ends without any clear delineation in the lateral lumbar aortic chain of nodes.
- The *middle* or *intermediate chain* comprises three to four nodes which are usually concealed on the posteromedial side of the artery. On the left side, they can be situated on the anterior aspect of the vein. Topographically, these retrovascular nodes are located in Cunéo's and Marcille's triangular lumbosacral fossa which is bounded medially by the body of the fifth lumbar vertebra, laterally by the medial border of the psoas and inferiorly by the upper border of the sacral wing. Usually the common iliac vessels cross the anterior surface of the fossa which is filled with adipose tissue and which contains the nodes superiorly and the lumbosacral and obturator nerves inferiorly.
- The *medial chain* runs along the inner side of the common iliac arteries. Together with those of the other side, its nodes constitute an uneven group located on the midline just below the aortic bifurcation in front of the fifth lumbar vertebra. Usually known as the *subaortic group of nodes*, the latter is sometimes divided into two distinct subgroups: the right subgroup, located below the left common iliac vein contains the *subvenous nodes*; the left subgroup, which lies in front of the same vein, contains the *prevenous nodes* (Figs. 1.7, 1.8).

Respectively constituting the terminal routes of the external and internal iliac chains, the lateral and intermediate common iliac chains do not receive any direct afferent vessels from the pelvic viscera. On the contrary, some lymphatics originating from the neck of the bladder, the cervix uteri and the posterior aspect of the rectum directly enter the median group of subaortic nodes. All these vessels follow the same course in the lower part of the sacrorectogenitopubic septum and superiorly, in the sacro-uterine folds, in the female. Closely linked to the pelvic diaphragm at their origin, they then ascend into the sacral concavity and join the lateral sacral chains. Some of them pass through the lymph nodes of the promontory; the others terminate in the subaortic nodes.

1.7.3 Functional Drainage Pathways

Spread around the iliac vessels or closely related to the pelvic organs, the lymph nodes of the pelvis are connected to one another by a large number of afferent or efferent vessels which constitute eight different drainage pathways. All these streams which traverse specific perivascular and fatty spaces of the pelvis share the same *main terminal route*, derived from the efferent pathway of the lower limbs. Comprising three lateral, intermediate and medial chains, the latter pass successively through the lacunar, external iliac and common iliac nodes to finally reach finally the lateral aortic nodes and the lumbar trunks entering the lower pole of the cisterna chyli. Connected to this common terminal route, the lymphatic pathways of the pelvis can be described as including three main anterior, middle and posterior pelvic pathways and five accessory pelvic pathways (Fig. 1.8).

- The *main anterior pelvic pathway* is constituted by the lymph vessels originating from the anterior pelvic viscera which drain into the medial external iliac nodes. Located in front of the ureter, the vessels and nodes of this *external iliac pathway* mainly occupy the subperitoneal adipose tissue of the obturator fossa. Surgically they correspond to the structures that are excised in obturator lymph node clearance. Clinically they are involved in the lymphatic spread of tumours of the fundus of the urinary bladder, lateral prostatic lobes, cervix uteri and fornix vaginae.
- The *main middle pelvic pathway* follows the route of the lymphatics of the *internal iliac chain*. Topographically located on the posterior aspect of the pelvic ureter, this pathway then runs superiorly along the sacro-iliac joint, exactly following the course of the internal iliac vessels. Its metastatic involvement is common in cases of prostatic and vesical malignancies, but also in cancer of the uterine body or of the middle part of the rectum.
- The *main posterior pelvic pathway* follows the *presacral chain*. Collecting vessels arising from the posterior parts of the prostate, urinary bladder, cervix uteri or from the posterior aspect of the rectum, this pathway has a fairly regularly curved course above the levator ani, along the lateral walls of the rectal compartment, then in front of the sacral concavity, after which it reaches the lateral or less frequently the median sacral nodes. Because some of its lymphatic vessels originating from the abovementioned organs terminate in the subaortic nodes, this posterior presacral pelvic pathway explains the

possible presence of subaortic skip metastases as a primary site of lymph node involvement in the case of pelvic tumours which usually first invade the external or internal iliac lymph node groups of the anterior and middle main pelvic chains.

- The *internal pudendal accessory pelvic pathway* follows the course of the internal pudendal vessels below the level of the levator ani muscle. Originating in Retzius's prevesical space, it drains descending lymph vessels arising from the neck of the urinary bladder, the apex of the prostate and the lower part of the vagina, and which pass in the narrow space between both medial sides of the puborectalis muscles. Thereafter following the lateral wall of the ischio-anal fossa, this pathway is connected behind the ischial spine with the middle internal iliac main pathway and constitutes an alternative route of lymphatic spread for malignant tumours of the prostate, the cervix uteri or the proximal part of the anal canal above the ano-cutaneous junction.
- The *gonadic ascending accessory pelvic pathway* runs along the gonadic vessels to reach the inferior group of lateral aortic nodes. Located on the lateral side of the abdominal part of the ureter in front of the psoas muscle, this ascending lymphatic plexus is the usual route of lymphatic spread for ovarian tumours. It also represents an alternative pathway of lymph node involvement for cancers of the uterine fundus, since some lymphatics originating from that area run alongside the uterine tube in the mesosalpynx and join the ovarian vascular pedicle. Some other lymph vessels of the uterine tube may also accompany the round ligament, thereby resulting in secondary metastatic nodes in the superficial inguinal area. Finally, it should be noted that at the point where they cross the external iliac vessels, the lymphatics of the gonadic accessory pathway seem to create several anastomosing channels with the large collectors of the external iliac chain. These few bypass connections may well explain the occasional occurrence of secondary lateral aortic metastatic nodes at the L3 level associated with primarily invaded external iliac nodes, but without any enlarged nodes in the common iliac or subaortic areas.
- The *inferior mesenteric accessory pelvic pathway* only involves the drainage of the rectal pelvic compartment. Originating from the upper part of the intramuscular and submucous networks of the rectum, this lymphatic chain accompanies the inferior mesenteric vessels on the left side of the abdomen and terminates in the preaortic nodes at the L3 level. Its potential neoplastic involvement should be considered in cancers of the rectal ampulla.
- The *superficial perineal accessory pelvic pathway* should finally be considered as a route of lymphatic spread for tumours of the perineal cutaneous part of the anal canal and the vulva. Located anteriorly, this subcutaneous pathway ends in the superficial inguinal nodes and through the deep inguinal nodes becomes connected to the common terminal pelvic route of the external and common iliac chains.

According some observations, the superficial inguinal nodes also drain lymph vessels arising from the uterine fundus and horns. Running along the round ligament of the uterus, these vessels pass through the inguinal canal and so give rise to a *last inguinal accessory pelvic pathway* which ends in the groin area.

Practically each organ within the pelvis thus contains its own primary dense submucosal lymphatic plexus which is then relayed by secondary intramuscular and perivisceral or subperitoneal networks, the density of which decreases progressively and which are finally connected to several of the above-mentioned main and accessory efferent lymphatic pathways. According to its location within the pelvic cavity and its vascular connections, each organ thus has a complex pattern of lymphatic drainage which usually involves at least two major efferent pathways and one or more accessory streams. The lymphatic spread of prostatic cancer may thus involve four alternative pathways: the external iliac, internal iliac, presacral and internal pudendal pathways. Tumours of the rectum preferentially invade the internal iliac and presacral chains, but may also spread via the inferior mesenteric and superficial perineal routes if the lesion extends near its proximal or distal extremities. Another example is that of uterine carcinomas in which lymphatic metastases may extend along six possible pathways mainly passing through the external iliac and internal iliac lymph nodes, but also including additional potential relays in the presacral nodes or along the lymphatic bypasses between the internal pudendal, inguinal and gonadic chains.

1.7.4 Delineation of Lymph Node Areas

Pelvic lymph node areas cover the anterior, lateral and posterior walls of the pelvic cavity, and can be differentiated as follows into ten volumes (Fig. 1.9):

- The three *median volumes* occupy the centre of

the pelvis and respectively include the juxtavisceral perivesical (V), parauterovaginal (G) and pararectal (R) groups of nodes. These correspond to the fatty tissue surrounding each organ, and their lateral, anterior and posterior boundaries are delineated by the right and left sacrorectogenitopubic septa, then by the successive prevesical, prevaginal, prerectal and sacrorectal fasciae.

- The seven *lateral paired volumes* are present on both sides and it is proposed that they should be distinguished as the external iliac, internal iliac, common iliac, subaortic, presacral and internal pudendal areas. On transverse CT or MR sections, their boundaries can be described as follows:

– The *external iliac lymphatic area* (level I) comprises a pyramidal volume with the external iliac vessels circumscribing its base. Laterally it is bounded by the medial side of the psoas muscle and medially by the peritoneal lining of the pelvic inlet. Its posterior border is delineated by the pelvic part of the ureter, and anteriorly its limit corresponds to the femoral septum where it continues within the deep inguinal lymphatic area. Downwards, this area extends into the pelvis, on the inner surface of the iliopubic branch of the upper part of the obturatorius internus and of the levator ani. Its lowest narrow part corresponds to the inferior free edge of the levator ani. This area contains the external iliac artery and vein as well as the lymphatic vessels and nodes of the main anterior pelvic pathway, and also includes the proximal part of the gonadic accessory pathway, the anterior parietal branches of the internal iliac vessels and the obturator nerve. The so-called 'obturator' lymph nodes are located at its centre and on the left side of the pelvis the interiliac nodes occupy its highest narrow apical part. On the right pelvic walls, this node is placed behind the ureter which crosses the iliac vessels more anteriorly than on the left side. However, it belongs to the external iliac chain; the right interiliac node thus becomes included in the next radiological volume.

– The *internal iliac lymphatic area* (level II) is located immediately behind the former one. It is also triangular in shape, is centred on the internal iliac artery and becomes enlarged caudally around its different visceral branches. Anteriorly, this volume is bounded by the pelvic part of the ureter and its posterior limit runs along the lateral edge of the sacrum then along the sacro-iliac joint. Inferiorly, the base of the triangle corresponds to the lower free edge of the levator ani downwards to the apex of the coccyx dorsally. The lateral wall is lined superiorly by the ischium, then by the medial surface of the piriformis and levator ani more caudally. Its medial wall extends towards the plane of the sacrorectogenitopubic septum. This area contains in the adipose tissue surrounding the internal iliac vessels most of their posterior parietal and visceral branches but also the lymphatic pathways of the middle main pelvic pathway, the proximal part of the posterior presacral pathway, the efferent pelvic nerves of the hypogastric plexus and the origin of the sciatic nerve.

– The *common iliac lymphatic area* (level III) is an upward extension of the two above-mentioned volumes, around the common iliac vessels. Its three-dimensional space corresponds to the lumbosacral fossa which is bounded laterally by the medial edge of the psoas muscle and medially by the lateral aspect of the L5 vertebra. Usually the blood vessels run along the anterior limit of this triangular volume which is based caudally on the upper surface of the sacral wing and contains the common latero- and retrovascular iliac lymph nodes as well as the lumbosacral nervous trunk and the origin of the obturator nerve.

– The *presacral lymphatic area* (level IV) corresponds to a triangular strongly curved volume which posteriorly faces the presacral concavity. Bounded anteriorly by the fascia recti, its extends laterally towards the lateral borders of the sacrum where it encounters the posterior limit of the internal iliac volume. Its apex is directed caudally and corresponds to the coccyx, while its base is delineated by the sacral promontory. Within this volume run the median and lateral sacral vessels, the lymphatics of the presacral chains, the anterior branches of the sacral nerves and the inferior hypogastric plexus.

– The *subaortic lymphatic area* (level V) continues superiorly the previous one and extends along the anterior aspect of the body of the L5 vertebra. Its apex is in the narrow space superiorly between both crura of the aortic bifurcation and its base, located at the upper border of S1 is contiguous with that of the presacral area. This short triangular almost planar volume includes the origin of the median sacral artery, the subaortic group of nodes and the superior sympathetic hypogastric plexus.

– The *internal pudendal lymphatic area* – VI) includes the prevesical fatty space and courses along the corresponding artery, on the lateral wall of the ischio-anal fossa in the narrow angle between the levator ani and the obturatorius internus muscles. Its posterior limit is marked by

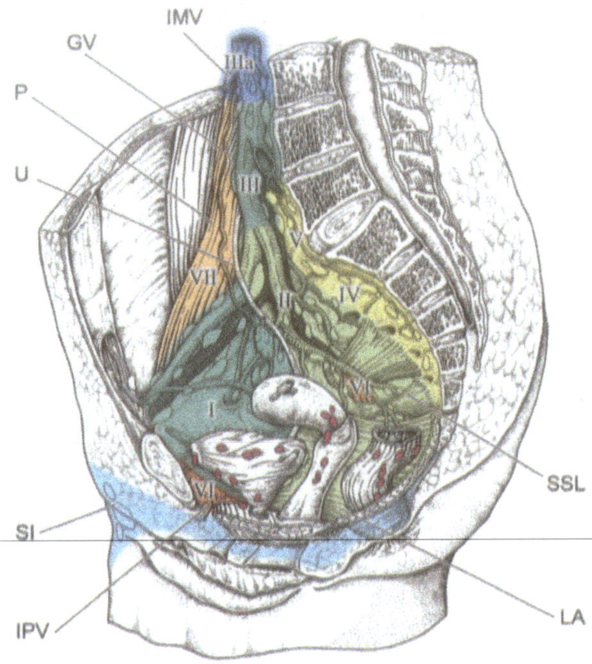
IMV
GV
P
U
IIIa
III
VII
II
V
IV
I
VI
SSL
SI
IPV
LA

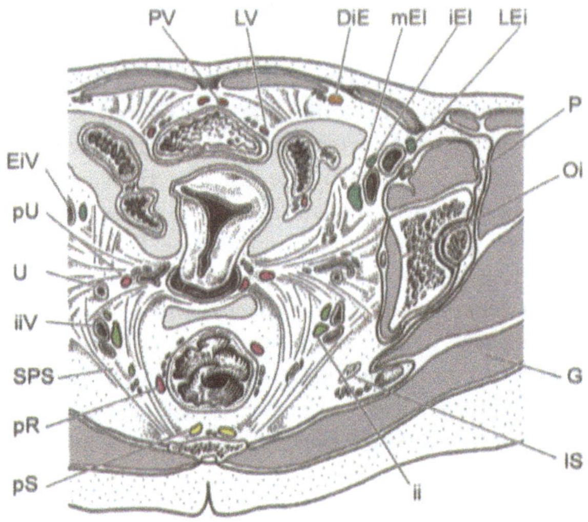
PV
LV
DiE
mEI
iEI
LEi
P
Oi
EiV
pU
U
iiV
SPS
pR
pS
G
IS
ii

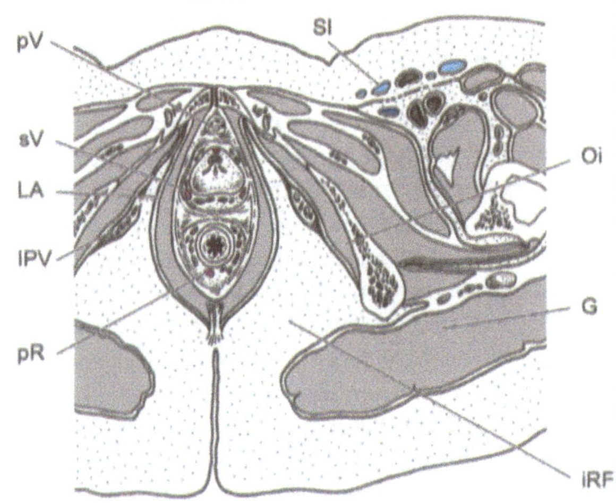
pV
SI
sV
LA
IPV
pR
Oi
G
iRF

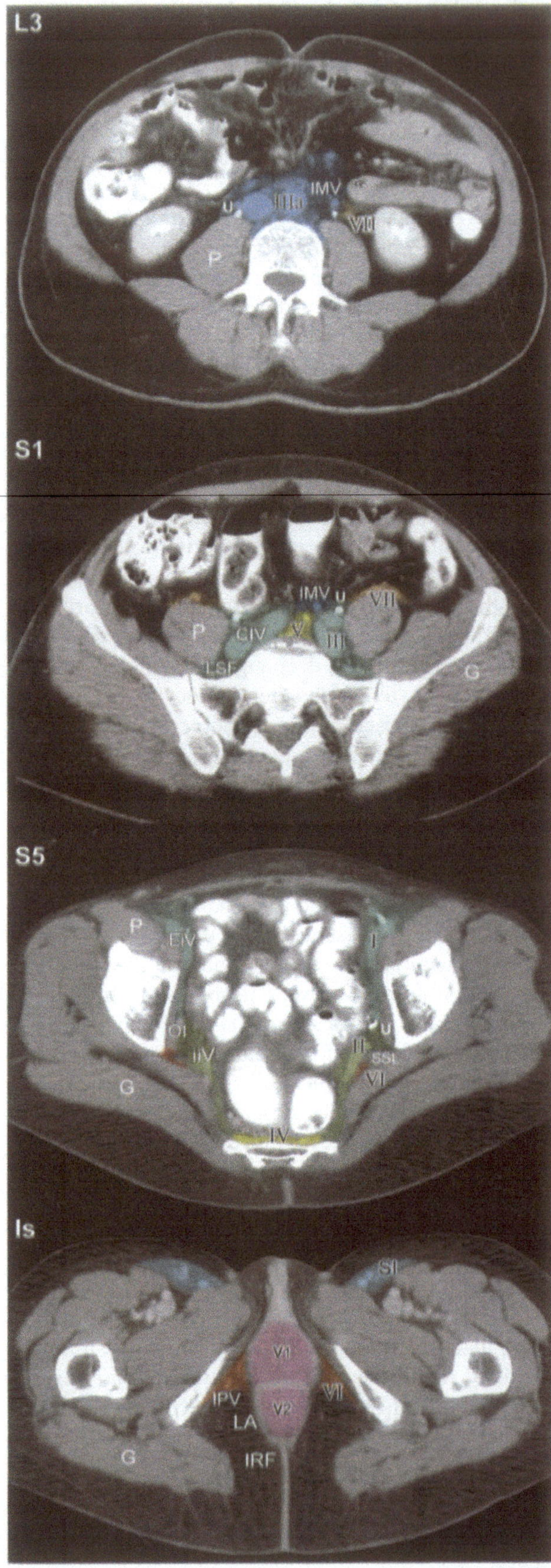
L3
IMV
IIIa
u
VII
P
S1
IMV
u
VII
P
CIV
V
III
LSF
G
S5
P
EiV
I
Oi
iiV
II
u
SSL
VI
G
IV
Is
SI
VI
IPV
LA
VI
IRF
G

the ischial spine where it joins the middle part of the internal iliac lymphatic area.
- The *gonadic lymphatic area* (level VII) finally occupies the lateral aspect of the common iliac area. Located in front of the psoas muscle, on the lateral side of the ureter, it extends from the L5 vertebra inferiorly, upwards to the L3 vertebra, where it fuses with the lateral part of the lower abdominal level IIIb. Centred on the gonadic vessels, this volume contains the distal part of the gonadic accessory pelvic pathway and also includes the proximal course of the genitofemoral nerve and of the lateral cutaneous nerve of the thigh.

At the end of the inferior mesenteric, inguinal and superficial perineal accessory pathways, two *extrapelvic areas* have also to be considered as target volumes in the treatment of intrapelvic tumours:

- The first one is the *inferior mesenteric area*. Arising from the upper limit of the rectal visceral volume, it follows the inferior mesenteric vessels within the left mesocolon, and continues superiorly with the central part of the lower abdominal volume (level IIIa), in front of the L3 vertebra.
- The second extrapelvic area corresponds to the *superficial inguinal volume* described with the lymphatics of the lower limb. Located in the groin, it contains the superficial perineal lymph vessels, in the lengthening of the soft tissues of the perineum, below the muscles of the urogenital diaphragm.

1.8 Lymphatics of the Lower Limbs

The lymphatic vessels of the lower limbs consist of two networks, one superficial and one deep, which are segregated by the deep fascia and remain completely independent of one another, although they finally converge in the popliteal fossa and proximally in the groin area. During their course, they are interrupted by several groups of nodes which are fewer in number in the lower limbs than elsewhere. The terminal groups, located on the anterior root of the thigh, comprise the superficial and deep inguinal lymph nodes. The outlying nodes, deeply located on the interosseous membrane of the leg or on the posterior aspect of the knee, are known as the anterior tibial and popliteal nodes (Fig. 1.10).

1.8.1 Lymph Node Groups

The *superficial inguinal lymph nodes* constitute one of the most important lymphatic centres of the body. They are usually from ten to 12 in number and are frequently larger than nodes from other lymphatic areas. They are all scattered in front of Scarpa's femoral triangle in a space which is bounded superiorly by the inguinal ligament, laterally by the medial border of the sartorius muscle, and medially by the upper border of the adductor longus. Topographically the nodes are situated under the subcutaneous tissue and the superficialis fascia, and lie posteriorly on the cribriform fascia which separates them from the femoral vessels and nerve, and from the nodes of the deep inguinal group. Due to their large number, the extensive space they occupy and their different drainage territories, they are usually divided into two groups and four subgroups. A horizontal line drawn through the terminal arch of the great saphenous vein separates the superior and inferior superficial inguinal groups. The latter groups are then subdivided into two secondary subgroups, i.e. a medial and a lateral group. In the former group, the nodes are usually arranged in a chain of five to six nodes parallel to the inguinal ligament. On the contrary, the latter group includes four to five elongated nodes set vertically along the terminal part of the great saphenous vein. According to several authors, additional small round nodes located in the saphenous opening are interposed between the previous nodes and constitute a supplementary central group. However, although this subdivision may have certain clinical implications, it remains purely relative from an anatomical point of view since a large number

Fig. 1.9. Radiological delineation of the pelvic lymph node areas. In addition to three central visceral volumes (V_1–V_3), seven lateral paired areas (levels I–VII) are defined on the pelvic walls. The corresponding target volumes are indicated by different *colours* on anatomical and CT sections performed through the upper-female and lower-male parts of the pelvis and also include additional extrapelvic superficial inguinal (*SI*) and lower abdominal (IIIA) areas. The key landmarks used to delineate the volumes are as follows: the ureter (*U*), internal iliac (*iiV*) external) iliac (*EiV*), gonadic (*GV*), inferior mesenteric (*IMV*) and internal pudendal (IPV) vessels, ischial spine (*IS*), sacrospinus ligament (*SSL*), sacrorectogenitopubic septa (*SPS*) and the psoas (*P*), levator ani (*LA*), obturatorius internus (*Oi*) and gluteal muscles (*G*). Legend and *colours* used to indicate the node groups are identical to those in Fig. 1.8 and the main fatty spaces are indicated as ischiorectal (*IRF*) and lumbosacral (*LSF*) fossae

of connections are present between the nodes from different subgroups, and also since their prefential tributaries are subject to numerous variations.

The afferent vessels of the *superolateral group* originate from the integuments of the gluteal region and the adjacent lateral part of the lower anterior abdominal wall below the umbilicus. The lymph nodes of the *superomedial group* receive afferent vessels from the hypogastric area of the abdominal wall, but also a large number of collecting vessels originating from the external genitalia including the skin of the penis, the scrotum, the vulva and the distal parts of the vagina and anal canal below the anocutaneous junction. As previously stated, they constitute the terminal relay of the superficial perineal alternative pathway for the lymphatic drainage of the lower pelvis. Furthermore, they also receive some afferent vessels from the uterine horns that run through the inguinal canal with the round ligament of the uterus. In the lower groups, both *inferomedial* and *inferolateral nodes* drain the terminal superficial lymphatic vessels of the lower limb, except those from the lateral edge of the foot and the posterolateral aspect of the leg.

Efferent vessels from all the groups of superficial inguinal nodes converge towards the central nodes when these are present, then extend towards the deep inguinal nodes. To reach them, they usually pass through the saphenous opening along the saphenous vein, while others pass through the cribriform fascia, thereby creating its multiperforated aspect. Among the efferent vessels arising from the lower nodes, some large collectors directly enter the pelvic cavity through the femoral ring. Running alongside the femoral vessels, either in front of them, but with the majority on the inner side of the vein, they end in the lower pole of the lateral and intermediate lacunar nodes.

The *deep inguinal lymph nodes*, which are embedded in the subfascial adipose tissue of the femoral canal, are located on the medial side of the femoral vein. They vary in number from one to three, and when three of them are present, the lowest node is always situated against the femoral vein just below the point where the terminal arch of the great saphenous vein opens into its anterior wall. When present, the highest node occupies the lateral part of the femoral ring. It can often protrude into the pelvis, and is known as Cloquet's node by French authors and is referred to as Rosenmüller's node in the German literature. Afferent vessels to the deep inguinal nodes mostly issue from the terminal collectors of the deep network of practically the whole lower limb, which accompany the femoral vessels. Nevertheless, they also receive some afferents from the superficial inguinal nodes and few lymphatic vessels from the glans penis in the male and the clitoris in the female. Their efferents penetrate the pelvis through the femoral canal, and join the lacunar nodes of the external iliac group.

The *popliteal lymph nodes* are from four to six in number, always small in size and are embedded in the loose adipose tissue within the popliteal fossa. Mainly located around the popliteal vessels, they form a chain around the vertical axis of the losangic space bounded superiorly by the hamstring muscles and inferiorly by the medial and lateral heads of the gastrocnemius. From the upper to the lower part, these nodes usually occupy three distinct locations:

- The most superficial node is situated just beneath the popliteal fascia against the termination of the small saphenous vein and its entry into the popliteal vein. Invariably located on the medial side of the tibial nerve, it drains the superficial lymphatic vessels of the calf and those of the lateral edge of the foot.
- The middle nodes are spread around the popliteal vessels, either on their lateral side or on their medial edge. Mainly linked to the popliteal vein, they drain the deep lymphatic collectors originating from the foot and the leg, coursing alongside the anterior tibial, posterior tibial and fibular vessels.
- The deepest node is located on the anterior aspect of the popliteal artery and lies against the oblique popliteal ligament. In close relation with the knee, it receives lymphatics from the joint, which accompany the genicular arteries.

The efferent vessels of the popliteal nodes mainly follow the popliteal vessels, pass through the adductor canal and then course alongside the femoral vessels before ending in the deep inguinal nodes. Some efferent vessels, however, remain at a more superficial level and have a different outcome. Running alongside anastomotic veins which unite the small saphenous vein with the great saphenous vein, they terminate in the inferomedial group of superficial inguinal nodes. This route is not as important as the former and may frequently be absent.

The *anterior tibial lymph node* is usually unique and lies close to the anterior tibial vessels on the anterior aspect of the interosseous membrane of the leg. Receiving afferents from the ascending collectors of the dorsum of the foot and the muscles of the anterior crural compartment, it gives off a single efferent channel which terminates in the middle popliteal lymph nodes.

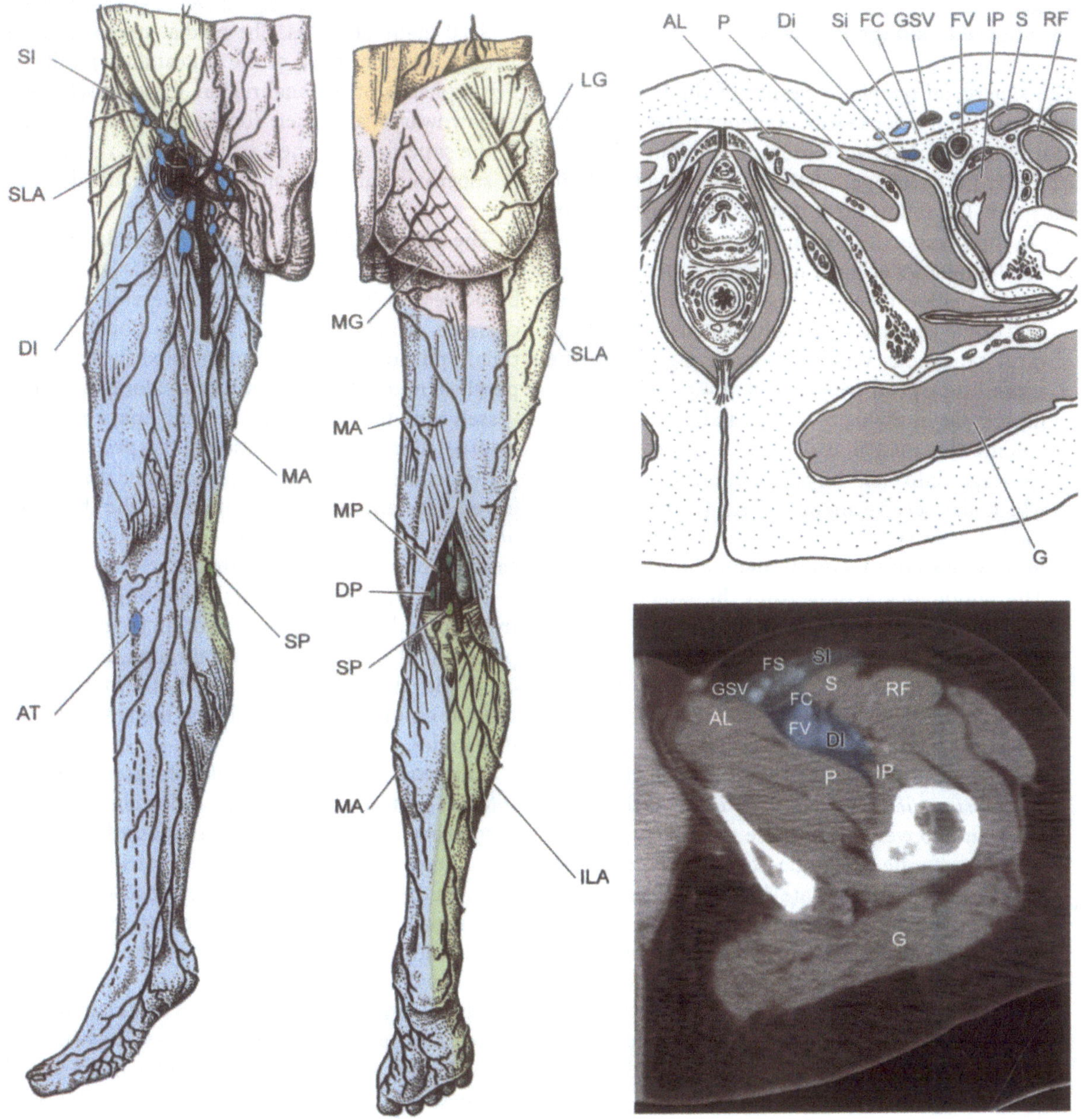

Fig. 1.10. Lymphatic pathways and target volumes of the lower limbs. Anterior and posterior anatomical views of the lower limb showing the distribution of lymph vessels and nodes. Node groups are identified as follows: superficial inguinal (*SI*), deep inguinal (*DI*), superficial popliteal (*SP*), middle popliteal (*MP*), deep popliteal (*DP*) and anterior tibial (*AT*) nodes. Collecting vessels of the superficial system give rise to the medial (*MA*), inferior lateral (*ILA*) and superior lateral (*SLA*) ascending pathways and to the medial (*MG*) and lateral gluteal (*LG*) pathways. The inguinal target volume is delineated on anatomical and CT sections of the groin area. Key anatomical landmarks indicating its boundaries are as follows: the femoral vessels (*FV*), great saphenous vein (*GSV*), cribriformis (*FC*) and superficialis (*FS*) fasciae, and the pectineus (*P*), adductor longus (*AL*), sartorius (*S*), rectus femoris (*RF*) and iliopsoas (*Ip*) muscles

1.8.2 Functional Drainage Pathways

The *superficial lymphatic vessels* of the lower limbs originate from a dense subcutaneous network which has its maximum development in the foot. The collecting trunks arising from this plexus all converge in the groin, but follow three distinct pathways according to their respective origins (Fig. 10):

- The lymphatics originating from the medial side of the foot follow an ascending course on the medial side of the leg which is closely related to that of the great saphenous vein. Thereby giving rise to the *medial superficial lymphatic pathway* of the lower limb, some of them are located in front and others behind the medial malleolus, and progressively converge into ten large longitudinal collectors which also receive afferents from the anterior and medial aspects of the thigh and terminate in the lower groups of superficial inguinal nodes.
- The lymphatics arising from the lateral part of the foot and the posterolateral part of the ankle progressively become satellites of the small saphenous vein. Following this venous channel, they initially course between the lateral malleolus and the calcaneal tendon and then ascend along the posterior aspect of the calf. They thus constitute the *lateral superficial lymphatic pathway* of the lower limb and converge into three terminal collectors which perforate the fascia covering the popliteal fossa and then terminate in the superficial and middle popliteal nodes. From this point, the lymphatic drainage of the posterolateral cutaneous cover of the leg and foot follows thus the deep lymphatic pathway, ending in the deep inguinal nodes. However, some superficial subcutaneous lymph vessels bypass the popliteal nodes, running alongside anastomosing veins that connect the great and small saphenous veins. Crossing the medial edge of the thigh, they finally reach the medial group of lower superficial inguinal nodes. This rare alternative route mentioned by Sappey can explain the fact that the sentinel node of a skin tumour located on the lateral edge of the calf may be identified in the superficial inguinal nodes, whereas it should theoretically be found among the popliteal or deep inguinal nodes.
- Finally, the collecting trunks from the cutaneous layer of the gluteal region are divided into *two superficial gluteal pathways*. The lateral stream usually constitutes the main pathway, drains the ascending lymph vessels from the outer two-thirds of the buttock, and turns around the greater trochanter to terminate in the superolateral group of superficial inguinal nodes. The medial stream concerns only the inner third of the gluteal area. Joining the lymphatics of the anal region, these vessels course downwards and then forwards, thereby entering the superficial perineal pathway which ends in the superomedial group of superficial inguinal nodes.

The *deep lymphatics* of the lower limbs drain the subfascial tissues and course as satellites of the main blood vessels. They thus comprise several converging channels which follow the anterior tibial, posterior tibial and fibular vessels. Interrupted by the middle popliteal nodes, they thereafter run along the femoral vessels until they reach the deep inguinal and lacunar external iliac nodes. In addition to this *principal channel* which drains all the deep tissues of the foot and leg and the anterior compartment of the thigh, *deep accessory channels* are present along the obturator and superior or inferior gluteal arteries.

Among these, the *obturator collecting trunks* arise from the adductor muscles and drain the medial compartment of the thigh. Passing through the obturator canal with their companion vessels, they terminate in the true obturator lymph node and then in the internal iliac nodes.

The *inferior gluteal lymphatics* accompany the inferior gluteal blood vessels and mainly drain the hamstring muscles and soft tissues of the posterior compartment of the thigh. Entering the pelvis through the lower part of the greater sciatic foramen, they usually end in a specific small node of the internal iliac group which is situated on the lower border of the piriformis.

The *superior gluteal lymphatics* originate from the gluteal and pelvitrochanteric muscles. They run along the superior gluteal vessels and then pass into the pelvis through the upper part of the greater sciatic foramen. Their terminal node usually occupies the highest position in the internal iliac chain on the anterior aspect of the actual trunk of the superior gluteal artery above the upper edge of the piriformis.

Given these anatomical considerations, lymphophilic tumours of the distal part of the lower limb and the anterior part of the thigh invade the principal channel with primary metastases in the popliteal and deep inguinal nodes before involving the external iliac chain. The lymphatic spread of posteriorly located deep tumours of the thigh or the buttock on the contrary bypasses this usual route interrupted in the groin area, and is characterised by the primary involvement of intrapelvic nodes linked to the internal iliac chain.

1.8.3
Delineation of Node Areas

The lymph node areas of the lower limbs consist of two main volumes located respectively on the posterior aspect of the knee and in the groin area. They are well circumscribed by the main muscular groups of the thigh and the calf, and include all the nodes of the main ascending pathways of the superficial and deep lymphatic pathways (Fig. 1.10). They are easily identifiable on CT or MR transverse sections, and are delineated as follows:

- The *inguinal volume* corresponds to the anatomical boundaries of Scarpa's femoral triangle. Limited superiorly by the inguinal ligament, it extends laterally to the medial border of the sartorius and medially to the lateral border of the adductor longus. Pyramidal in shape, the inguinal volume is bounded on its anterior surface by the fascia superficialis of the groin area. Posteriorly, its deep walls are constituted by the outer surface of the iliopsoas muscle, laterally and medially, by the anterior aspect of the pectineus muscle. The base of the pyramid lies proximally and corresponds to the femoral septum. At this point underlined by the upper border of the pubis, it encounters the anterior extremity of the external iliac volume of the pelvic lymphatic chains. Caudally the apex of the inguinal volume is located in the narrow angle between the sartorius and adductor longus muscles. Surgically the inguinal volume is clearly divided into two topographical compartments respectively containing the saphenous vein and the superficial inguinal nodes on one side, and the femoral blood vessels accompanied by the deep inguinal nodes on the other. The cribriform fascia which covers the femoral canal constitutes the anatomical plane which segregates both these superficial and deep compartments which are cleared separately or in continuity in an inguinal dissection. Because of its low thickness and its multiple perforations, this plane is usually difficult to recognise on radiological images. The anterior limit of the inguinal volume therefore remains partially virtual, just as its subdivision into deep and superficial compartments. In addition to the femoral artery and vein, the deep part of the inguinal volume contains the deep inguinal lymph nodes, the origin of the external pudendal, superficial circumflex iliac and superficial epigastric vessels, and the common stem of the femoral nerve that runs on the surface of the iliopsoas muscle. The superficial part of the inguinal volume includes in the subcutaneous fat the superficial inguinal nodes, the terminal part of the great saphenous vein and the femoral branch of the genitofemoral nerve.
- The *popliteal volume* occupies the losangic space of the popliteal fossa. Superiorly it is then bounded by the medial (semitendinous and semimembranous) and lateral (biceps femoris) hamstring muscles. Inferiorly it extends between the medial and lateral heads of the gastronemius. Its anterior aspect corresponds to the posterior capsule of the knee joint covered by the popliteus, while its posterior surface extends between the four above-mentioned muscular edges, in order to virtually represent the anatomical plane of the popliteal fascia. In addition to the popliteal lymph nodes within the fatty tissue of the fossa, this volume contains the popliteal blood vessels and their articular branches, the terminal part of the small saphenous vein and the tibial nerve. The common fibular nerve, running along the lower border of the biceps femoris, should not be systematically included in the lymphatic volume. As previously stated, the popliteal lymph nodes indeed occupy the central axis of the fossa in the immediate vicinity of the veins. They thus have a close relation with the tibial nerve but are quite distant from the fibular terminal branch of the sciatic nerve.

1.9
Conclusions

The anatomical study of the lymphatic system shows that it consists of two superficial and deep networks of lymph vessels which converge within each part of the body into deep lymph node areas. Located in the lateral regions of the neck, the root of the limbs, the central part of the chest and along the large arteries and veins of the abdomen and pelvis, these lymph nodes areas share the common characteristics of being filled with fat, centred on large blood vessels, and well circumscribed by specific muscular bellies and fasciae. In most cases, the anatomical landmarks used to delineate these volumes on sequential radiological sections are quite similar to those used by surgeons during dissection procedures. However, the lymphatic drainage of each organ involves several functional pathways including the main collecting chains, but also alternative routes which are not always considered in current surgical practice. Taking this functional plasticity of the lymphatic system into account, the radiological delineation of the target volumes may thus exactly match their surgical boundaries in the case of specific tumour locations, but in other malignancies it should extend beyond these narrow limits to include the entire potential volume of their multidirectional lymphatic spread. In this respect, detailed anatomical knowledge of the dynamic lymphatic network associated with each area of the body is essential to define all the sites in which the presence of metastatic nodes should be investigated in tumour assessment and staging, but also to delineate on a rational morphological basis the optimal target volumes to be treated by conformal radiotherapy.

References

Berg JW (1955) The significance of axillary node levels in the study of breast cancer. Cancer 63:776–778

Bourgery J (1836) Les vaisseaux lymphatiques In: Bourgery J: Traité complet de l'anatomie de l'homme, vol 4. Delaunay, Paris, pp 147–158, pl 78–94

Candela FC, Kothari K, Shah JP (1990) Patterns of cervical node metastases from squamous carcinoma of the oropharynx and hypopharynx. Head Neck Surg 12: 197–203

Caplan I (1990) Anatomical review of the lymph nodes of the mediastinum. Surg Radiol Anat 12:9–18

Gabriel WB, Dukes C, Bussey HJR (1935) Lymphatic spread in cancer of the rectum. Br J Surg 23:395–413

Gregoire V, Coche E, Cosnard G et al (2000) Selection and delineation of lymph node target volumes in head and neck conformal radiotherapy. Proposal for standardizing terminology and procedure based on the surgical experience. Radiother Oncol 56:135–150

Haagensen CD, Feind CR, Herter TP et al (1972) The lymphatics in cancer. Saunders, Philadelphia

Hayman LA, Taber KH, Diaz-Harchan PJ et al (1998) Spatial compartments of the neck part III: axial sections. Int J Neuroradiol 4:393–402

Henriksen E (1949) The lymphatic spread of carcinoma of the cervix and the body of uterus. Am J Obstet Gynecol 58:924–942

Lindberg R (1972) Distribution of cervical lymph node metastases from squamous cell carcinomas of the upper respiratory and digestive tracts. Cancer 29:1446–1449

Pfrundner L, Pahnke J, Willner J (2000) Systematics in lymphatic tumor spread of carcinomas of the upper aerodigestive tract: a clinical study based on embryonic data. Eur Arch Otorhinolaryngol 257:561–569

Plentl AA, Friedman EA (1971) Lymphatic system of the female genitalia. The morphologic basis of oncologic diagnosis and therapy. Saunders, Philadelphia

Poirier P, Cuneo B, Delamere G (1903) The lymphatics. Archibald Constable & Co, Westminster

Richter E, Feyerabend T (1991) Normal lymph node topography. CT atlas of lymphatics. Springer, Berlin Heidelberg New York

Riquet M, Le Pimpec-Barthes, Hidden G (2001) Lymphatic drainage of the pericardium to the mediastinal lymph nodes. Surg Radiol Anat 23:317–319

Robbins KT (1999) Integrating radiological criteria into the classification of cervical lymph node disease. Arch Otolaryngol Head Neck Surg 125:385–387

Robbins KT, Medina JE, Wolfe GT et al (1991) Standardizing neck dissection terminology. Official report of the Academy's Committee for Head and Neck Surgery and Oncology. Arch Otolaryngol Head Neck Surg 117:601–605

Rouviere H, Tobias MJ (1938) Anatomy of the human lymphatic system. Edwards, Ann Arbor

Saito H, Sato T, Yamashita Y, Amagase T (2002) Topographical analysis of lymphatic pathways from the meso- and hypopharynx based on minute cadaveric dissections: possible application to neck dissection in pharyngeal cancer. Surg Radiol Anat 24: 38–49

Sappey PC (1888) Des vaisseaux lymphatiques. In: Sappey PC, Traité d'anatomie descriptive, vol 2. Delahaye A, Lecrosnier E, Paris, pp 731–842

Shah JP (1990) Patterns of cervical lymph node metastasis from squamous carcinomas of the upper aerodigestive tract. Am J Surg 160:405–409

Testut L (1893) Des lymphatiques. In: Testut L, Traité d'anatomie humaine, vol 2. Doin, Paris, pp 267–308

Verge P, Vanneuville G, Escande VG et al (1982) A study of lymph drainage of the larynx. Folia Morphol 30:173–178

Vidic B, Suarez-Quian C (1998) Anatomy of the head and neck. In: Harrison LB, Session SRB, Ki Hong W (eds) Head and neck cancer. A multidisciplinary approach. Lippincott-Raven, Philadelphia, pp 79–114

Warwick R, Williams P (1973) Topography of the lymph nodes and vessels. In: Gray's anatomy, 35th edn. Longman, Edinburgh pp 727–744

Whitmore I (1998) Lymphoid system. In: Federative Committee on Anatomical Terminology – terminologica anatomica. Thieme Verlag, Stuttgart, pp 100–103

2 Imaging the Lymph Nodes: CT, MRI, and PET

E. E. Coche, T. Duprez, M. Lonneux

CONTENTS

2.1 Introduction

The detection of malignant lymph nodes remains a major challenge in spite of the marked improvement in currently available imaging modalities (Van den Brekel and Castelijns 1999). Cross-sectional techniques capable of 3D reconstruction such as computed tomography (CT) and magnetic resonance imaging (MRI) are now in standard use for the radiological staging of nodal status. However in spite of improved technology regarding the speed of image acquisition, spatial resolution, 3D image post-processing and even tissue contrast modulation, their capacity for tissue characterization is limited (Carrington 1998). Integrating other modalities to obtain additional information on e.g. the vascular architecture of the nodes (color Doppler ultrasound), or on metabolic indexes such as glucose uptake [positron emission tomogra-

E. E. Coche, MD; T. Duprez, MD; M. Lonneux, MD, PhD
Cliniques Universitaires Saint-Luc, Université Catholique de Louvain, Avenue Hippocrate, 10, 1200 Brussels, Belgium

phy (PET)] is essential to achieve increased sensitivity and specificity of the pre- and post-treatment nodal work-up of patients with neoplastic disease (Jabour et al. 1993; Moritz et al. 2000). Vast research areas are being explored in the field of MRI on intrinsic tissue parameter measurements and organ-targeted contrast agents (Anzai and Prince 1997; Dooms et al. 1985; Hoffman et al. 2000). The combined anatomical (CT/MR) and metabolic (PET) data provided in a single view through image fusion is being increasingly used, as this technological refinement has been reported to provide enhanced sensitivity and specificity thresholds in malignant lymph node depiction (Wahl et al. 1994).

2.2 Computed Tomography Imaging

2.2.1 Hardware/Software Requirements for High-Quality CT

Computed tomography technology has continued to improve over the past decades. The first CT mode introduced in the early 1970s by Godfrey Hounsfield was *sequential,* i.e., the patient remained stationary while transverse slices were acquired but with a spatial table incrementation between slice acquisitions (Hounsfield 1973). The main limitations to this initial approach were the time required to perform the examination and the gap between two slices, possibly resulting in lesion misregistration. For several years, *spiral/helical* (Towers 1993) or *volumetric* CT has been used in clinical practice; data recording is obtained during the continuous rotation of a set of detectors while the table undergoes continuous motion at a predetermined speed (Brink 1995; Kalender et al. 1990). This new approach has several advantages when compared to the conventional CT mode. Among these, the following should be emphasized: shortened acquisition time (under one minute to obtain a complete volume of 30 cm FOV in the Z-axis with intermediate spatial resolution), optimization of the intravenous injection of iodinated contrast medium, acquisition of an uninterrupted volume of data which can subsequently be post-processed, and a substantial decrease in patient irradiation. It has recently been demonstrated that for a given X-ray dose and using overlapping reconstruction, the spiral CT technique has a better longitudinal resolution than the conventional CT technique (Kalender et al. 1994; Wang and Vannier 1994; Wang et al. 1994). Recently spiral CT technology has further improved with the incorporation of multiple rows of detectors instead of a single row (*"multislice"* or *"multirow"* CT) (Fuchs et al. 2000; Klingenbeck-Regn et al. 1999). With the recent decrease in gantry rotation time, multislice helical CT is now up to eight times faster than conventional single-slice helical CT. The concurrent acquisition of multiple slices results in a significant reduction in scanning time, permitting one-step acquisition of large volumes, a procedure which was previously unfeasible. In a similar manner, given volumes can be scanned using narrower beam collimation, resulting in a higher transverse spatial resolution without additional time loss. Both high-resolution and standard images can be reconstructed in the so-called *"combi-mode"* from data acquired using narrow collimation. On the one hand, patient dose exposure is reduced because repeated scanning is no longer required. On the other hand, narrow collimation is beneficial to standard reconstructions, as partial volume artifacts are drastically reduced.

2.2.2 Basic Tissue Contrast on CT Images

Spontaneous tissue contrast on CT images is directly related to the X-ray characteristics. Only thin tissue slices are irradiated, without subsequent deleterious superimposition or blurring of structures located outside the selected slice planes (Petterson 1995). Each detector rotating around the patient during data acquisition receives a variable amount of X-rays depending on the physical parameters of the incidental beam [kilovoltage (kV), milliamperes per second (mAs)], and on the specific attenuating characteristics (tissue volume, physical composition) of the patient's tissues. The CT system measures the tissue attenuation coefficient which has a diagnostic value. Attenuation is quantified by a numerical value ranging from approximately −1,000 to 3,000 Hounsfield units (HU). The system is calibrated so that water has an attenuation value of 0 HU, and air an attenuation value of −1,000 HU. A normal lymph node is a soft tissue structure with spontaneous intermediate density of 30–50 HU. The node hilum density may be negative when it contains fatty tissue. However, calcifications have a high attenuation value and therefore appear very bright on CT images. The CT technique is far more sensitive than MRI in depicting calcifications (Naidich et al. 1999). When necrosis occurs, the lymph node may show low attenuation values due to the fluid content. To better characterize a normal or abnormal structure and differentiate it from its environment, intravenous contrast medium may be injected before or during the CT procedure. Most CT contrast media contain iodine (I). After a rapid intravenous bolus injection, contrast medium molecules rapidly diffuse through most capillary membranes from the intravascular to the extravascular space, allowing the detection of necrotic areas within the nodes and/or tumor (Figs. 2.1, 2.3a) which contain less contrast medium-filled blood vessels than the surrounding normally vascularized tissues. The intensity of nodal contrast enhancement after contrast medium perfusion depends on the degree of vascularization (Sakai et al. 2000). Nodal enhancement is a non-specific finding, as inflammatory or tumoral nodes may have similarly higher attenuation values due to contrast medium uptake by the feeding vessels.

2.2.3 CT Image Acquisition Parameters

2.2.3.1 *Kilovoltage, Milliamperes per Second*

The kV reflects the energy level of the incidental X-ray beam. Higher energies result in an increased penetration through the tissues so that a greater number of photons can reach the detectors on the opposite side. Subsequent reduction in quantum noise leads to smoother images. The mAs value quantifies the number of emitted X-ray photons. The quantum noise value is inversely proportional to the mAs number. Increasing the mAs decreases the quantum noise value and increases contrast resolution. In selecting the mAs value, the radiologist must take into account the overall image quality, the radiation dose, and ultimately the impact of the image quality on the final diagnosis. The standard values used at our institution are 120 kV and 150 mAs for cervical region imaging and 100 kV and 165 mAs for the chest and abdomen imaging. The mAs value must be significantly increased for conformal radiotherapy (CRT) planning. For example, in the case of whole-body scanning, imaging must be performed at 120 kV and at around 300 mAs.

2.2.3.2 *Beam Collimation*

Beam collimation designates the actual width of the incidental X-ray beam. In sequential CT, the basic slice thickness is defined as follows: a 5-mm wide beam leads to the acquisition of a 5-mm thick section, and a 10-mm wide beam to a 10-mm thick section. In spiral CT, slice thickness is increased by image distortion due to the continuous motion of the patient through the gantry during scanning. Selecting the beam collimation (the nominal slice thickness) is one the first parameters to define, since it has a major impact on the sensitivity of lesion detection. For detecting small nodes, it would be inappropriate to choose a thick slice section since a thin lesion could be missed because of the partial volume averaging effects. Usually, lymph node staging using CT requires a 3–5 mm slice thickness in the neck area (van den Brekel and Castelijns 2000) and 5–10 mm in the chest and abdomen.

2.2.3.3 *Rotation Time*

Rotation time designates the length of time necessary for the beam source to complete one full 360° rotation. Until recently, this took one second for all spiral scanners. Nowadays the *multislice* CT (MSCT) mode has enabled this to be reduced to a sub-second rotation time (Klingenbeck-Regn et al. 1999), i.e. from one to 0.5 second. With this kind of CT system, four contiguous slices may be obtained during one rotation with eight images acquired in one second. For oncology patients, this new approach limits the time the patient has to spend in an uncomfortable position, reduces the need for repeated breath-holding and for repeated contrast medium injections (Rydberg et al. 2000). The image quality of spiral CT with a sub-second gantry rotation period is better than that obtained with a one-second rotation time, particularly for mediastinal examinations (Rubin et al. 1998). In the near future, MSCT systems will be introduced with a rotation time of less than 0.5 second, enabling the acquisition of 38 images per second.

2.2.3.4 *Pitch*

In sequential scanning, the patient remains stationary during acquisition of the multiple projections needed to reconstruct the transaxial image. In spiral CT, the patient is continuously moved through the gantry during data acquisition. In single-slice spiral scanning, the pitch is determined by the ratio of the table movement per each 360° gantry rotation to the beam collimation. The pitch equals 1 if the beam collimation is 10 mm and the patient is moved into the gantry by 10 mm during every 360° rotation. If the beam collimation is 10 mm, with the patient being passed through the gantry at a speed of 20 mm/rotation, the pitch value increases to 2. Increasing the pitch leads to an overall decrease in the delivered radiation dose (with all other imaging parameters remaining unchanged), since the overall scanning time is shortened as a result of the faster passage of the patient through the gantry. A pitch value greater than 1 can be selected if the area of interest is too large to be covered by the prescribed collimation when using a pitch of 1. The use of a greater pitch increases the distortion along the z-axis and also increases the noise. This distortion may impact on the delineation of the target volume in CRT. Image quality in this case would be preserved with a pitch value of around 2 (Wang and Vannier 1997).

2.2.3.5
Matrix and Field of View

The image matrix quantifies the number of pixels of the image grid. The spatial volume represented by an individual pixel depends on the size of the field of view (FOV). Current spiral CT scanners reconstruct standard images with a 512×512 display matrix. As the total number of pixels in each image is limited, the selection of a larger FOV results in a larger volume of each pixel with a concomitant loss of spatial resolution. The optimal FOV depends on the size of the region being explored, with the most appropriate FOV being around 230–250 mm for the neck, and about 400–500 mm for the chest and abdomen.

2.2.3.6
Contrast Medium

All intravenous contrast agents currently approved for CT imaging contain iodine atoms bound within complex organic vector molecules. The protocol for contrast medium injection varies according to the explored area.

For *neck* examination, most authors (Mancuso et al. 1983; Som 1987) recommend biphasic injection. At our institution, the first 50–60 cc of contrast medium (300–350 mg I/ml) are injected as a drip perfusion to impregnate the interstitial compartment. The other 50–60 cc of contrast medium are injected at a rate of 2 cc/s approximately 2 minutes after the first drip perfusion injection. The delay before imaging is 30 seconds after administering the second injection. This protocol usually provides an adequate opacification of the different vascular structures, thereby allowing an accurate interpretation of head and neck CT images. A recent report has highlighted the value of delayed scans in head and neck spiral CT examination (Harris et al. 1996). The latter authors have demonstrated a greater definition of some neck lesions on images obtained 10–15 minutes after contrast medium injection. Although slightly less spatial resolution is obtained with spiral CT than with the conventional serial CT due to the reduced scanning times, the spiral technique usually permits better vessel opacification. When using a faster CT technique and a power injector, asymmetric or heterogeneous opacification of the internal jugular veins is frequently observed, which may mimic venous thrombosis or nodal necrosis when viewed as a single slice (Sakai et al. 1997).

For *chest* imaging, 80–120 cc of a concentrated iodinated agent (100–150 mg I/ml) are injected through an antecubital vein at a rate of 1–2 cc/s. The delay before imaging is 35–50 seconds depending on the circulation time. Leung has recommended the intravenous injection of 100 ml of 150 mg I/ml contrast medium at a rate of 2.5 ml/s with a delay before scanning of 25 seconds (Leung 1997). For abdominal examination, the maximum contrast enhancement of the vessels mainly relies on the volume of the contrast medium injected and on the time to peak enhancement, which is determined by the injection rate (Han et al. 2000). Our current abdominal injection protocol for lymph node assessment consists of the perfusion of 100 ml of contrast agent (300 mg I/ml) at a rate of 2 ml/s and a delay before scanning of 35 seconds.

2.2.4
Post-processing of CT Images

2.2.4.1
Window Setting

The full range of attenuation values cannot be displayed on the CT images due to the limitation in the number of gray scale levels detectable by the human eye. A single window setting cannot properly display all the information contained in the CT image. The optimal window width and window level (W/L) settings for soft tissues such as lymph nodes may vary according to the CT system, the monitor, the printer and the type of film. The optimal window setting is approximately 400/50 HU for soft tissue and lymph node analysis. However, a bone window setting of 1,700/300 HU may be used to better identify nodal calcifications.

2.2.4.2
Reconstruction Interval

Data are volumetrically acquired by the spiral CT technique, and axial transverse images may be subsequently reconstructed at any point throughout the volume. Images may be reconstructed at intervals which are smaller than the initial nominal slice thickness. When images are reconstructed at smaller increments than the beam collimation, they "overlap" one another. The creation of overlapping sections improves the longitudinal resolution of reformated images in the z-axis (Kalender et al. 1994). This property allows the reconstruction of high-resolution 2D or 3D images. Overlapping slices also improve the detection of small structures.

2.2.4.3
2D and 3D Reconstructions

Both kinds of reconstruction require the acquisition of only one data set, thus avoiding additional examination time and/or an increase in radiation exposure. High-quality orthogonal and 3D reconstructions are obtainable without the step borders artifact observed in standard incremental scans. The topographical relationships between the lymph nodes and any other tissues or vessels can then be evaluated in sagittal, axial, coronal, or oblique views. Multiplanar reformation (MPR) creates images along arbitrary straight or curved planes of at least one voxel in thickness. MPR images can be created in any plane with the same spatial resolution as the original axial transverse sections (*"isotropic"* viewing). MPR ignores all data except those along the single voxel path defining the reformation plane. This technique is easy to use and facilitates the assessment of the relationship between lymph nodes, vessels and other anatomical structures (Fig. 2.1). True 3D rendering techniques consider the entire data set or an edited subset of data for the generation of images. Shaded surface display (SSD) and volume rendering (VR) are the two existing algorithms for 3D image rendering using spiral CT. With the VR technique, the processing method is based on the use of a linear projection of virtual rays through the data set to create a projectional image of the pixel of interest. The relative density information is preserved by this technique, since it is not surface-dependent. The other technique, i.e. the SSD, uses intensity thresholding of the CT data so that all values within a defined range are selected for rendering and the remainder are removed from the data set (Cline et al. 1991; Magnusson et al. 1991). These two 3D reconstruction techniques

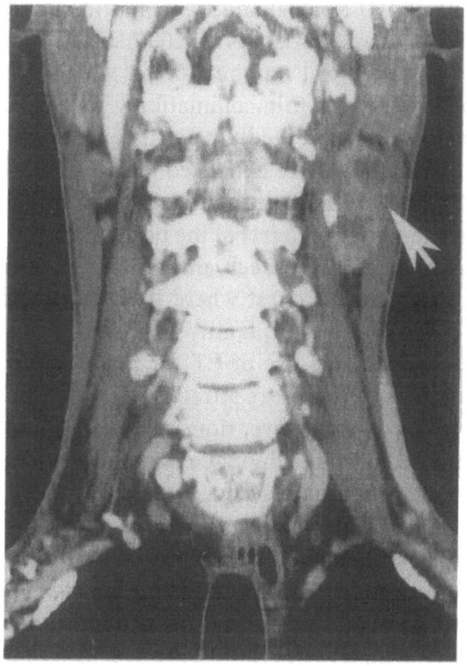

Fig. 2.1. Coronal CT reformatted image of the cervical area: 40-year-old man with an ulcerated epiglottis tumor. Data were obtained by contrast-enhanced MSCT using the following parameters: FOV: 230 mm; slice thickness: 2 mm; reconstruction interval: 1 mm; table speed: 6.7 mm/s; kV: 120; mAs: 150; matrix: 512×512. Frontal reformation demonstrated the posterior location of necrotic lymph nodes (*arrow*) between the posterior scalene and the sterno-cleido-mastoid muscles on the left side

are rarely used in clinical practice because the nodal density is too close to that of the surrounding muscles or viscera to obtain accurate nodal definition. Further software improvements are needed before an accurate 3D nodal display can be obtained.

2.2.5
Normal Lymph Nodes on CT Images

Computed tomography imaging permits an adequate assessment of the lymphatic system in almost all parts of the body. The high tissue contrast between the lymph nodes and the surrounding fatty tissue is usually sufficient to delineate normal or enlarged lymph nodes. The injection of intravenous iodinated contrast medium usually helps to differentiate the lymphatic structures from the adjacent vascular structures. Its use is mandatory for lymph node assessment in the cervical region because of the poor fatty interfaces in this area. On unenhanced CT images, normal lymph nodes display the same intermediate density as the muscles at 30–40 HU. Normal nodes are elliptic, round or triangular in shape (Sakai et al. 2000). The node hilum may contain small amounts of fat which are sometimes detectable on thin collimation CT images. After intravenous contrast medium perfusion, normal nodes become slightly more enhanced than the muscles. Both CT and MR modalities are suited to nodal status assessment in most parts of the body. MRI performance is highest in the neck and abdomen, and to a lesser extent in the chest where it is restricted by the presence of a large quantity of air. In terms of cost effectiveness, the use of CT for nodal status assessment seems to be a more attractive proposition than MRI which is expensive, time-consuming and more often used for parenchymal examination than for "pure" nodal status assessment.

The *cervical lymph nodes* are divided into four to five groups, all being contiguous to one another. Most classification systems are based on the studies of Rouvière (1948). The TNM system divides the head and neck lymph nodes into 12 groups. In recent studies (Grégoire et al. 2000; Som et al. 1999) the neck has been divided into six levels including eight nodal groups (Fig. 2.2a, b).

The *thoracic lymph nodes* are usually classified into parietal and visceral groups. Different classifications based on location and drainage routes have been proposed by various authors. For the past 10 years, two systems of nodal classification for lung cancer staging have been commonly used (Cymbalista et al. 1999): that of the American Joint Committee on Cancer (AJCC 1992) and that of the American Thoracic Society (ATS) together with the North American Lung Cancer Study Group (American Thoracic Society 1983) (Fig. 2.2c).

The *abdominal lymph nodes* are usually classified either according to the course of the major vessels and the ligaments, or to their location within the peritoneal or the retroperitoneal cavities. Lymph nodes are located e.g. within the subdiaphragmatic area, the gastrohepatic ligament, the retrocrural space, the upper paraaortic area (from the celiac to the renal arteries), the lower paraaortic area (from the renal arteries to the iliac bifurcation), the porta hepatis, the portacaval space, and the internal or external iliac area (Fig. 2.2d–f).

2.2.6 Pathological Lymph Nodes on CT Images

Many different radiological criteria are used to assess the presence or absence of metastatic tissue within the lymph nodes. These include the axial diameter, the pattern of enhancement, the spheroid shape and the grouping of the nodes. The size and shape of normal lymph nodes vary according to their different locations in the body, and therefore different criteria must be used for each location to characterize nodes as benign, normal sized or abnormally enlarged.

In the *head and neck*, any combination of shape and minimum or maximum axial diameter seems to be a less valid indicator than minimum axial diameter alone (van den Breckel et al. 1990a). Cervical lymph nodes with a diameter greater than 10 mm in the short axis should be considered as abnormal. The dimension in the axial plane should not exceed 11 mm in the jugulodigastric subanatomy and 10 mm in the other locations (Mancuso et al. 1983; Som 1992; van den Breckel et al. 1990a). In a recent study, CT was reported to perform slightly better than MRI in the detection of squamous cell carcinoma (SCC) nodal metastases in neck nodes on the basis of the size of the nodes and the presence of central necrosis (Curtin et al. 1998). With the use of a 1-cm cut-off size or the presence of an internal abnormality to indicate a positive node, CT had a negative predictive value of 84% and a positive predictive value of 50%.

On *chest* CT, a short-axis nodal diameter exceeding 1 cm is considered abnormal, except in the subcarinal space (Naidich et al. 1999). The diameter of the node usually parallels its likelihood of harboring active disease. For example, in patients with bronchogenic carcinoma, the likelihood of mediastinal node involvement is directly proportional to nodal size. In a prospective study including 143 patients with bronchogenic carcinoma, the sensitivity of CT in detecting a malignant lymph node on a per patient basis was 64%, with a specificity of 62% (McLoud et al. 1992). In this study a lymph node measuring between 1 to 1.9 cm and 2 to 2.9 cm was found to be malignant in 25% and 62% of cases, respectively.

On *abdominal* CT scan, reports on the upper limits of normal node size vary from 6 to 20 mm, also depending on their location. Some authors have found that a short-axis nodal diameter exceeding 6 mm in the retrocrural space, 8 mm in the paracardiac and gastrohepatic ligament areas, 10 mm in the porta hepatis, 9 mm in the upper paraaortic region, and 11 mm in the lower paraaortic area is indicative of abnormality, particularly if multiple nodes are present (Dorfman et al. 1991).

It should be emphasized that the simple assessment of lymph node size is not in itself a sufficiently accurate method for determining whether nodes are normal or abnormal. During the early stages of vari-

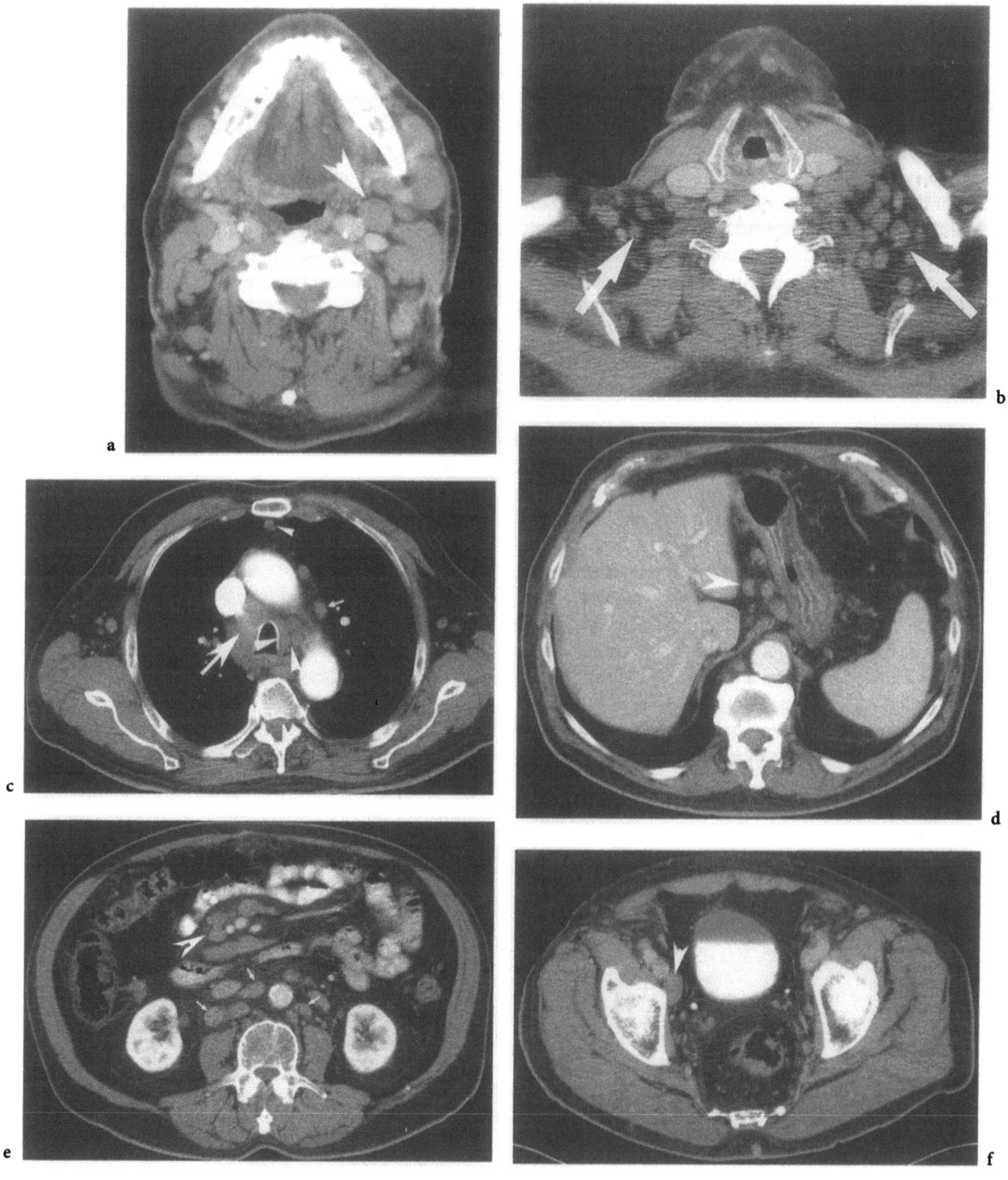

Fig. 2.2a–f. The ability of spiral CT to accurately depict lymph nodes in almost all areas of the body: examples of lymph nodes within the neck, the chest and the abdomen. **a** Axial contrast-enhanced MSCT view at upper neck level in a 73-year-old man with a lymphoma. The following parameters were used: FOV: 250 mm; slice thickness: 3.2 mm; table speed: 16.7 mm/s; kV: 120; mAs: 214; matrix: 512×512. Bilateral homogeneous lymph nodes are visible, mainly in zone II (*arrow*). **b** Axial CT view at lower neck level shows numerous small lymph nodes in zone V (*arrows*). **c** Axial contrast-enhanced MSCT view at lower tracheal level using the following parameters: FOV: 430 mm; slice thickness: 5 mm; table speed: 17.5 mm/s; kV: 120; mAs: 149; matrix: 512×512. A homogeneous lymph node of 12 mm in the short axis is depicted on station nr 4 R (*arrow*). Small lymph nodes are visible on station nr 4 L (*arrowhead*), 5 (*short arrow*), 6 (*small arrowhead*) and in both axillae. **d** Axial contrast-enhanced MSCT view obtained at upper abdominal level using the following parameters: FOV: 430 mm; slice thickness: 5 mm; table speed: 16.7 mm/s; kV: 120; mAs: 214; matrix: 512×512. Small sub-centimeter lymph nodes are seen in the left gastric artery area (*arrowhead*). **e** Axial CT image at mid-abdomen level showing numerous lymph nodes located in the mesenterium (*arrowhead*) and in the retroperitoneal spaces (*short arrows*). **f** A lymph node measuring 15 mm in the short axis was present in the right external iliac vein area (*arrowhead*)

ous pathological processes, significant nodal involvement may be present in the absence of macroscopic enlargement of the nodes. Other morphological criteria may help the radiologist to accurately classify the type of lymph nodes. It has also been reported that the nodal enhancement pattern may be helpful in differentiating benign from malignant nodes. On contrast-enhanced CT, until proven otherwise, a central zone of low attenuation within the node reveals the presence of tumoral cells and/or necrosis, regardless of nodal size (Sakai et al. 2000; Yousem et al. 1992) (Figs. 2.1, 2.3a). The presence of extranodal tumor extension is depicted on contrast-enhanced CT as an irregular and usually thick enhanced rim infiltrating the adjacent fatty planes (Fig. 2.3b). The presence of nodal calcification is indicative of disease, which may be at an active stage or not. Nodal calcification is common in many non-malignant conditions such as sarcoidosis, tuberculosis, histoplasmosis, coccidioidomycosis and other infectious diseases (Sakai et al. 2000). Inflammatory diseases such as rheumatoid arthritis, scleroderma and amyloidosis may also result in nodal calcium deposits. Pneumoconiosis used to be the most common cause of benign lymph node calcification in previous decades. Nodal calcifications are also present in neoplastic conditions such as Hodgkin's lymphoma, treated metastatic nodes arising from primary prostate carcinoma, testis, colon, thyroid primary neoplasms, and neuroblastoma (Dolan 1963; Eisenkraft and Som 1999; Ghahremani and Straus 1971). Calcifications may appear in the metastatic nodes before any therapeutic intervention takes place, i.e. in patients with malignancies originating from primary lung, testicular, breast, colonic, ovarian neoplasms, and head and neck SCC (Eisenkraft and Som 1999).

2.3 Magnetic Resonance Imaging

2.3.1 Hardware/Software Requirements for High-Quality MRI

2.3.1.1 Strength of the Basic Magnetic Field

In an MR system the strength of the basic magnetic field is expressed in Tesla (T), with 1 T being equivalent to 10^4 Gauss. The higher the magnetic field, the higher the signal-to-noise ratio (SNR) of the images ("higher, faster, stronger"). 1.5-T systems

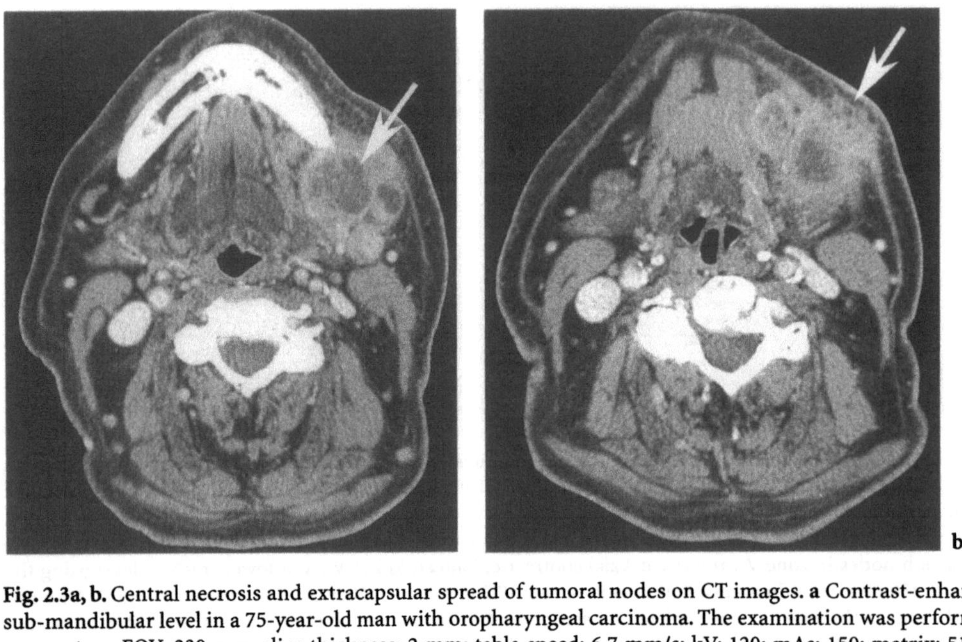

a b

Fig. 2.3a, b. Central necrosis and extracapsular spread of tumoral nodes on CT images. **a** Contrast-enhanced axial CT section at sub-mandibular level in a 75-year-old man with oropharyngeal carcinoma. The examination was performed using the following parameters: FOV: 230 mm; slice thickness: 2 mm; table speed: 6.7 mm/s; kV: 120; mAs: 150; matrix: 512×512. A large nodular mass consistent with clustered lymph nodes is well depicted on the left side, at level I. The central area of the mass shows low attenuation (*arrow*), indicative of necrosis. **b** Contrast-enhanced axial CT section obtained 2 cm below the level of the previous view (**a**) using the same parameters. The margins of the lymph nodes show an irregular, thick enhanced rim which infiltrates the adjacent fatty tissue. This findings reflects macroscopic extracapsular tumoral spread

are currently standard for "high-field" MR scanners, although others use "intermediate" to "low" fields at 1, 0.5, or even 0.2 T. "Ultra-high" whole-body 3-T systems are now entering clinical practice. Higher SNR can be of value in four ways when examining patients with neoplastic disease:

A reduction in examination time for patients who are intolerant to the MRI procedure: images of diagnostic quality can more easily be obtained within shortened acquisition times when using higher-field systems.

An increase in spatial resolution of the images either by increasing the matrix size or decreasing the slice thickness, or incorporating both for a similar acquisition time, with only one restriction to time-saving: the need to increase the number of slices when decreasing the slice thickness to cover a similar volume.

An increase in temporal resolution of serial images after intravenous bolus injection of paramagnetic contrast agent: analysis of the temporal pattern of contrast enhancement has been applied to nodal imaging with promising results (Laissey et al. 1994). In this respect, higher-field systems allow repeated acquisitions within shortened time periods, resulting in an improved analysis of the enhancement profile.

Motion artifacts "freezing" is a critical measure when examining severely ill patients who are unable to remain immobile and/or refrain from swallowing for a few minutes while under examination. The higher the strength of the basic field, the better the quality of the image obtained with ultra-short acquisition times: about 150 ms/slice in echo-planar imaging (EPI) and 6–7 s/slice by gradient-recalled echo (GRE) technique using start-of the-art systems. But the fastest sequences are also the most sensitive to many artifacts (e.g. field inhomogeneity, magnetic susceptibility, chemical shift, motion). Freezing may be therefore be obtained at the expense of clarity, and critical image degradation may occur when examining small structures such as the lymph nodes. Physiological motion, e.g. that of the heart and lungs or the bowels, are other aspects of the same issue, and can be partially managed by pharmacological means or by breath-holding for short acquisition periods, by cardiac gating, or by respiratory triggering. Finally, motion freezing is more effectively achieved by ultra-short spiral CT acquisition (see 2.2) than by MRI, which still suffers from significant limitations in speed/quality correlation, in spite of recent technological advances.

Significant material drawbacks paralleling an increase in field strength limit recourse to increasingly higher strengths, i.e.:

- an increase in all hardware and software constraints and requirements.
- an increase in all artifacts (e.g. motion, magnetic susceptibility, chemical shift).
- an increase in the T1 relaxation time in all tissues, which results in slightly degraded fatty tissue contrast on T1-weighted images.

1.5 T has become the standard value in oncological imaging, an excellent trade-off between the pros and cons of field strength increase. For several months the major manufacturers of MR systems have been advocating the use of their new 3-T whole-body system and have indicated that it could well replace older systems, but this new technology needs to be fully evaluated.

2.3.1.2 Magnetic Field Gradients

Magnetic field gradients are additional magnet coils which are repeatedly switched during data acquisition to generate spatial encoding of the magnetic resonance signal. Major improvements in gradient technology, i.e. strength (nowadays up to 60 mT/m) and technical performance (e.g. decreased rise times, active shielding, non-resonant properties) have led to a marked improvement in image quality, both as regards spatial resolution and acquisition speed at all fields.

2.3.1.3 Anatomically Adapted Coils

Since the intensity of the MR signal decreases with the square of the distance between the explored (or "emitting") area and the receiving device (or "coil"), the design of receiving coils has been adapted as closely as possible to the anatomy of the investigated areas. Additional refinements in coil technology (e.g. preamplification, quadrature design, phased-array multiple components) have led to improved signal reception and processing. All MRI manufacturers currently propose a wide variety of anatomically adapted coils. The use of a specifically designed neck phased-array coil and a thoraco-abdominal phased array multi-coil system is currently advocated for lymph node imaging, instead of the outdated "body-coil" included in the system.

2.3.1.4 Access to Off-line Workstations

Image data acquisition, image reconstruction and image post-processing – serial steps in the MR procedure – can be performed at different times and locations. The imaging system usually acquires raw data and performs standard image reconstruction online to allow real-time optimized management of the current examination. The transfer of images (or even the raw data) to an independent workstation should then be made to avoid time-wasting interference with the ongoing examinations on the clinical imager. Powerful workstations are required to perform complex image processing, e.g. 3D/multiplanar reformation, segmentation, parametric quantitative analysis, or image fusion to other imaging modalities such as CT, PET and others.

2.3.1.5
The Fast Spin Echo Technique

The fast spin echo (FSE) technique, based on the rapid acquisition with relaxation enhancement (RARE) approach defined by JÜRGEN HENNIG in 1986, made a major contribution to the clinical application of MRI in the early 1990s, not only because of increased acquisition speed and subsequent time-saving, but also because of the specific characteristics of the technique which allow a significant reduction of many artifacts (HENNIG et al. 1986). This became the standard technique in T2-weighted imaging of the cervical nodal regions shortly after its introduction in clinical practice (FULBRIGHT et al. 1994; HELD and BREIT 1994; YOUSEM and HURST 1994). FSE is currently included in all clinical imagers at all field strengths and has replaced conventional spin echo (CSE) in the investigation of almost all parts of the body, including the nodal areas.

2.3.2
Basic Tissue Contrast on MR Images

2.3.2.1
Introduction

The tissue signal intensities on MR images reflect their differences in physico-chemical composition and magnetic properties. A vast number of intrinsic (tissue) and extrinsic (e.g. magnetic field properties, pulse sequence data, etc.) parameters influence MRI rendering of tissue contrast. The main parameters, however, are the density of hydrogen nuclei (protons) and the relative proportion of the latter with free-water properties (a long longitudinal "T1" relaxation time and a long transversal "T2" relaxation time), or bound properties (short T1 and T2 relaxation times) such as the fatty tissue protons (MITCHELL 1999). As water and fat are the main components of the body and contain a large number of hydrogen nuclei, it can be said that MRI is the hydrogen nucleus ("proton") imaging of these major components. The pulse sequence parameters may be optimized to express either the short T1 relaxation times of the bound protons as a high signal intensity ("T1-weighted" sequences), or the long T2 relaxation times of the free-water protons as a high signal intensity ("T2-weighted" sequences). T1- and T2-weightings provide the basic contrasts in MR images. CSE, FSE, GRE, or EPI are only different technical modalities by which T1- and T2-weightings are obtained (RINCK 1993).

2.3.2.2
The Lymph Nodes on T1-weighted MR Images

The adipose tissue which contains a majority of bound protons appears very bright on T1-weighted images. In turn, tissues which contain a majority of free-water protons with longer T1 and T2 relaxation times display intermediate to low signal intensity. Normal pathological but non-necrotic nodes display this low/intermediate T1 signal intensity (Fig. 2.4a, c). As most of the nodes are embedded within a fatty environment, the spontaneous contrast between the nodes and the surrounding tissues is excellent. Although the delineation of the nodal contours is extremely clear on T1-weighted images, the low/intermediate signal intensity of normal nodes may be similar to that of numerous other normal (e.g. muscles) or abnormal tissues (e.g. metastatic or reactive inflammatory nodes). The only determinant feature is that necrotic-cystic nodes have a very low T1 signal intensity due to an increase in free-water proton content.

2.3.2.3
The Lymph Nodes on T2-weighted MR Images

The fatty tissue usually displays a lower signal intensity on T2-weighted than on T1-weighted images, but to a lesser degree when FSE is utilized which results in a significant residual T1-weighting responsible for high signal intensity of the fat despite overall T2-weighting of the image (Fig. 2.4b, d). The major difference between T1- and T2-weightings is that water-containing tissue displays a higher signal intensity in the latter which is proportional to the amount of free-water protons present. Tumoral tissues with a high degree of cellularity and a high nucleo-cytoplasmic ratio with a resulting low "cytoplasmic water" content but a high density of lipidic membrane interfaces

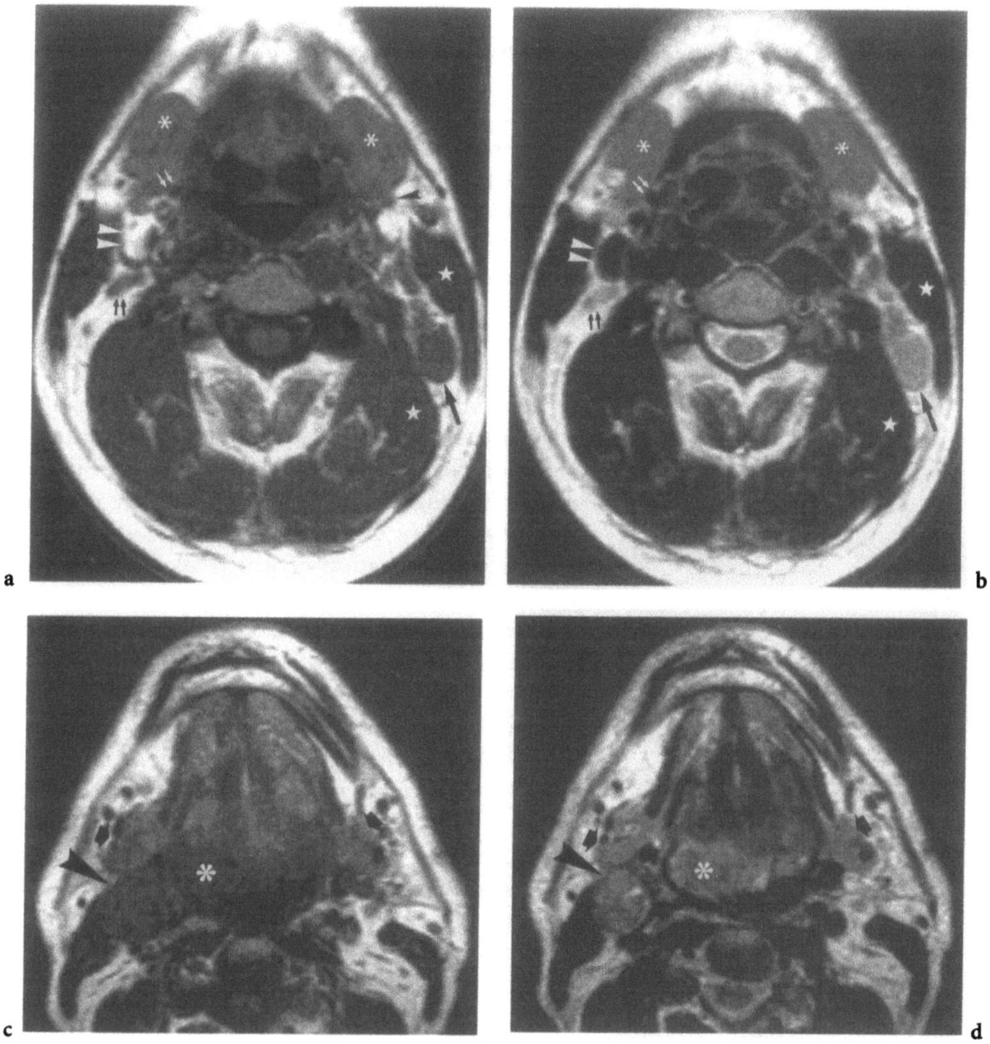

Fig. 2.4a–d. The potential of unenhanced MRI to differentiate lymph nodes from muscles, vessels, and glands by comparing "native" (unenhanced) T1- and T2-weighted images. **a, b** Posterior jugular node involvement in a case of oropharyngeal SCC (the primary tumor is not seen on these views). **a** Precontrast CSE transverse T1-weighted image without FS at a three-fold level displays tumoral lymph node involvement (*black arrow*) with a similar low signal intensity to muscles (*white stars*), some vessels (*thin black arrowhead*) and submandibular glands (*white notches*), contrasting well with the bright signal intensity of the surrounding fatty tissue. Vessels may display either low signal intensity due to the "flow void" phenomenon (*double thin white arrows*) or very bright signal intensity due to flow artifacts (*double white arrowheads*). Bright artifacts within the flow vessel lumen are increased when using the GRE technique, which has been advocated for differentiating nodes from vessels. **b** FSE transverse T2-weighted image without FS in a similar slice location to **Fig. 2.1a** clearly differentiates the different structures, with an intermediate signal intensity shown by the tumoral node, and a very low signal intensity of the muscles and all the vessels due to the flow-void phenomenon. Fatty tissue remains very bright on these T2-weighted images obtained via the FSE technique without FS, due to the "shine-through" effect of residual T1-weighting. An almost isosignal intensity between the enlarged node (*black arrow*) and normal sized contralateral nodes (*thin black double arrows*) on both weightings may be observed. **c, d** SCC of the base of the tongue with jugular lymph node involvement. **c** Precontrast CSE transverse T1-weighted image without FS through the level of the primary tumor (*white notch*) and that of a homolateral jugular lymphadenopathy (*black arrowhead*). Both sites display a similar low signal intensity. In turn, the submandibular glands exhibits slightly higher signal intensity due to physiological fatty infiltration in this elderly patient (*black arrows*). **d** FSE T2-weighted transverse image without FS in a similar slice location: all three structures display a similar intermediate signal intensity. Contrary to the previous case, the T2-weighting seems more "confusing" as all three structures exhibit a similar signal intensity, but the comparison of both weightings allows an accurate identification of the nodes

display a low T2 signal intensity. Normal nodes usually display a low to intermediate T2 signal intensity. Tumoral nodes may exhibit a low to high signal intensity depending on the balance between cellular density (decrease in signal intensity) versus stromal inflammatory changes and necrosis (increase in signal intensity) (Fig. 2.5).

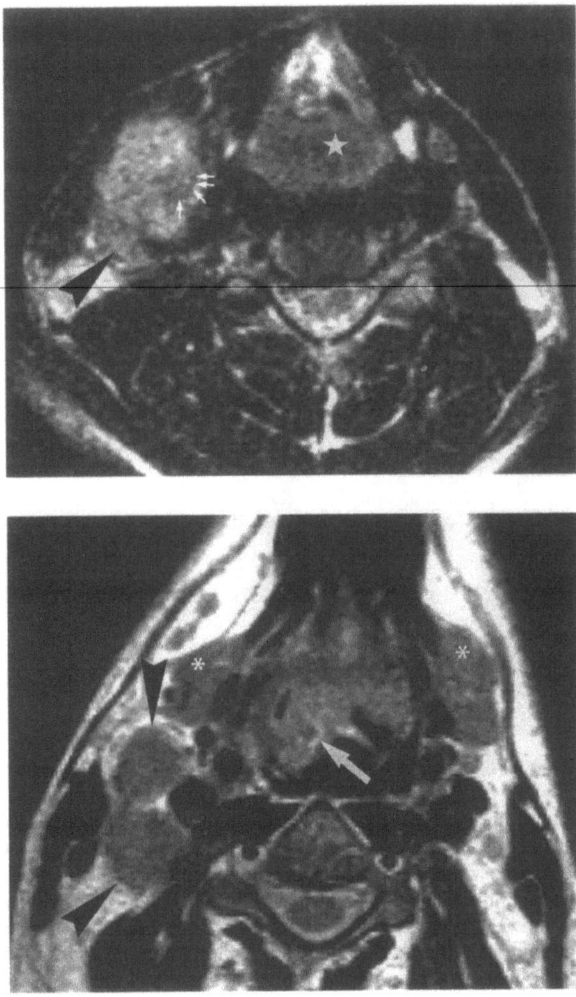

a

b

Fig. 2.5a, b. Variability in the pretreatment T2 signal intensity of the primary neoplasm and the metastatic nodes. **a** FSE T2-weighted transverse image without FS in a case of posterior laryngeal SCC where the primary tumor (*white star*) displays a lower signal intensity than the metastatic homolateral jugular nodes (*black arrowhead*); however, sub-areas of lower signal intensity are present within the nodes (*thin white arrows*). Low SNR due to the use of a head coil to explore the neck results in the "noisy" appearance of this image (obtained seven years ago). Currently available specifically adapted neck coils ensure routine optimized image quality. **b** FSE T2-weighted transverse image without FS in a case of SCC of the base of the tongue (*white arrow*) where the primary tumor displays a slightly higher signal than the metastatic jugular nodes (*black arrowheads*). As in **Fig. 2.1d**, the isointensity between node metastases and submandibular glands (*white notches*) may be confusing

2.3.2.4
Standard Contrast Procedures

2.3.2.4.1
T1 Contrast-enhancement by Paramagnetic Contrast Agent Perfusion

Paramagnetic contrast agents are in standard use for the routine MR examination of patients with neoplastic diseases. These agents consist of macromolecular chelates carrying a few gadolinium (Gd) atoms with a strong paramagnetic effect, resulting in a marked decrease in T1 and T2 relaxation times of the surrounding free-water and fat protons. Reducing the T1 relaxation time has a major impact on the T1-weighted images, as an increase in signal intensity is observed in the vascularized areas the permeative vasculature of which allows interstitial leakage of the contrast medium molecules. However, contrast enhancement suffers from certain limitations and drawbacks:

- contrast enhancement highlights the lesional vasculature and permeable properties of the vessel walls, but this feature is non-specific with respect to the inflammatory or tumoral nature of the lesion.
- if the lesion is embedded within the fatty tissue – as in the vast majority of lymph nodes – the contrast between the lesion and the surrounding adipose tissue decreases on post-contrast T1-weighted images, since white on white provides a lower contrast than gray on white. This drawback may be overcome by using the fat saturation (or fat suppression) option – designated by the acronym "FS" – which decreases the brightness of the fat on MRI without decreasing that due to contrast enhancement (see below).

Paramagnetic agents reduce the T1 and the T2 relaxation times of the surrounding protons. The reduction in T2 relaxation time only has a theoretical impact on the image, since the decrease in signal intensity due to T2 reduction is not visible to the human eye on T2-weighted images with a standard window setting, and the pre- and post-contrast T2-weighted images therefore look similar. Our approach, like that of many others, is as follows: we first acquire the pre-contrast T1-weighted images, perfuse the paramagnetic contrast agent (always at a standard dose of 0.1 mM Gd/kg), then immediately after perfusion acquire the T2-weighted images which are unaffected by the contrast agent. As sufficient time for T2-weighted image acquisition has elapsed, high-quality T1-weighted post-contrast images are obtained with adequate contrast diffusion and deposition within the tissues due to a sufficient time lapse between perfusion and image acquisition. If additional T1-weighted sequences are acquired later, the interpretation of these images must take into account the time lapse between contrast agent perfusion and image acquisition, as contrast enhancement characteristics evolve over time.

2.3.2.4.2
Suppression of Fat Signal Intensity

The high signal intensity of fatty tissue both on T1-weighted and on FSE T2-weighted images may hinder the detection of small enhanced foci (on T1-weighted images), or small amounts of abnormally hydrated tissue (on T2-weighted images) within the fat. By decreasing the "flashy" brightness of the adipose tissue, the detection of small structures embedded within it can be improved. In the early 1990s, FS prepulses with a specific frequency-selective spectral saturation of the fatty protons were introduced in clinical imagers, and could be combined with all kinds of sequences independently of the weighting (T1/T2) or the technique used (CSE, FSE, GRE, EPI). These procedures have rapidly replaced the short tau inversion recovery (STIR) sequence aimed at suppressing fat signal intensity. However, the significant drawbacks of the FS prepulses must be considered:

- FS prepulse application requires time within the time of repetition (TR) of pulse sequence data. Therefore prolonged TRs are necessary, few of which have an impact on long TR sequences (such as T2-weighted sequences), but which nevertheless have a marked effect on short TR sequences (such as the T1-weighted sequences) both as regards the decreased number of slices obtainable within a defined TR or the need to increase the latter so that the number of slices remains unchanged, thereby prolonging the acquisition times and modifying the T1-weighting characteristics of the sequence.
- FS may be heterogeneous throughout the image, to a higher degree if large FOVs are used which include a number of air/bone/soft tissue interfaces and structures of different shape/size (e.g. the neck versus the shoulder).
- theoretically the comparison between pre- and post-contrast T1-weighted images should be made between strictly similar images except for contrast agent perfusion, which means that a comparison should be made between pre- and post-contrast T1-weighted FS images. As "native" unenhanced pre-contrast T1-weighted images without fat saturation seem mandatory, fat saturated pre-contrast images should be obtained in addition to "normal" T1-weighted images, resulting in a significant increase in examination time.

In our experience, the FS option is invariably activated for the T2-weighted sequences (exclusively using the FSE technique). Pre- and post-contrast T1-weighted images are obtained in the reference plane (usually transverse) without FS. If a specific question remains unanswered regarding these "standard" post-contrast images which could be addressed by using FS, then an additional FS sequence – similar to the unsuppressed pre- and post-contrast sequences – is obtained in the reference plane. In the second (usually coronal) or even third (usually sagittal) "extra" planes (in addition to the reference plane), only FS post-contrast T1-weighted images are acquired.

2.3.3
Clinical Trade-offs in MR Nodal Imaging

2.3.3.1
Nodal Imaging as Ancillary to Primary Tumor Staging

Magnetic resonance nodal status is frequently interpreted as an "extra" item of information displayed on images which are aimed at the optimal depiction of the primary tumor. This means that node depiction may be limited to fewer incidences and/or weightings than the primary neoplasm, since optimized tumoral investigation requires specifically adapted and centered sequences (e.g. thin slices, limited FOVs). The complete set of pre- and post-contrast T1-weighted and T2-weighted images is thus rarely available for all nodal areas. At our institution, we include an additional large FOV coronal sequence at the end of the examination if all nodal areas have not been covered by the initial primary-targeted sequences. Post-contrast T1-weighting is the method of choice for this ultimate "nodal" sequence (Fig. 2.6c), but coronal large FOV pre-contrast T1-weighted images obtained at the beginning of the examination could constitute a viable alternative to this approach.

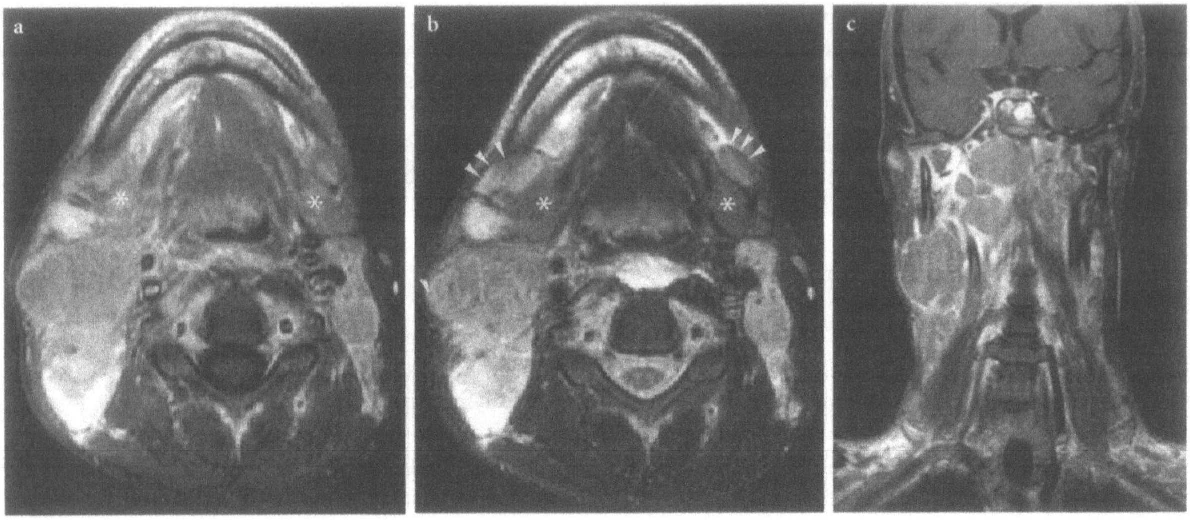

Fig. 2.6a–c. The fat suppression option: Undifferentiated carcinoma of the rhinopharynx with diffuse nodal involvement. **a** Post-contrast CSE T1-weighted transverse image with FS: the suppression of the fat signal results in good delineation of enhanced nodal masses and inflammatory/infiltrative environment (i.e. in the right spinal area) **b** FSE T2-weighted transverse image with FS in a similar slice location to Fig. 2.5a: lymph node contours appear more accurately delineated (*white arrowheads*), and the differentiation between nodes and salivary glands (*notches*) seems better than on the previous image even though a global similarity between both is obvious, except for the discriminating signal intensity of the cerebrospinal fluid (CSF) surrounding the spinal cord. **c** Post-contrast CSE T1-weighted coronal image with FS: adenomegalies are well delineated and surrounded by highly enhanced areas. The high-quality image has been obtained using an up-to-date specifically adapted phased-array neck coil

2.3.3.2
Reduction of Acquisition Times

Reducing the duration of the MR sequences leads to a reduction in patient discomfort and in a decreased risk of motion artifacts. However, reduced acquisition times may result in critical image degradation. In turn, long acquisition times may result either in unnecessary pictorial quality of the images or in insufficient quality due to motion artifacts introduced by patients who are unable to keep still, refrain from swallowing, or hold their breath. Finding the optimal trade-off between time and diagnostic relevance is the most commonly encountered challenge in MRI clinical practice, and is a crucial factor in examining oncology patients.

2.3.3.3
MR Nodal Staging with or without Contrast Agent Perfusion?

The comparison of T1- and T2-weighted images in the same plane provides relevant information on tissue characteristics (Figs. 2.4, 2.5). The "basic" unenhanced images allow a clear delineation of the nodes and their differentiation from other structures such as vessels and muscles, thereby avoiding the need for contrast agent perfusion even for head and neck imaging. However, improved MRI performance in nodal examination when paramagnetic contrast agents are used has repeatedly been reported (Chong et al. 1996; Som 1992; Van den Brekel et al. 1990b). Post-contrast images of the nodal areas are frequently available, since accuracy in the delineation of the primary tumor requires contrast agent perfusion. But information on the high or low degree of vascularization per se does not result in significantly increased specificity regarding the normal, inflammatory or neoplastic nature of the nodes. The true advantage of post-contrast T1- compared to T2-weighted images appears to lie in the depiction of non-cystic nodal necrosis. By interpreting only unenhanced images there is a risk that non-cystic nodal necrosis may remain undetected (Van den Brekel and Castelijns 1999). However, in our experience this seems to occur less frequently than cystic necrosis which is well depicted on T2-weighted images (Fig. 2.7).

2.3.3.4
3D Acquisition vs 3D Post-processing

Routine MR images are contiguous (or not) 2D slices. These images can be subsequently loaded in a 3D post-processing program which can reformat views in all planes. Acceptable image quality of the refor-

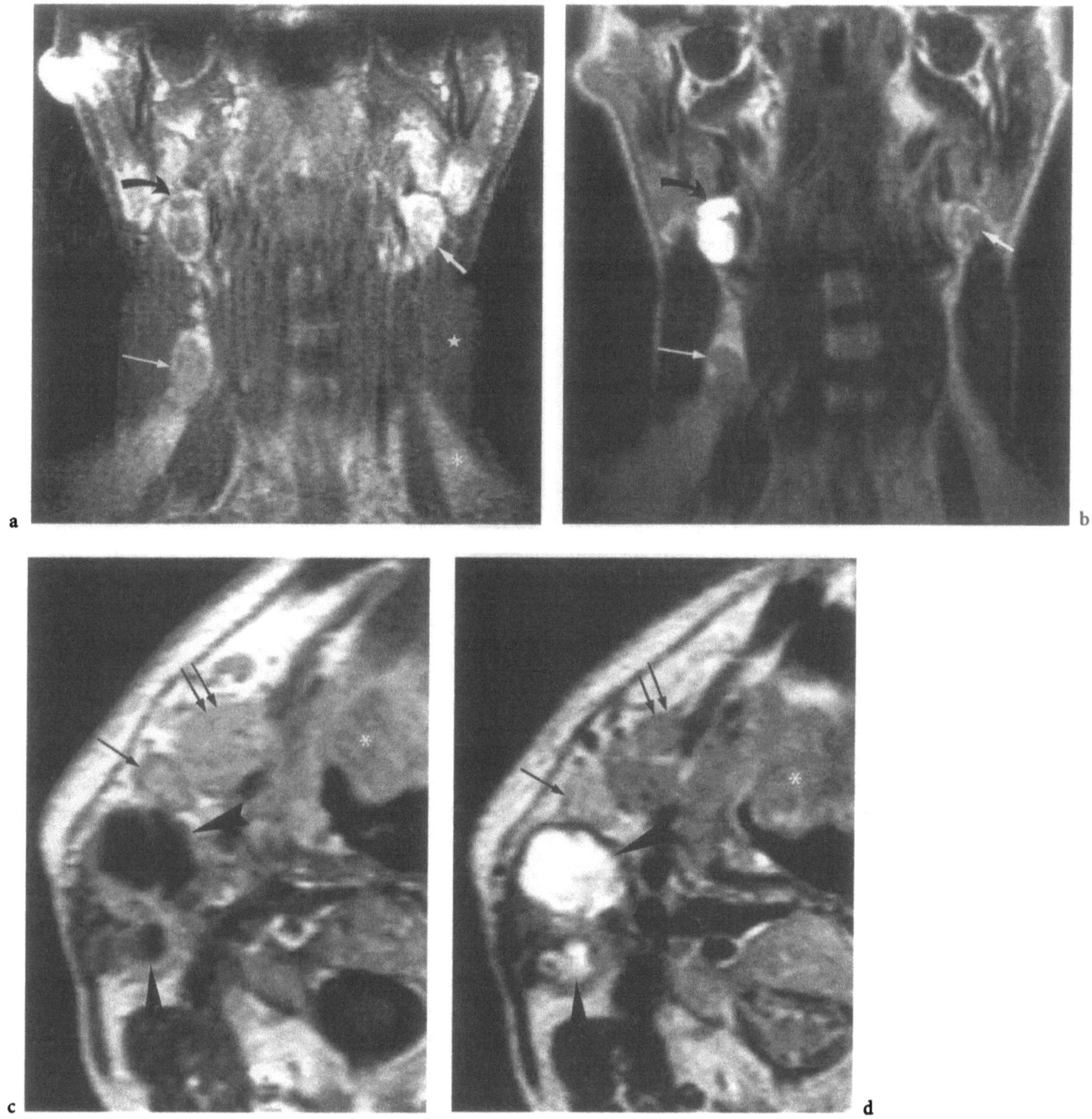

Fig. 2.7. Central necrosis of metastatic lymph nodes. **a, b** Bilateral nodal metastases of oropharyngeal SCC. **a** Post-contrast CSE T1-weighted coronal image with FS shows three different metastatic nodal patterns: (1) an area of low signal intensity surrounded by an intensely contrast-enhanced rim (*black curved arrow*); (2) an area of intermediate signal intensity with a bright rim (*thin white arrow*); (3) an area of intermediate signal intensity partially "obscured" by an intensely "flashing" rim (*thick white arrow*). Fat is well suppressed at the level of the *white star*, but less satisfactorily so at the level of the *white notch*. **b** FSE T2-weighted coronal image without FS in a strictly similar slice location to **3a** clearly reveals central necrosis as a very bright cystic area within the node displaying the lowest T1 signal intensity (*black curved arrow*), whereas the other nodes are not necrotic-cystic. **c, d** Close-ups of metastatic jugular nodes of an infiltrating SCC of the right vallecula (*white notch*). **c** Post-contrast CSE transverse T1-weighted image without FS. Necrotic areas within the nodes display very low signal intensity (*arrowheads*). A non-necrotic lymph node (*arrow*) and submandibular gland (*double arrows*) exhibit similar signal intensity. **d** FSE T2-weighted transverse image without FS in a similar slice location to that in **3c** shows very bright signal intensity of the nodal necrotic-cystic areas. Signal intensities of the non-necrotic node and the submandibular gland are significantly different

matted views may be obtained if the original slices were acquired without interslice gaps, and were not excessively thick when compared to the FOV and the matrix size, the main parameters of final voxel size. In cases of excessive voxel volume and/or a discrepancy between the three main parameters (thickness, FOV, matrix), the reformatted images exhibit the well-known "staircase" phenomenon. In true 3D mode, the area of interest is acquired as a volume and the raw data are processed using volumetric reconstruction algorithms which result in better multidirectional reformatting possibilities. However, 3D acquisition suffers from a major drawback, as it demands an excessive amount of time. The GRE technique introduced in the late 1980s has resulted in a significant increase in acquisition speed, thereby allowing 3D acquisition within an acceptable time frame. Up to now, the GRE technique still remains the method of choice for 3D volume imaging, albeit with an accompanying increase in artifacts connected with its use (e.g. motion and flow sensitivity, magnetic susceptibility) which limit image quality in heterogeneous regions such as the head and neck, where numerous interfaces are present between the bone, soft tissue and air. For large volume imaging, the time-saving GRE technique should be used. But the unavoidable trade-offs involved in maintaining acquisition time within an acceptable range could affect optimal spatial resolution, which is too high a price to pay when analyzing structures as small as nodes. Therefore 3D MRI is only of limited interest for nodal imaging, except for co-registration purposes. 3D GRE imaging of brain or neck volumes requiring 10 minutes (or more) acquisition time were used during the initial period when we co-registered MR and PET data at our institution. At present, usual FSE 2D sequences utilizing standard parameters (5 mm slice thickness, no interslice gap, matrix 256×512, FOV 24×24 cm) and requiring less than 3 minutes are co-registered with PET data with sufficient spatial resolution and anatomical depiction to identify structures with increased amounts of glucose uptake.

2.3.4 In the Research Field

2.3.4.1 *Lymphophilic Experimental MR Contrast Agents*

MR contrast agents with preferential uptake within the reticular tissues are currently under investigation. MR "lymphography" involves the use either of "negative" contrast agents (dark areas on T2-weighted images), or "positive" contrast agents (bright areas on T1-weighted images) for the normal nodes which take up the contrast agent. The most frequently investigated negative contrast agent introduced in clinical practice contains dextran-coated ultra-small superparamagnetic iron oxide (USPIO) particles, and has shown promising early results, i.e. increased sensitivity and specificity in nodal metastases detection (Anzai and Prince 1997; Harika et al. 1996; Hoffman et al. 2000). Gadofluorine 8, tyrosine-GDTA, and perfluorinated Ga chelates are positive contrast agents that have been experimentally evaluated in animal models, again with promising early results (Fujimoto et al. 2000; Misselwitz et al. 1999; Staatz et al. 2001). However, whether the crucial goal of detecting small metastatic deposits within unenlarged nodes could be truly addressed by this technique is uncertain as long as MRI spatial resolution remains such a limiting factor.

2.3.4.2 *In Vivo Measurements of Intrinsic Physical Properties of the Tissues*

Different magneto-physical properties of the tissues can be determined using the MR technique. Multi-echo sequences allow precise measurements in milliseconds of the *T1 and T2 relaxation times* (Dooms et al. 1985). Adequate comparative measurement and mathematical treatment of the voxel signal intensities with and without application of an off-resonance prepulse saturating the restricted proton pool (immobile water protons surrounding macromolecules) allow the *magnetization transfer ratio* (MTR) to be calculated between the restricted proton pool and the free-water proton pool (water molecule protons, the movement of which is unrestricted by interaction with the adjacent macromolecules (Grossman et al. 1994). The *apparent diffusion coefficient* (ADC) which can be calculated after the application of diffusion-sensitizing gradients in the so-called "diffusion-weighted" (DW) sequences reflects the restriction of free-water molecular movement (Le Bihan and Turner 1991). Attempts have been made to measure the relaxation times (Dooms et al. 1985; Wiener et al. 1986) and the MTR (Yousem 1999) within the nodes. The time parameters may have a low impact on differentiating tumoral from non-tumoral nodes since a wide overlap between normal, reactive and tumor categories has been observed. MTR measurements within the nodes have demonstrated a better performance, with statistically significant differences in mean MTR between malignant and benign adenopathies (Gillams et al. 1996; Sheppard and Yousem 1994). However, these studies suffered from certain weaknesses such as the absence of comparison between MTR values and size criteria in the same nodes, or the presence of a wide standard deviation in MTR values within malignant nodes due to the inclusion of necrotic-cystic nodes. But the accuracy of statistically significant thresholds issued from large normative databases suffers from limited power in individual cases due sensitivities and specificities of less than 100%. Moreover, the limited spatial resolution of MRI techniques does not enable accurate analysis or biophysical measurements to be made within very small volumes, which restricts the applicability of this method to only a limited number of nodal areas.

2.3.4.3 Perfusion-weighted Imaging

Perfusional parameters may be obtained using different MRI techniques such as bolus tracking T2* susceptibility imaging or arterial spin labeling (ASL) (Petrella and Provenzale 2000). Again, the node size may restrict the applicability of this technique to a limited number of nodal areas. To our knowledge, the specificity of the perfusional parameters in differentiating benign from malignant nodes has yet not been investigated.

2.3.5 Neoplastic Lymph Nodes: Specific MR Targets

2.3.5.1 Introduction

Detecting malignant lymph nodes still remains a major challenge due to two inherent limitations present in all morphological imaging techniques: (a) the failure to detect small metastatic deposits within macroscopically unenlarged nodes; and (b) the inability to differentiate between inflammatory nodal response and tumor invasion within enlarged nodes. Improved criteria for the semiological evaluation of nodal images have been developed which, however, remain limited to probabilities without giving a 100% confidence level (Curtin et al. 1998). Critical evaluation of the nodal images must be made by including the normal range of size and number for each location to reach the best confidence level in lymph node status interpretation (Carrington 1998). Basic concepts regarding nodal size, shape, site, number, fatty core and central necrosis are applicable to both MRI and CT with minor differences between the two techniques, such as the unsurpassed ability of CT in detecting calcium deposits within (or outside) nodes. The specific features of the MR technique have been described below.

2.3.5.2 Extracapsular Tumoral Spread

The irregular margins of an enlarged node suggest tumoral spread beyond the nodal capsule. It has generally been considered that CT is more accurate in depicting extracapsular spread (Chong et al. 1996; Yousem et al. 1992). In our experience, however, we have found that MRI performs well in this respect (Fig. 2.8) although experienced investigators have stated that preoperative imaging techniques may only detect the presence of major macroscopic extranodal spread. As even pathologists do not always agree on the presence of microscopic nodal spread, the radiological assessment of extracapsular spread should be considered as being unreliable, even when using MRI (van den Brekel and Castelijns 1999).

2.3.5.3 Contrast Enhancement

All nodes become enhanced after perfusion of paramagnetic contrast medium. Tumoral nodes may become enhanced to a different degree which is not predictive of the histological content of the involved nodes. By whitening the nodes, the administration of contrast agent decreases the spontaneous contrast between the nodes and the fatty environment. The FS option must therefore be used, with the subsequent drawbacks of time loss and increase in artifacts. Moreover, post-contrast T1-weighted and T2-weighted information is often redundant, except in the specific case of non-cystic necrosis within the nodes which remains undetected or is only poorly detected on T2 images (van den Brekel and Castelijns 1999). The incidence of this condition seems low in our clinical experience. Whether paramagnetic contrast agent perfusion is an absolute requirement in a "pure" nodal MR setting is open to question. In routine practice the issue does not arise, since MR examination addresses both aims of primary and nodal staging.

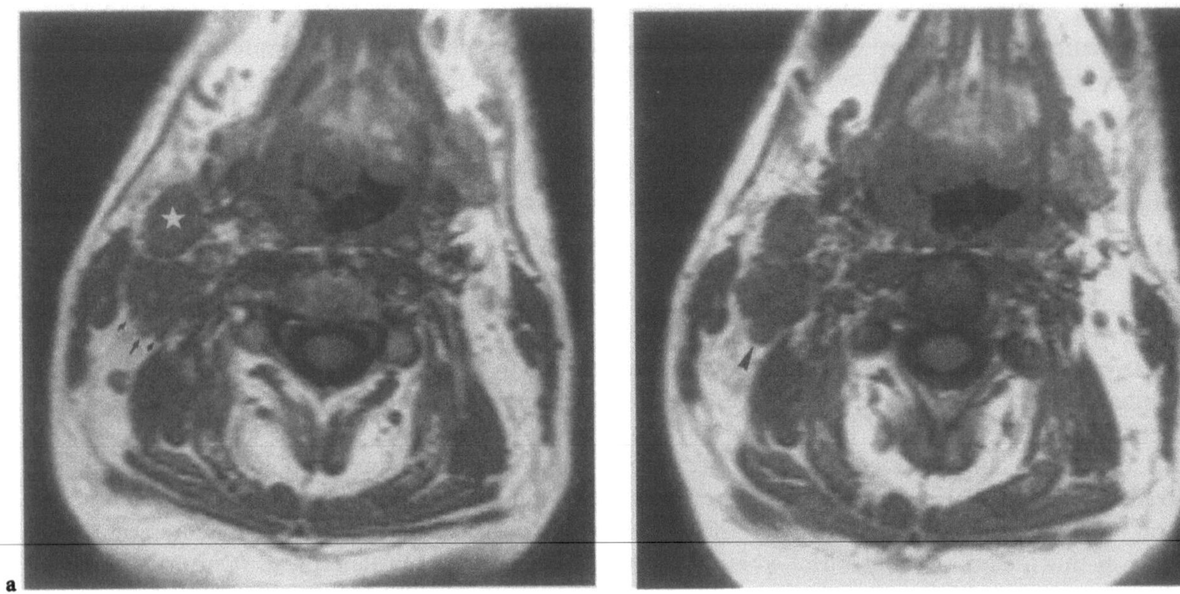

Fig. 2.8a, b. Suspected extracapsular tumoral spread. Contiguous pre-contrast CSE T1-weighted transverse images without FS in a case of SCC of the base of the tongue and the right vallecula. **a** Lower slice: two enlarged tumoral nodes are present in the homolateral jugular area. The anterior node (*white star*) has smooth contours, suggesting the absence of extranodal spread. The posterior node exhibits suspicious irregularities in its posterior aspect (*thin black arrows*). **b** Contiguous slice in upper location: pseudopodal tumoral extrusion (*arrowhead*) reinforces the suspicion for extranodal tumoral spread

2.3.5.4
Post-treatment Nodal Status

Increased accuracy in the assessment of post-treatment nodal status is obtained when strictly similar images are compared, both as regards weightings and slice locations (Fig. 2.9). In our clinical approach, the pretreatment examination is always reviewed before planning the follow-up to ensure optimal reproducibility between examination protocols. Adequate timing of the first "baseline" post-treatment examination is a controversial issue, with the contradictory demands of detecting tumor residue/relapse as soon as possible, and waiting for the resolution of disturbing inflammatory post-treatment reactions. But there seems to be general consensus that a delay of 3–4 months after completion of radiation therapy (RT) is optimal to perform control imaging (Van den Brekel and Castelijns 1999). The main observations on post-therapeutic examination have been listed below:

- *Complete disappearance:* in Fig. 2.9, enlarged nodes suspected of harboring macrometastases on the basis of pretreatment images are no longer detectable.
- *Normalized appearance:* enlarged nodes exhibit a normalized size. They usually appear to be intensely vascularized, possibly indicative of inflammatory changes (not illustrated).
- *Evolution to shrunk fibrous scar:* the nodes appear to be shrunk, hypovascularized on post-contrast T1-weighted images and hypointense on T2-weighted images. which is considered to reflect fibrotic evolution. This pattern usually takes more time than the standard 3–4 months delay after treatment completion (Fig. 2.10).

2.3.5.4
Nodal Relapse

Neither CT nor MRI have performed well in the early detection of recurrent/residual disease due to confusing post-therapeutic inflammatory changes in the treated areas. The results of meticulous attempts at the early detection of nodal relapse have been frustrating (Dillon and Harnsberger 1991; Gussack and Hudgins 1991). However, recent studies have demonstrated the impact of the PET technique in determining disease-free post-treatment status in patients with head and neck neoplasms (Mukherji et al. 2000).

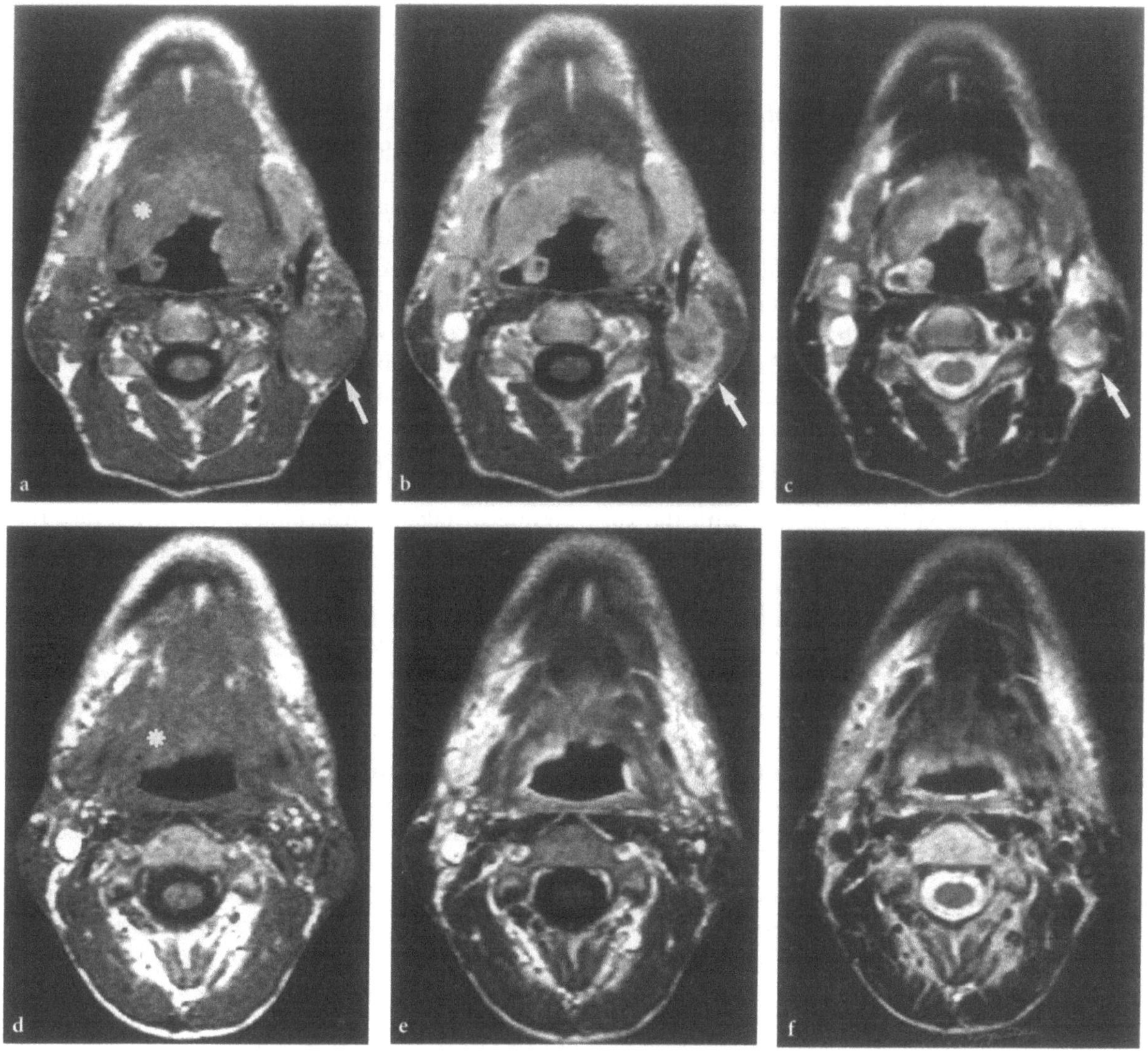

Fig. 2.9a–e. Comprehensive MR setting of pre- and post-treatment status. All slice locations are similar in all weightings in both studies to ensure accurate intra- and inter-examination comparison. **a–c** Upper row: pre-contrast T1(**a**), post-contrast T1 (**b**), and T2 (**c**) images prior to RT. **d-f** Similar views 3 months after completion of RT. Both the vallecular primary tumor (*white notches*) and the nodal metastases (*arrows*) completely disappeared after treatment. The availability of the three "colors" (pre- and post-contrast T1, and T2) in strictly similar plane and slice locations on the pre- and post-therapeutic examination allows confirmation of the complete disappearance of the lesions

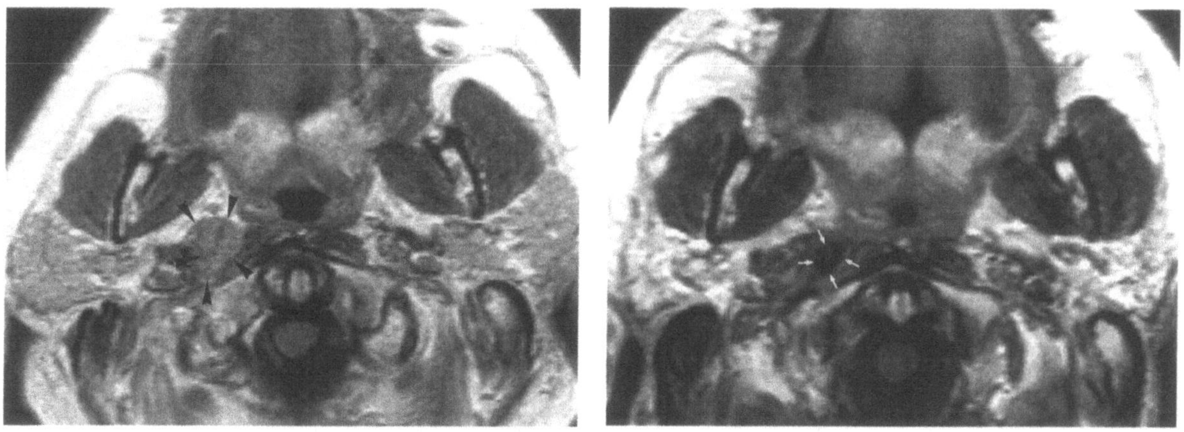

Fig. 2.10a, b. Post-RT metastatic lymph node scarring. **a** Post-contrast CSE T1-weighted transverse image of the pre-RT MR examination: a right lateral-retropharyngeal lymph node metastasis can be clearly seen (*arrowheads*). **b** Post-contrast CSE T1-weighted transverse image in a similar slice location 8 months after completion of RT: a residual nodule exhibits very low signal intensity without contrast enhancement (*arrows*), corresponding to fibrous scarring

2.4 Positron Emission Tomography Imaging

2.4.1 Physical Principles of PET Imaging

Positrons are electron anti-particles. A positron is produced during the decay of a nuclide having an excess of protons within the nucleus when compared to the number of neutrons. Positron emitters are obtained by bombarding nuclides with a cyclotron-generated proton beam. Like the electrons, the positrons may have different energy levels, ranging from 0 to a specific value. After emission, the positron is slowed down by interaction with the surrounding matter and ultimately hits an electron, which results in the *"annihilation"* reaction. This occurs after a short distance of a few millimeters, the precise length of which depends on the positron energy. For example, the average traveling distance of a positron is 0.35 mm for ^{18}F (maximum distance: 2.3 mm) and 1.1 mm for ^{15}O (maximum distance: 8.1 mm). The annihilation reaction results in the production of a pair of photons both energized at 511 keV. Positron emitters allow the labeling of biomolecules without modifications in their chemical and biological properties, e.g. ^{15}O, ^{11}C or ^{13}N can be used as direct substitutes for ^{16}O, ^{12}C or ^{14}N, and ^{18}F can replace ^{1}H. Another characteristic of positron emitters is their short physical half-life compared to other nuclides used in nuclear medicine imaging such as ^{99m}Tc or ^{201}Tl. Their half-lives range from 2 minutes for ^{15}O to 110 minutes for ^{18}F, which reduces their availability for PET systems not equipped with an on-site cyclotron.

The detection of radioactivity within the patient's body is carried out by scintillators which produce visible light when hit by an incident photon. Photons resulting from the annihilation reaction have two major characteristics: first a high energy level of 511 keV, which requires crystals with a high stopping power for detection. If the stopping power is too low, the probability of detecting a photon by interaction with the crystalline material will be lessened and the event may not be detected. Sodium iodine (NaI) is the most commonly used scintillation material in nuclear medicine, with a high photon yield at 40 scintillation photons/keV when compared to other materials such as bismuth germanium oxide (BGO) with 4.8 scintillation photons/keV. In spite of a lower photon yield, BGO is better suited for 511 keV photon detection because of its higher stopping power. PET detectors are typically made of BGO crystals 4 mm in cross-section and 20–30 mm in length, arranged in groups and connected to photomultiplier tubes. Blocks of detectors are arranged in rings, covering an axial FOV of 10–16 cm. The second major characteristic of the annihilation photons is that they are emitted in opposite directions, and therefore require a pair of crystals placed at an angle of 180° so they can be detected. A given pair of detectors selectively detects events occurring along a single line connecting them. The site of photon production (annihilation reaction) can be localized by analyzing multiple lines of response crossing each other at the production point. Only photons that hit the pair of detectors within a definite time frame are taken into account by the PET system (the "true" coincidences), and coincidental events occurring too late in time from one another are rejected. Both constraints of coincidental emission and time frame ensure the accurate spatial localization of the radioactivity within the body (electronic collimation), without the need for external collimators which would reduce the sensitivity of the system.

Up to 80% of the gamma radiation can be absorbed by the patient's body: the so-called "attenuation" phenomenon. In PET imaging, attenuation does not depend on the location in depth of the decay event, since event detection relies on a pair of photons travelling along a line. Attenuation can be quantified by measuring the absorption of the 511 keV photons produced by an external radiation source through each line of response. This is commonly obtained by rotating a ^{68}Ge external radiation source around the patient. Correction for attenuation allows the measurement of quantitative indexes, which are ancillary for diagnostic purposes but necessary for the assessment of the tumoral response to therapy.

2.4.2 Metabolic Imaging of Tumors

Tumoral cells undergo changes involving many metabolic pathways. A particular metabolic function within the cells can be measured in vivo by detecting specific radio-labeled molecules. A large number of metabolic characteristics of tumoral cells have been studied using radiotracers labeled with positron emitters: blood flow (with $H_2{}^{15}O$ as tracer), protein synthesis (with labeled amino acids such as ^{11}C-methionine or ^{11}C-tyrosine), DNA synthesis (with labeled DNA precursors such as ^{11}C thymidine) and glucose consumption (with labeled glucose analogs). Static (after a period of radiotracer incorporation) as well as dynamic (during radiotracer incorporation) images can be obtained, depending on which clinical issue has to be investigated. Functional imaging has become the necessary complement to anatomical imaging in a number of medical domains, especially in oncology where glucose metabolism imaging using 2-[^{18}F]-fluoro-2-deoxy-D-glucose (FDG) combined with PET has proven to be a powerful diagnostic and staging tool. Several changes in glucose metabolism are responsible for the increased accumulation of labeled glucose in tumoral cells (Vuilliez 1998). The increase in lactate production within tumors is first evidenced by an increase in tumoral anaerobic glycolysis, as observed by Warburg in the 1930s (Warburg 1930). The overexpression of glucose transporters on the cell membrane, mainly subtypes 1 and 3 (Brown et al. 1993, 1996; Mellanen et al. 1994; Reske et al. 1997; Younes et al. 1995), as well as their upregulation by hypoxia which is frequently observed in tumors (Burgman et al. 2001) first account for increased glucose uptake. Moreover, intracellular enzyme characteristics are altered: hexokinase, the first-step phosphorylating enzyme, is overexpressed in tumoral cells (Bustamente and Pedersen 1977) and becomes less sensitive to downregulation. Glucose-6-phosphatase, the reverse enzyme of hexokinase, is underexpressed or absent in tumors (Weber and Cantero 1955), so that incoming glucose is rapidly phosphorylated and further metabolized. An increase in glucose uptake and consumption is observed in tumoral cells compared to adjacent cells. This metabolic phenomenon is related to cell multiplication and therefore is also present in non-neoplastic proliferative cells, e.g. inflammatory cells (Kubota et al. 1992) such as macrophages or granulocytes. Malignant transformation leads to a permanent dysregulation of the rate of proliferation, which boosts the mechanisms of increased glucose uptake. FDG is the analog of choice for PET imaging since, contrary to native glucose which is rapidly metabolized into CO_2, deoxyglucose is trapped in its monophosphorylated form after the action of hexokinase. The next glycolytic enzyme, glucose-6-isomerase, does not recognize FDG as substrate. This leads to the accumulation of labeled deoxyglucose in the tumoral cell, with the result that tumoral foci are easily detected throughout the body (high tumor-to-background ratio) apart from the brain where the normal high cortical glucose uptake hampers the detection of tumoral lesions within the gray matter.

2.4.3 FDG-PET Acquisition Protocols in Oncology

Specifically adapted PET scanners are BGO-based systems (see above) with a resolution of 5 mm in the axial plane. Since they are expensive, alternative methods for FDG imaging have been developed using modified but standard gamma cameras with NaI crystals and electronic or external collimators, or incorporating specific electronics for the detection of coincidence photons. Such modified systems suffer from lower sensitivity for the detection of annihilation photons, and thus have a lower diagnostic capacity, especially for small lesions (<1.5 cm) and/or abdominal foci (Delbeke et al. 1999; Landoni et al. 1999; Lonneux et al. 1998; Martin et al. 1995; Shreve et al. 1998). Although the clinical usefulness of modified systems has been established in lung (Tatsumi et al. 1999; Weber et al. 1999) and in head and neck cancers (Stokkel et al. 2000), more studies are needed before the equivalence of modified and PET-specifically adapted systems for cancer detection and staging can be determined. This point is crucial for nodal staging, since the cut-off size of positive nodes is often close to or less than 1.5 cm.

2.4.3.1 Patient Preparation

Patients must have fasted for at least 6 hours prior to examination to ensure that they are in a euglycemic state (no competition between labeled and native glucose) with normal insulin levels. This is of importance, since elevated insulin levels result in increased muscular and cardiac glucose uptake at the expense of tumoral uptake (Langen et al. 1993; Torizuka et al. 1998). For imaging cervical malignancies (head and neck SCCs, thyroid tumors or lymphomas), the oral administration of 10 mg diazepam 30 minutes before injection of the tracer is advisable to decrease the cervical muscular uptake occurring in some patients, which interferes with the interpretation of the cervical lymph node stations (Barrington and Maisey 1996) (Fig. 2.11).

2.4.3.2 Tracer Injection

370 MBq (10 mCi) FDG are injected intravenously. Oral or intravenous hyperhydration is necessary to accelerate urinary excretion of the unbound fraction of tracer, thereby reducing the radioactive load and increasing the tumor-to-background ratio, especially

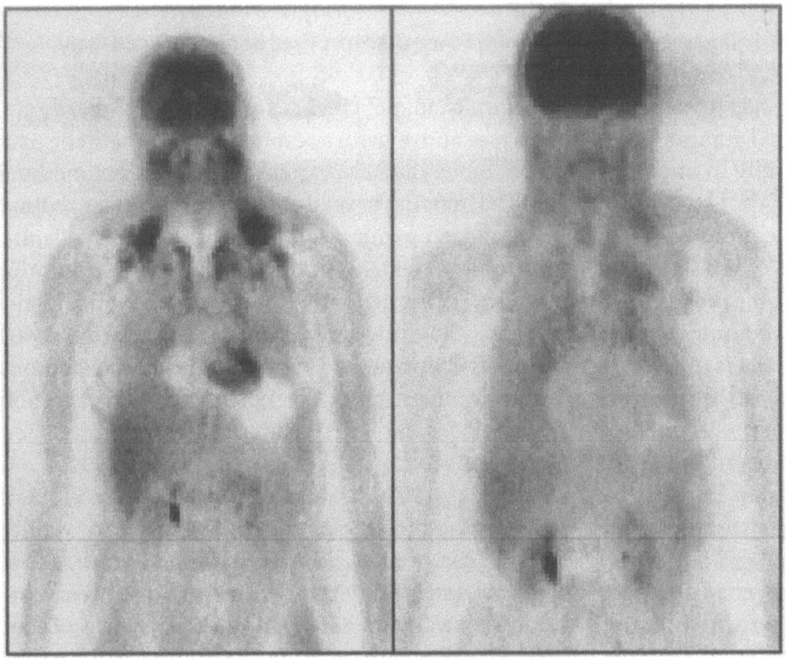

Fig. 2.11. Coronal whole-body FDG-PET view. High muscular uptake is observed in the cervical area precluding the detection of metastatic lymph nodes (*left*). A similar view in the same patient obtained one week later, after the administration of 10 mg diazepam 30 min before FDG injection (*right*): pre-medication with diazepam is advisable when assessing head and neck tumors

in the abdomen and pelvis. Urinary excretion can be further stimulated by intravenous administration of diuretic drugs 15 minutes after tracer injection. During the 1-hour incorporation period, patients are instructed to remain quiet and calm to minimize uptake by the laryngeal and skeletal muscles.

2.4.3.3 Imaging and Data Processing

Immediately after the bladder has been emptied, the patient is positioned in the PET system. The standard FOV usually covers the upper part of the body from the pelvis to the top of the head. This common procedure is referred to as a *"whole-body"* examination. If necessary, e.g. in the case of melanoma or sarcoma, the lower limbs are included in the FOV. Consecutive emission scans of 5 minutes each over seven bed positions are acquired in 2D mode followed by transmission scans of 1 minute each for attenuation correction purposes. Specifically adapted regional acquisition protocols can be introduced for particular clinical problems, such as for the staging of the head and neck region where a longer acquisition time in 3D mode increases the image quality. At our institution, images are reconstructed by iterative algorithm (Lonneux et al. 1999) and segmented attenuation correction. The advantages of whole-body attenuation correction are the following: better spatial localization, accurate lesion geometry (essential for further image co-registration with CT or MRI), and the possibility of quantifying tracer uptake, which can be helpful in some instances (see above). The sensitivity is also increased by correction for attenuation, especially for abdominal lesions (Hustinx et al. 2000).

2.4.4 FDG-PET Imaging of Cancer

A unique feature of FDG-PET imaging is the possibility of obtaining information on both locoregional and distant tumoral spread in a single imaging procedure. FDG-PET is therefore viewed as a sensitive tool for cancer staging in many clinical situations: the initial staging of cancer (lung cancer, lymphoma, melanoma), restaging after induction therapy (lung cancer, lymphoma, breast cancer), evaluation of residual mass (lymphoma, testicular cancer) or the detection of recurrence (colorectal, breast, head and neck cancer). As far as RT is concerned, the potential value of FDG-PET imaging is two-fold. First, PET could help in better delineating the active fraction of the tumor in order to deliver an extra dose to this region or reduce the total target field. This approach needs further validation, since only preliminary results have been reported so far. Second, the ability of PET to correct the pretreatment staging of tumors obviously has a major impact on patient management. For example, PET represents a breakthrough in nodal staging since it allows the characterization of lymph nodes as benign or malignant independent of their size, although one should not forget that this technique has limitations as regards spatial resolution. PET findings may change tumoral N staging by detecting increased metabolism within normal-sized lymph nodes (upstaging) or conversely, by showing that enlarged benign lymph nodes do not concentrate FDG (downstaging). Of course PET sensitivity and specificity are not totally satisfactory, as the limited spatial resolution of the system impedes the detection of micrometastases, and since benign but highly inflammatory lymph nodes can display increased FDG uptake. In many instances, structural imaging should be considered as a complement to FDG-PET, because multimodal image registration allows a more accurate localization of highly metabolic foci (Fig. 2.12).

2.4.4.1 Lung Cancer

The use of FDG-PET in the examination of lung tumors has significantly increased the accuracy of the preoperative staging of patients with non-small cell carcinoma. Table 2.1 summarizes the published data.

PET leads to a significant increase in the sensitivity and specificity of preoperative N staging, resulting in a 50% reduction of invasive staging procedures, e.g. mediastinoscopy (Vansteenkiste and Mortelmans 1999). As PET has a very high negative predictive value, a PET-negative mediastinum allows curative surgery to be performed without prior mediastinoscopy. In turn, PET-positive homolateral mediastinal involvement (N2 disease) requires invasive confirmation to avoid refusal of surgery

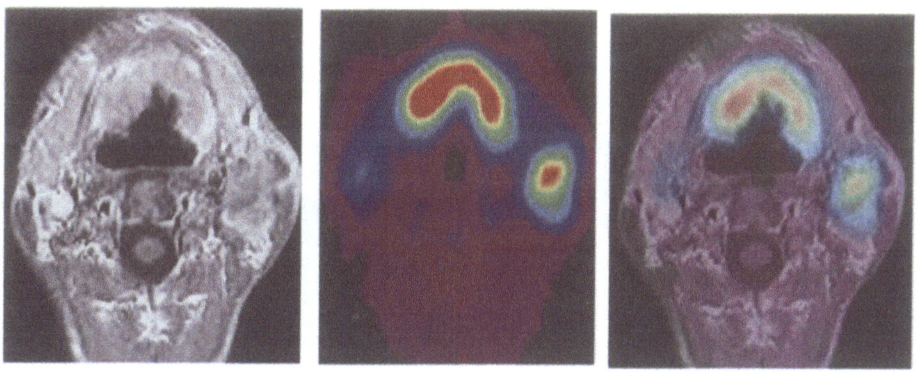

Fig. 2.12. Multimodal image fusion (*right*) using MR (*left*) and FDG-PET (*middle*) images of a hypopharyngeal SCC with metastatic cervical lymph nodes. Anatomical data are of assistance in precisely delineating the topographical location of the hot spots observed on the FDG-PET images

Table 2.1. Comparison of FDG-PET and CT for the nodal staging of non-small-cell lung cancer

Reference	No. of patients	PET Sensitivity	PET Specificity	CT Sensitivity	CT Specificity
Chin et al. (1995)	30	78	81	56	86
Patz et al. (1995)	42	83	82	43	85
Sasaki et al. (1996)	29	76	98	65	87
Sazon et al. (1996)	32	100	100	81	56
Scott et al. (1996)	27	100	98	60	93
Steinert et al. (1997)	47	89	99	57	94
Valk et al. (1995)	76	83	94	63	73
Wahl et al. (1994)	23	82	81	64	44
Vansteenkiste et al. (1998a)	68	93	95	75	63
Bury et al. (1996)	50	90	86	72	81
Guhlmann et al. (1997)	32	80	100	50	75
Total	456	87	92	62	76

by a patient with a false-positive PET scan. The lack of anatomical landmarks on PET images often interferes with the precise localization of the most appropriate nodal station to be sampled. Therefore, PET-CT image co-interpretation or fusion increases the diagnostic accuracy of the imaging examination (Vansteenkiste et al. 1998b) by indicating the best-suited nodal site for biopsy (Fig. 2.13).

In the field of RT, some reports have suggested that the metabolic information provided by PET could help in delineating the active fraction of the tumor, resulting in narrowed irradiation fields (Giraud et al. 2001; Vanuystel et al. 2000). Similarly, it has been also stated that PET could help in differentiating tumoral tissue from benign atelectasis in central lung neoplasms (Nestle et al. 1999). However, published studies in the field have mainly been retrospective, and further data are needed to validate these promising hypotheses. Correction for tumor movement during breathing is also being developed at the technical level, which would increase the accuracy of the metabolic data provided by PET examination (Nehmeh et al. 2001).

2.4.4.2
Head and Neck Tumors

The advantage of FDG-PET in the N staging of SCC tumors of the head and neck region is not clearly established when compared to morphological CT and MR modalities (Table 2.2).

It has been suggested that PET is of greater accuracy in predicting the absence of nodal involvement (higher negative predictive value than CT-MR), which could reduce the indications for bilateral neck dissec-

Table 2.2. Comparison of FDG-PET and CT/MRI for the nodal staging of head and neck squamous-cell carcinoma

		PET		MRI or CT	
	n	Sens	Spec	Sens	Spec
Laubenbacher et al. (1995)	22	89	100	72	56
Braams et al. (1995)	12	91	88	36	94
Adams et al. (1998)	60	90	94	82	85
Benchaou et al. (1996)	48	72	99	67	97
Stokkel et al. (2000)	54	96	90	85	86
Di Martino et al. (2000)	37	83	91	86	97
Paulus et al. (1998)	25	50	100	40	100

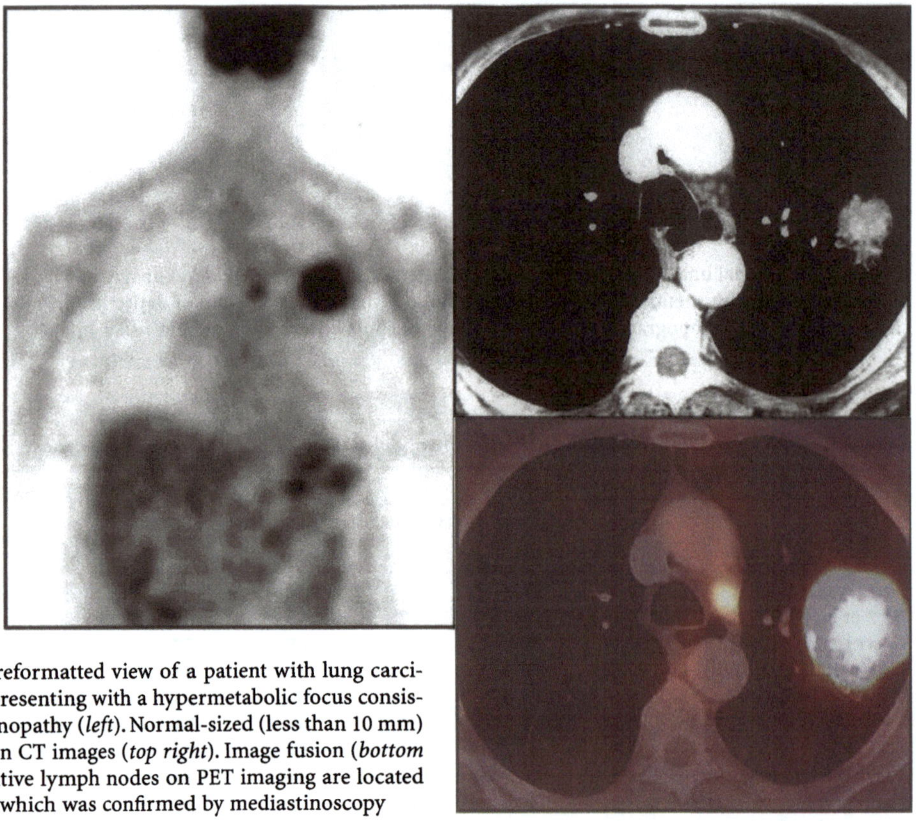

Fig. 2.13. Coronal FDG-PET reformatted view of a patient with lung carcinoma of the left upper lobe presenting with a hypermetabolic focus consistent with left mediastinal adenopathy (*left*). Normal-sized (less than 10 mm) lymph nodes are visualized on CT images (*top right*). Image fusion (*bottom right*) demonstrates that positive lymph nodes on PET imaging are located within the left mediastinum, which was confirmed by mediastinoscopy

tion (Braams et al. 1995; Myers et al. 1998). One of the most interesting applications of PET is that concerning the detection of the primary tumor in the presence of cervical metastatic adenopathy from unknown SCC. Indeed, with an identification rate of up to 40% in patients with a previously negative standard examination (including CT, US and panendoscopy) PET contributes positively to patient management by allowing selective treatment of the primary, instead of irradiating large volumes if the primary tumor remains unidentified (Aassar et al. 1999; Bohuslavizki et al. 2000; Hanasono et al. 1999) (Fig. 2.14).

2.4.4.3 *Lymphomas*

PET-FDG has proven to be very effective in the staging of both Hodgkin's and non-Hodgkin's lymphomas. PET is highly sensitive in detecting nodal and bone marrow involvement, resulting in disease upstaging in about 10% of patients (Moog et al. 1997, 1998a,b). Again, the ability of PET to detect active disease in unenlarged lymph nodes explains these results. PET has been shown to modify patient management in about 25% of cases (Shah et al. 2000), e.g. by indicating a switch from RT to systemic chemotherapy in patients initially classified as stage I and who were subsequently upstaged by PET (Fig. 2.15).

2.4.4.4 *Esophageal Cancer*

PET has demonstrated promising results in the pretreatment evaluation of esophageal tumors. The sensitivity of PET in tumoral node detection is similar to that of CT and endoscopic ultrasound, but its specificity is higher (Flamen et al. 2000; Lerut et al. 2000). It is also useful in detecting distant lymph node or non-nodal metastases (Block et al. 1997), but nodal involvement adjacent or close to the primary tumor cannot be differentiated from uptake within the latter. The detection by PET of non-palpable metastases within the jugular lymph nodes can be of major importance in treatment planning (Figs. 2.16, 2.17).

2.4.4.5 *Testicular Tumors*

No data are currently available on the use of FDG-PET in the preoperative staging of testicular tumors, although its use in the assessment of viable tumor tissue after therapy has been recognized (Cremerius et al. 1998). In the pretreatment setting, the sensitivity of this method for nodal involvement detection is close to that of CT (around 60%). In non-seminomatous tumors, PET information could avoid retroperitoneal lymph node resection if high sensitivity was demonstrated, which has not been observed in the few published cases. In seminomatous tumors, RT of the lymph outflow is an established standard procedure in early tumoral stages which does not require positive imaging.

2.4.4.6 *Breast Tumors*

The detection of micrometastases within axillary lymph nodes is not possible by FDG-PET due to

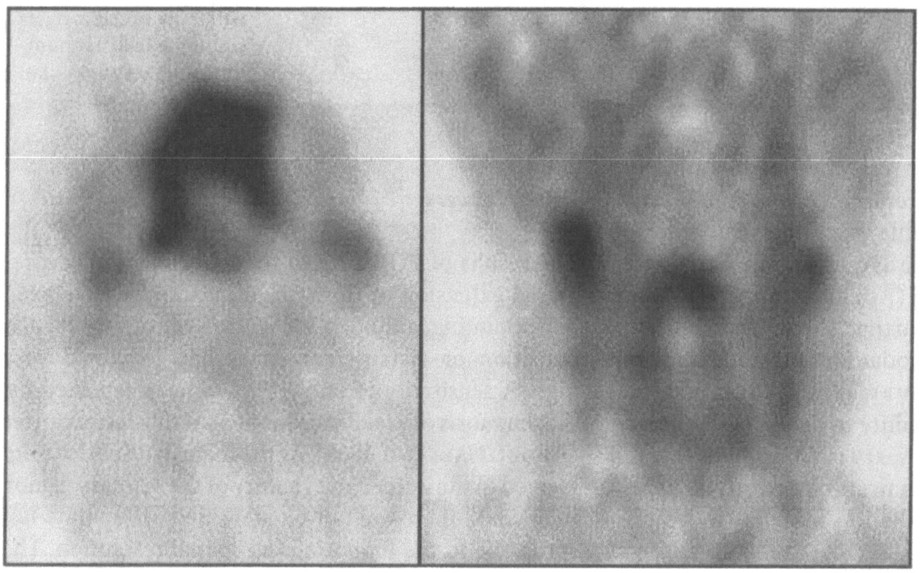

Fig. 2.14. Whole-body FDG-PET: axial (*left*) and coronal (*right*) views of bilateral nodal metastases of hypopharyngeal SCC. The right adenopathy measured less than 10 mm and was therefore incorrectly rated as benign on the CT images

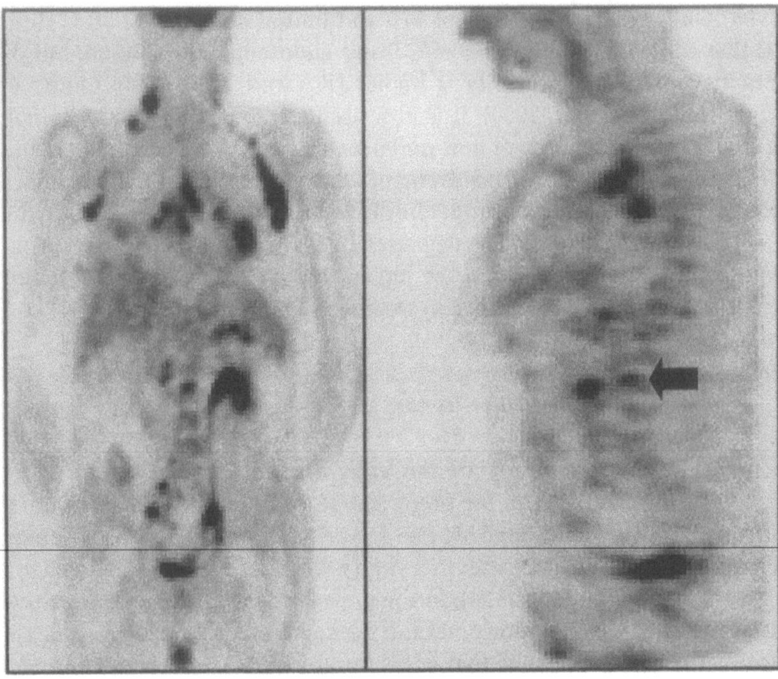

Fig. 2.15. FDG-PET coronal (*left*) and sagittal (*right*) reformatted views in a patient with non-Hodgkin's lymphoma. PET depicts tumoral lymph nodes on both sides of the diaphragm, as well as a bone lesion within a vertebral body (*arrow*). Blind bone marrow biopsy performed in the posterior left iliac crest was negative. Vertebral bone marrow involvement was later confirmed by MR examination (not illustrated)

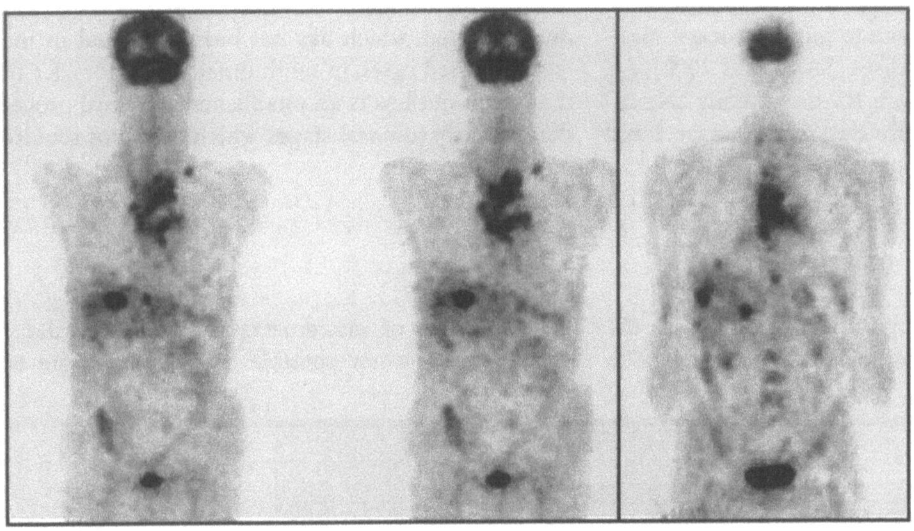

Fig. 2.16. Three adjacent coronal reformatted views featuring typical FDG-PET findings in esophageal carcinoma with bulk nodal metastases in the mediastinum, liver, and left supra-clavicular nodal area

the limitations in spatial resolution of this method. Therefore, PET cannot replace conventional surgical exploration of the axilla using the sentinel node technique. Reported sensitivities for N staging were initially good (80–95%) (Adler et al. 1997; Avril et al. 1996) but it was further shown that sensitivity dropped to 33% for nodal metastases from small primary tumors (pT1) (Avril et al. 1996). A potential advantage of PET is its ability to detect nodal metastases in the internal mammary chain, as illustrated in Fig. 2.18. However, the clinical impact of this aspect on delineation of the radiation field has to be prospectively studied.

2.4.4.7
Other Cancers

The results of FGD-PET in the assessment of locoregional extension of digestive tract tumors have been disappointing, although the overall sensitivity for the detection of distant metastases has remained very high. A sensitivity of only 25% has been reported for the diagnosis of nodal involvement in colorectal cancer (Abdel-Nabi et al. 1998). As the metastatic nodes were located in the immediate vicinity of the primary tumor, they could therefore not be identified as separate hot spots due to the limitations in spatial resolution. The

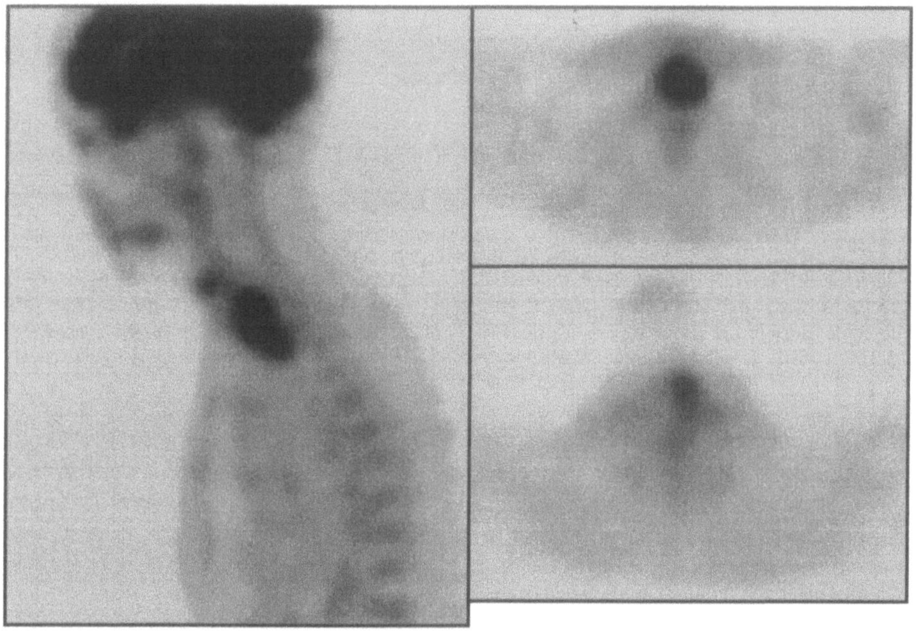

Fig. 2.17. Sagittal view (*left*) and axial views (*right*) at the level of the esophageal primary tumor (*top*) and left paratracheal metastatic lymph node (*bottom*), found to be negative on CT examination but later confirmed as positive by ultrasound and biopsy

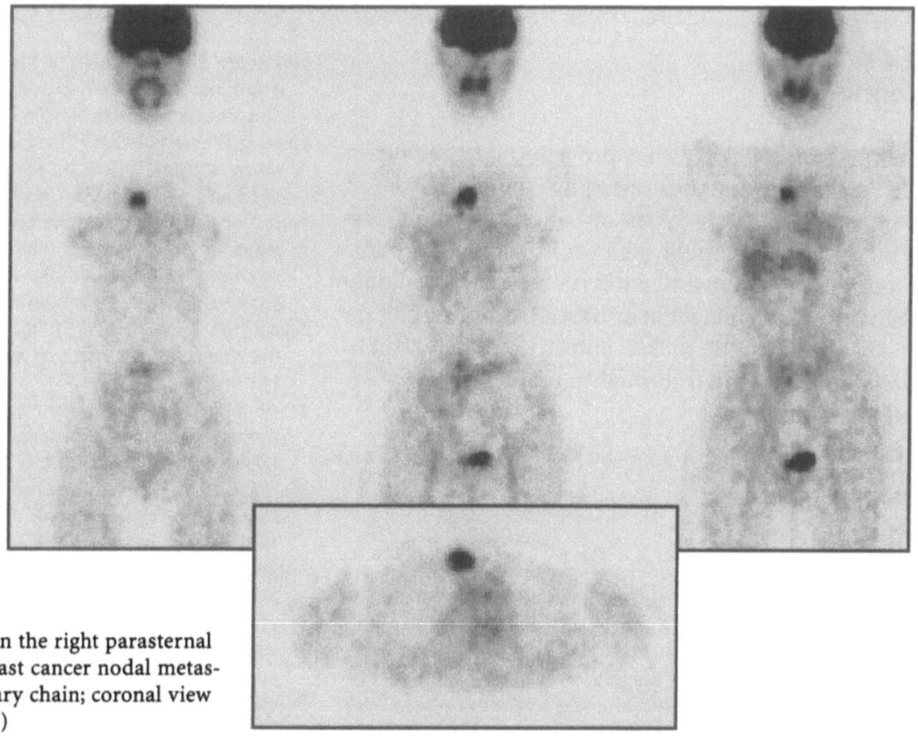

Fig. 2.18. High FDG uptake in the right parasternal region corresponding to breast cancer nodal metastases in the internal mammary chain; coronal view (*top*) and axial view (*bottom*)

use of FDG-PET can reasonably be advocated for the preoperative staging of rectal tumors when enlarged lymph nodes are visualized on CT or EUS, since this could influence the therapeutic decisions. In pancreatic cancer, a sensitivity of 49% and a specificity of 63% have been reported for metastatic lymph node detection, while the sensitivity for detection of metastases is about 80% (Diederichs et al. 2000).

In the gynecological domain, PET has recently been proposed as a technique for assessing the lymphatic extent of uterine cervical cancers, and has shown higher sensitivity and specificity than CT (Sugawara et al. 1999). By detecting metastatic lymph nodes, PET could play a role in indicating adjuvant RT (Fig. 2.19).

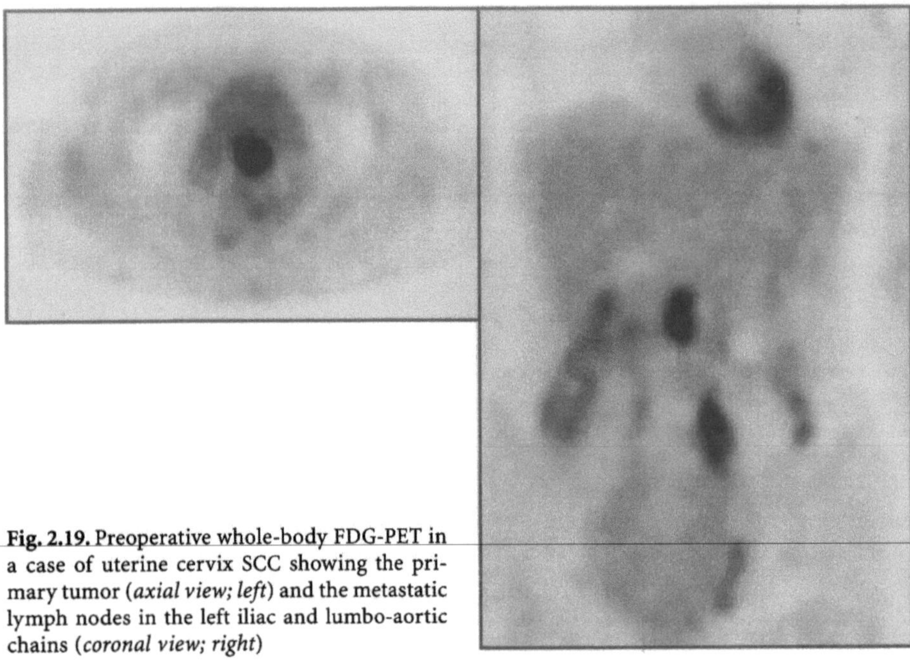

Fig. 2.19. Preoperative whole-body FDG-PET in a case of uterine cervix SCC showing the primary tumor (*axial view; left*) and the metastatic lymph nodes in the left iliac and lumbo-aortic chains (*coronal view; right*)

2.4.5 Conclusion

Whole-body PET-FDG has proven to be effective in the diagnosis, staging, restaging and detection of recurrence in many types of cancer. Although few studies have been published on its role in RT planning and further investigation is necessary to validate the concept of "metabolism-based" conformal RT, in many instances PET makes a positive contribution to patient management through a more accurate staging of the disease.

References

Aassar et al (1999) Metastatic head and neck cancer: role and usefulness of FDG PET in locating occult primary tumors. Radiology 210:177–181

Abdel-Nabi H et al (1998) Staging of primary colorectal carcinomas with fluorine-18 fluorodeoxyglucose whole-body PET: correlation with histopathologic and CT findings. Radiology 206:755–760

Adams S et al (1998) Prospective comparison of 18F-FDG PET with conventional imaging modalities (CT, MRI, US) in lymph node staging of head and neck cancer. Eur J Nucl Med 25:1255–1260

Adler L et al (1997) Axillary lymph node metastases: screening with [F-18]2-deoxy-2-D-glucose (FDG) PET. Radiology 203:323–327

American Joint Committee on Cancer (1992) Lung. In: Beahrs OH, Henson DE, Hutter RVP et al (eds) Manual for staging cancer, 4th edn. Lippincott, Philadelphia, pp 115–121

American Thoracic Society (1983) Medical Section of the American Lung Association. Clinical staging of primary lung cancer. Am Rev Respir Dis 127:659–664

Anzaï Y, Prince MR (1997) Iron-oxide enhanced MR lymphography: the evaluation of cervical lymph node metastases in head and neck cancer. J Magn Reson Imag 7:75–81

Avril N et al (1996) Assessment of axillary lymph node involvement in breast cancer patients with positron emission tomography using radiolabelled 2-(fluorine-18)-fluoro-2-deoxy-D-glucose. J Natl Cancer Inst 88:1204–1209

Barrington S, Maisey M (1996) Skeletal muscular uptake of fluorine-18-FDG: effect of oral diazepam. J Nucl Med 37: 1127–1129

Benchaou M et al (1996) The role of FDG-PET in the preoperative assessment of N-staging in head and neck cancer. Acta Otolaryngol 116:332–335

Block M et al (1997) Improvement in staging of esophageal cancer with the addition of positron emission tomography. Ann Thorac Surg 64:770–776

Bohuslavizki KH et al (2000) FDG PET detection of unknown primary tumors. J Nucl Med 41:816–822

Braams J et al (1995) Detection of lymph node metastases of squamous-cell cancer of the head and neck with FDG-PET and MRI. J Nucl Med 36:211–216

Brink J (1995) Technical aspects of helical (spiral) CT. Radiol Clin North Am 33:834–851

Brown R, Wahl R (1993) Overexpression of GLUT-1 glucose transporter in human breast cancer. An immunohistochemical study. Cancer 72:2979–2985

Brown R et al (1996) Intratumoral distribution of tritiated FDG in breast carcinoma: correlation between Glut-1 expression and FDG uptake. J Nucl Med 37:1043–1047

Burgman P et al (2001) Hypoxia-induced increase in FDG uptake in MCF7 cells. J Nucl Med 42:170–175

Bury T et al (1996) Staging of the mediastinum: value of positron emission tomography imaging in non-small cell lung cancer. Eur Respir J 9:2560–2564

Bustamente E, Pedersen P (1977) High aerobic glycolysis of rat hepatoma cells in culture: role of mitochondrial hexokinase. Proc Natl Acad Sci USA 74:3735–3739

Carrington B (1998) Lymph nodes. In: Husband JHS, Reznek RH (eds) Imaging in oncologic. Isis Medical Media, Oxford, pp 729–748

Chin R et al (1995) Mediastinal staging of non-small-cell lung cancer with positron emission tomography. Am J Respir Crit Care Med 152:2090–2096

Chong VFH et al (1996) MR features of cervical node necrosis in metastatic disease. Clin Radiol 51:103–109

Cline HE et al (1991) 3D surface rendered MR images of the brain and its vasculature. J Comput Assist Tomogr 15:344–351

Cremerius U et al (1998) FDG-PET for detection and therapy control of metastatic germ cell tumor. J Nucl Med 39: 815–822

Curtin HD et al (1998) Comparison of CT and MR imaging in staging of neck metastases. Radiology 207:123–130

Cymbalista M et al (1999) CT demonstration of the 1996 AJCC-UICC regional lymph node classification for lung cancer staging. Radiographics 19:899–900

Delbeke D et al (1999) FDG PET and dual-head gamma camera positron coincidence detection imaging of suspected malignancies and brain disorders. J Nucl Med 40:110–117

Diederichs C et al (2000) Values and limitations of 18F-fluorodeoxyglucose-positron-emission tomography with preoperative evaluation of patients with pancreatic masses. Pancreas 20:109–116

Dillon WP, Harnsberger HR (1991) The impact of radiologic imaging on staging of cancer of the head and neck. Semin Oncol 18:64–79

DiMartino E et al (2000) Diagnosis and staging of head and neck caner. Arch Otolaryngol Head Neck Surg 126: 1457–1461

Dolan PA (1963) Tumor calcification following therapy. Am J Roentgenol 89:166–174

Dooms GC et al (1985) Characterization of lymphadenopathy by magnetic resonance relaxation times: preliminary results. Radiology 155:691–697

Dorfman RE et al (1991) Upper abdominal lymph nodes: criteria for normal size determined with CT. Radiology180: 319–322

Eisenkraft BL, Som PM (1999) The spectrum of benign and malignant etiologies of cervical node calcification. Am J Roentgenol 172:1433–1437

Flamen P et al (2000) Utility of positron emission tomography for the staging of patients with potentially operable esophageal carcinoma. J Clin Oncol 18:3202–3210

Fuchs T et al (2000) Technical advances in multi-slice spiral CT. Eur J Radiol 36:69–73

Fujimoto Y et al (2000) Magnetic resonance lymphography of profundus lymph nodes with liposomal gadolinium diethylenetriamine pentaacetic acid. Biol Pharm Bull 23: 97–100

Fullbright et al (1994) MR of the head and neck: comparison of fast spin-echo and conventional spin-echo sequences. Am J Neuroradiol 15:767–773

Ghahremani GG, Straus FH (1971) Calcification of distant lymph node metastases from carcinoma of colon. Radiology 99:65–66

Gillams et al (1996) Magnetization transfer contrast MR in lesions of the head and neck. Am J Neuroradiol 17: 355–360

Giraud P et al (2001) CT and (18)F-deoxyglucose (FDG) image fusion for optimization of conformal radiotherapy of lung cancers. Int J Radiat Oncol Biol Phys 49:1249–1257

Grégoire V et al (2000) Selection and delineation of lymph node target volumes in head and neck conformal radiotherapy. Proposal for standardizing terminology and procedure based on the surgical experience. Radiother Oncol 56:135–150

Grossman RI et al (1994) Magnetization transfer: theory and applications in neuroradiology. Radiographics 14:279–90

Guhlmann A et al (1997) Lymph node staging in non-small cell lung cancer: evaluation by [F]FDG positron emission tomography (PET). Thorax 52:438–441

Gussack GS, Hudgins PA (1991) Imaging modalities in recurrent head and neck tumors. Laryngoscope 101:119–124

Han JK et al (2000) Factors influencing vascular and hepatic enhancement at CT: experimental study on injection protocol using a canine model. J Comput Assist Tomogr 24:400–406

Hanasono MM et al (1999) Uses and limitations of FDG positron emission tomography in patients with head and neck cancer. Laryngoscope 109:880–885

Harika et al (1996) Macromolecular intravenous contrast agent for MR lymphography: characterization and efficacy studies. Radiology 198:365–370

Harris EW et al (1996) Enhanced CT of the neck: improved visualization of lesions with delayed imaging. Am J Roentgenol 167:1057–1058

Held P, Breit A (1994) MRI and CT of tumors of the pharynx: comparison of two imaging procedures including fast and ultrafast MR sequences Eur J Radiol 18:81–89

Hennig J et al (1986) RARE-imaging. A fast imaging method for clinical MR. Magn Reson Med 3:829–833

Hoffman HT et al (2000) Functional magnetic resonance imaging using iron oxide particles in characterizing head and neck adenopathy. Laryngoscope 110:1425–1430

Hounsfield GN (1973) Computerized transverse axial scanning (tomography). Description of system. Br J Radiol 46: 1016–1022

Hustinx R et al (2000) Impact of attenuation correction on the accuracy of FDG-PET in patient with abdominal tumors: a free-response ROC analysis. Eur J Nucl Med 27:1365–1371

Jabour BA et al (1993) Extracranial head and neck: PET imaging with 2-(18)fluoro-2-deoxy-D-glucose and MR imaging correlations. Radiology 186:27–35

Kalender WA et al (1990) Spiral volumetric CT with single-breath-hold technique, continuous transport, and continuous scanner rotation. Radiology 176:181–183

Kalender WA et al (1994) A comparison of conventional and spiral CT: an experimental study on the detection of spherical lesions. J Comput Assist Tomogr 18:167–176

Klingenbeck-Regn K et al (1999) Subsecond multi-slice computed tomography: basics and applications. Eur J Radiol 31:110–124

Kubota R et al (1992) Intratumoral distribution of fluorine-18-fluorodeoxyglucose in vivo: high accumulation in macrophages and granulation tissues studied by microautoradiography. J Nucl Med 33:1972–1980

Laissey JP et al (1994) Enlarged mediastinal lymph nodes in bronchogenic carcinoma: assessment with dynamic contrast-enhanced MR imaging. Radiology 191:263–267

Landoni C et al (1999) Comparison of dual-head coincidence PET versus ring PET in tumor patients. J Nucl Med 40: 1617–1622

Langen K et al (1993) The influence of plasma glucose levels on fluorine-18-fluorodeoxyglucose uptake in bronchial carcinomas. J Nucl Med 34:355–359

Laubenbacher C et al (1995) Comparison of fluorine-18-fluorodeoxyglucose PET, MRI and endoscopy for staging head and neck squamous-cell carcinomas. J Nucl Med 36: 1747–1757

Lebihan D, Turner R (1991) Intravoxel incoherent motion imaging using spin echoes. Magn Reson Med 19:211–227

Lerut T et al (2000) Hitopathologic validation of lymph node staging with FDG-PET scan in cancer of the esophagus and gastroesophageal junction. A prospective study based on primary surgery with extensive lymphadenectomy. Ann Surg 232:743–752

Leung AN (1997) Spiral CT of the thorax in daily practice: optimization of the technique. J Thoracic Imag 12:2–10

Lonneux M et al (1998) Can dual-headed 18F-FDG SPECT imaging reliably supersede PET in clinical oncology? A comparative study in lung and gastrointestinal tract cancer. Nucl Med Commun 19:1047–1054

Lonneux M et al (1999) Attenuation correction in whole body FDG oncological studies: the role of statistical reconstruction. Eur J Nucl Med 6:591–598

Magnusson M et al (1991) Evaluation of methods for shaded surface display of CT volumes. Comput Med Imaging Graphics 15:247–256

Mancuso AA et al (1983) Computed tomography of cervical and retropharyngeal lymph nodes: normal anatomy, variants of normal, and application in staging head and neck cancer. Radiology 148:715–723

Martin W et al (1995) FDG-SPECT: correlation with FDG-PET. J Nucl Med 36:988–995

McLoud TC et al (1992) Bronchogenic carcinoma: analysis of staging in the mediastinum with CT by correlative lymph node mapping and sampling. Radiology 182:319–323

Mellanen P et al (1994) Expression of glucose transporters in head and neck tumors. Int J Cancer 56:622–629

Misselwitz B et al (1999) Gadoflurorine 8: initial experience with a new contrast medium for interstitial MR lymphography. MAGMA 8:190–195

Mitchell DG (1999) MRI principles. Saunders, Philadelphia

Moog F et al (1997) Lymphoma: role of whole-body 2-deoxy-2-[F-18]fluoro-D-glucose (FDG) PET in nodal staging. Radiology 203:795–800

Moog F et al (1998a) 18-F-fluorodeoxyglucose-positron emission tomography as a new approach to detect lymphomatous bone marrow. J Clin Oncol 16:603–609

Moog F et al (1998b) Extranodal malignant lymphoma: detection with FDG PET versus CT. Radiology 206:475–481

Moritz JD, Ludwig A, Oestmann JW (2000) Contrast-enhanced color Doppler sonography of enlarged cervical lymph nodes in head and neck tumors. Am J Roentgenol 174: 1279–1284

Mukherji SK et al (2000) The ability of dual camera coincidence tomography 18F fluorodeoxyglucose imaging to differentiate recurrent head and neck SCC from post-treatment changes. The Radiological Society of North America, 88th annual scientific assembly, Chicago, paper 473

Myers L et al (1998) Positron emission tomography in the evaluation of the N0 neck. Laryngoscope 108:232–236

Naidich DP et al (1999) Computed tomography and magnetic resonance of the thorax. Lippincott-Raven, Philadelphia

Nehmeh SA, Ford E, Rosenzweig K et al (2001) Gated positron emission tomography: a technique for reducing lung tumor motion effect. J Nucl Med 42:34P

Nestle U et al (1999) 18F-deoxyglucose positrom emission tomogrpahy (FDG-PET) for the planning of radiotherapy in lung cancer: high impact in patients with atelectasis. Int J Radiat Oncol Biol Phys 44:593–597

Patz E et al (1995) Thoracic nodal staging with PET imaging with 18FDG in patients with bronchogenic carcinoma. Chest 108:1617–1621

Paulus P et al (1998) 18FDG-PET for the assessment of primary head and neck tumors: clinical, computed tomography and histopathological correlation in 38 patients. Laryngoscope 108:1578–1583

Petrella J, Provenzale J (2000) MR perfusion of the brain: techniques and applications. Am J Roentgenol 175:207–19

Petterson H (1995) The NICER centennial book. A global textbook of radiology. Nicer Institute, Oslo

Reske S et al (1997) Overexpression of glucose transporter and increased FDG uptake in pancreatic carcinoma. J Nucl Med 38:1344–1348

Rinck PA (1993) Magnetic resonance in medicine – the basic textbook of the European MR forum, 3rd edn. Blackwell Scientific, London

Rubbin GD et al (1998) Thoracic spiral CT: influence of subsecond gantry rotation on image quality. Radiology 208: 771–776

Rouvière H (1948) Anatomie humaine descriptive et topographique, 6th edn. Masson, Paris

Rydberg J et al (2000) Multisection CT: scanning techniques and clinical applications. Radiographics 20:1787–1806

Sakai O et al (1997) Asymmetrical or heterogenous enhancement of the internal jugular veins in contrast-enhanced CT of the head and neck. Neuroradiology 39:292–295

Sakai O et al (2000) Lymph node pathology. Benign proliferative lymphoma, and metastatic disease. Radiol Clin North Am 5:979–998

Sazaki M et al (1996) The usefulness of FDG positron emission tomography for the detection of mediastinal lymph node metastases in patients with non-small cell lung cancer: a comparative study with X-ray computed tomography. Eur J Nucl Med 23:741–747

Sazon D et al (1996) Fluorodeoxyglucose positron emission tomography in the detection and staging of lung cancer. Am J Respir Crit Care Med 153:417–421

Scott W et al (1996) Mediastinal lymph node staging of non-small cell lung cancer: a prospective comparison of computed tomography and positron emission tomography. J Thorac Cardiovasc Surg 111:642–648

Shah N et al (2000) The impact of FDG positron emission tomography imaging on the management of lymphomas. Br J Radiol 73:482–487

Sheppard LM, Yousem DM (1994) MTI of cervical adenopathies. ASNR, paper 130

Shreve P et al (1998) Oncologic diagnosis with 2-[fluorine-18]fluoro-2-deoxy-D-glucose imaging: dual-head coincidence gamma camera versus positron emission tomographic scanner. Radiology 207:431–437

Som PM (1987) Lymph nodes of the neck. Radiology 165: 593–600

Som PM (1992) Detection of metastasis in cervical lymph nodes: CT and MR criteria and differential diagnosis. Am J Roentgenol 158:961–969

Som PM et al (1999) An imaging-based classification for the

cervical nodes designed as an adjunct to recent clinically based nodal classifications. Arch Otolaryngol Head Neck Surg 125:388–396
Staatz G et al (2001) Interstitial T1-weighted MR lymphography: lipophilic perfluorinated gadolinium chelates in pigs. Radiology 220:129–136
Steinert H et al (1997) Non-small cell lung cancer: nodal staging with FDG PET versus CT with correlative lymph node mapping and sampling. Radiology 202:441–446
Stokkel M et al (2000) Preoperative evaluation of patients with primary head and neck cancer using dual-head 18-fluorodeoxyglucose positron emission tomography. Ann Surg 231:229–234
Sugawara Y et al (1999) Evaluation of FDG PET in patients with cervical cancer. J Nucl Med 40:1125–1131
Tatsumi M et al (1999) Feasibility of fluorodeoxyglucose dual-head gamma camera coinidence imaging in the evaluation of lung cancer: comparison with FDG PET. J Nucl Med 40: 566–573
Torizuka T et al (1998) Effect of insulin on uptake of FDG by experimental mammary carcinoma in diabetic rats. Radiology 208:499–504
Towers JM (1993) Spiral or helical CT? Am J Roentgenol 161(4):901–902
Valk P et al (1995) Staging non-small cell lung cancer by whole-body positron emision tomographic imaging. Ann Thorac Surg 60:1573–1582
Van den Brekel MWM, Castelijns JA (1999) New developments in imaging of neck node metastases. In: Mukherji SK, Castelijns JA (eds) Modern head and neck imaging. Springer, Berlin Heidelberg New York
Van den Brekel MWM, Castelijns JA (2000) Imaging of lymph nodes in the neck. Semin Roentgenol 1:42–53
Van den Brekel MWM et al (1990a) Cervical lymph node metastasis: assessment of radiologic criteria. Radiology 177:379–384
Van den Brekel MWM et al (1990b) Detection and characterization of of metastatic cervical adenopathies by MR imaging: comparison of different MR techniques. J Comput Assist Tomogr 14:581–589
Vansteenkiste JF, Mortelmans L (1999) FDG-PET in the locoregional lymph node staging of non-small cell lung cancer: a comprehensive review of the Leuven lung cancer group experience. Clin Pos Imaging 2:223–231
Vansteenkiste JF et al (1998a) Lymph node staging in non-small cell lung cancer with FDG-PET scan: a prospective study on 690 lymph node stations from 68 patients. J Clin Oncol 16:2142–2149
Vansteenkiste JF et al (1998b) FDG-PET scan in potentially operable non-small cell lung cancer: do anatomometabolic PET-CT fusion images improve the localisation of regional lymph node metastases? Eur J Nucl Med 25: 1495–1501
Vanuystel L, Vansteenkiste JF, Stroobants S et al (2000) The impact of (18)F-fluoro-2-deoxy-D-glucose positron emission tomography (FDG-PET) lymph node staging on the radiation treatment volumes in patients with non-small cell lung cancer. Radiother Oncol 55:317–324
Vuillez JP (1998) Métabolisme glucidique des cellules tumorales: conséquences pour l'utilisation de radiopharmaceutiques analogues du glucose. Med Nucl Imag Fonct Metab 22:9–29
Wahl RL et al (1994) Staging of mediastinal non-small cell lung cancer FDG PET, CT, and fusion images: preliminary prospective evaluation. Radiology 191:371–377
Wang G, Vannier MW (1994) Longitudinal resolution in volumetric X-ray CT-analytical comparison between conventional and helical CT. Med Phys 21:429–433
Wang G, Vannier MW (1997) Optimal pitch in spiral computed tomography. Med Phys 24:1635–1639
Wang G et al (1994) Theoretical FWTM values in helical CT. Med Phys 21:753–754
Warburg O (1930) The metabolism of tumors. Arnold Constable, London, pp 75–327
Weber G, Cantero A (1955) Glucose-6-phosphatase activity in normal, precancerous, and neoplastic tissues. Cancer Res 15:105–108
Weber W et al (1999) Assessment of pulmonary lesions with 18F-fluorodeoxyglucose positron imaging using coincidence mode gamma cameras. J Nucl Med 40:574–578
Wiener JI et al (1986) Breast and axillary tissue MR imaging: correlation of the signal intensities and relaxation times with pathological findings. Radiology 160:299–305
Younes M et al (1995) GLUT1 expression in human breast carcinoma: correlation with known prognostic markers. Anticancer Res 15:2895–2898
Yousem DM (1999) Magnetization transfer imaging of the extracranial head and neck. In: Mukherji SK, Castelijns JA (eds) Modern head and neck imaging. Springer, Berlin Heidelberg New York
Yousem DM, Hurst RW (1994) MR of cervical lymph nodes: comparison of fast spin echo and conventional T2 W scans. Clin Radiol 49:670–675
Yousem DM et al (1992) Central nodal necrosis and extracapsular neoplastic spread in cervical lymph nodes: MR imaging versus CT. Radiology 182:753–759

3 Selection and Delineation of Lymph Node Target Volumes in Head and Neck Conformal and Intensity-Modulated Radiation Therapy

V. Grégoire, E. Coche, G. Cosnard, M. Hamoir, H. Reychler

CONTENTS

V. Grégoire, MD, PhD
Associate Professor, Radiation Oncology Department, Université Catholique de Louvain, St-Luc University Hospital, 10 Ave Hippocrate, 1200 Brussels, Belgium
E. Coche, MD
Assistant Professor, Radiology Department, Université Catholique de Louvain, St-Luc University Hospital, 10 Ave Hippocrate, 1200 Brussels, Belgium
G. Cosnard, MD
Professor, Radiology Department, Université Catholique de Louvain, St-Luc University Hospital, 10 Ave Hippocrate, 1200 Brussels, Belgium
M. Hamoir, MD
Professor, ENT and Head and Neck Surgery Department, Université Catholique de Louvain, St-Luc University Hospital, 10 Ave Hippocrate, 1200 Brussels, Belgium
H. Reychler, MD, DMD
Professor, Oral and Maxillo-Facial Surgery Department, Université Catholique de Louvain, St-Luc University Hospital, 10 Ave Hippocrate, 1200 Brussels, Belgium

3.1 Introduction

The use of conformal and intensity-modulated radiation therapy to deliver the dose more precisely to the target volumes while protecting the normal tissues at risk obviously requires a proper knowledge of the volumes to be irradiated and an accurate delineation of these volumes on a 3D basis. These requirements have always existed, but were greatly simplified in 2D planning in the sense that one dimension was evidently missing or greatly minimized. For instance, in head and neck tumors irradiated, as still suggested in all major textbooks, by two opposed lateral fields, there was no need to define the tumor or lymph node extension in the medio-lateral direction. In some ways, conformal and intensity-modulated radiation therapy requires the radiation oncologist to approach this issue in the spirit of a surgeon planning and performing an operation. The surgical field is replaced by a computed tomography (CT) scan or a magnetic resonance (MR) image and the scalpel by a mouse or an electronic pencil. Without any doubt, this represents a new challenge for the radiation oncology community. Such a procedure requires a precise knowledge of CT- or MRI-based anatomy, as well as microscopic extension of the tumors and/or nodes in the fatty tissues, along the aponeurotic fascia and muscles, or around the blood vessels and nerves.

In this framework, this chapter proposes guidelines for the selection and delineation of target volumes in the neck of patients with head and neck squamous cell carcinomas (SCC). Such guidelines are based on the standardized neck dissection terminology adopted by head and neck surgeons. First, the terminology used for the lymph node levels and for node dissection is presented. Then information on metastatic nodal extension of major tumor sites is reviewed, from which guidelines for target volume extension are proposed. Last, following the surgical terminology, tentative rules are proposed for the delineation of the neck node levels based on modern imaging modalities. Such guidelines and rules could contribute to reducing the differences in treatment planning from patient to patient, and to making comparisons between clinical series, or the conducting of multicenter trials, much more accurate.

3.2 Classification of Neck Node Levels and Dissection Terminology

3.2.1 Anatomical Description and Nomenclature of the Neck Nodes

The head and neck region has a rich network of lymphatic vessels draining from the base of the skull through the jugular nodes, the spinal accessory nodes and the transverse cervical nodes to the venous jugulo-subclavian confluent or the thoracic duct on the left side and the lymphatic duct on the right side (Rouvière 1948; Vidic and Suarez-Quian 1998). A comprehensive anatomical description of this network was made by Rouvière more than 50 years ago (Rouvière 1948). The whole lymphatic system of the neck is contained in the cellulo-adipose tissue delineated by aponeurosis enveloping the muscles, the vessels and the nerves. The lymphatic drainage is mainly ipsilateral, but structures like the soft palate, the tonsils, the base of the tongue, the posterior pharyngeal wall and especially the nasopharynx have bilateral drainage. On the other hand, sites such as the true vocal cord, the paranasal sinuses and the middle ear have few or no lymphatic vessels at all.

The nomenclature of head and neck lymph nodes has been complicated by various confusing synonyms that are still in use in major textbooks and articles. More recently, several expert bodies have proposed the adoption of systematic classifications aimed at standardizing the terminology. Following the description by Rouvière, the TNM atlas proposed a terminology, dividing the head and neck lymph nodes into 12 groups (Spiessl et al. 1992). In parallel to this classification, the Committee for Head and Neck Surgery and Oncology of the American Academy for Otolaryngology-Head and Neck Surgery has been working on a classification (the so-called Robbins classification), dividing the neck into 6 levels including 8 node groups (Robbins et al. 1991). This classification is based on the description of a level system which has been used for a long time by the Head and Neck Service at the Memorial Sloan-Kettering Cancer Center (Shah et al. 1981). As one of the objectives of the Robbins classification was to develop a standardized system of terminology for neck dissection procedures, only the lymph node groups routinely removed during neck dissection were considered. For example, retropharyngeal and parotid nodes which are not removed during standard neck dissection are not included in Robbins's classification. The terminology proposed by Robbins was also accepted by representatives of the major European cancer centers (Milan, Villejuif, Amsterdam) and was recommended by the UICC (Hermanek et al. 1993). A comparison between the TNM and the Robbins terminology is shown in Table 3.1. The major advantage of the Robbins classification over the TNM terminology is the definition of the boundaries of the node levels. The delineation of these boundaries is based on anatomical structures such as major blood vessels, muscles, nerves, bones and cartilage that are easily identifiable by the surgeon during neck dissection procedures (Fig. 3.1). The orientation of these anatomical boundaries refers to a patient lying in a supine position with his neck in a surgical position, i.e. in hyperextension to better individualize the anatomical structures.

Level Ia is a unique median region which contains the submental nodes. The lymph nodes are located in a triangular region limited anteriorly by the platysma muscle, posteriorly by the mylohyoid muscles, cranially by the symphysis of the mandible, caudally by the hyoid bone, and laterally by the anterior belly of the digastric muscle. The medial limit of level Ia is virtual, as the region continues into the contralateral level Ia. Nodes in level Ia drain the skin of the chin, the mid-lower lip, the tip of the tongue, and the anterior floor of the mouth. Level Ia is at greatest risk for harboring metastases from cancer arising from the floor of the mouth, the anterior oral tongue, the anterior mandibular alveolar ridge, and the lower lip.

Level Ib contains the submandibular nodes. It is located within the boundaries of the anterior and posterior belly of the digastric muscle, the stylohyoid muscle and the body of the mandible. It is limited anteriorly by the stylohyoid muscle, posteriorly by a vertical plane defined by the spinal accessory nerve (SAN), medially (deeply) by the anterior belly of the digastric muscle, and laterally (superficially) by the

Table 3.1. Comparison between the TNM atlas terminology and the ROBBIN classification of the lymph nodes of the neck

TNM atlas for lymph nodes of the neck		ROBBINS classification	
Group No.	Terminology	Level	Terminology
1	Submental nodes	Ia	Submental group
2	Submandibular nodes	Ib	Submandibular group
3	Cranial jugular nodes	II	Upper jugular group
4	Medial jugular nodes	III	Middle jugular group
5	Caudal jugular nodes	IV	Lower jugular group
6	Dorsal cervical nodes along Spinal accessory nerve	V	Posterior triangle group
7	Supraclavicular nodes	V	Posterior triangle group
8	Prelaryngeal and paratracheal nodes	VI	Anterior compartment group
9	Retropharyngeal nodes	-	-
10	Parotid nodes	-	-
11	Buccal nodes	-	-
12	Retroauricular and occipital nodes	-	-

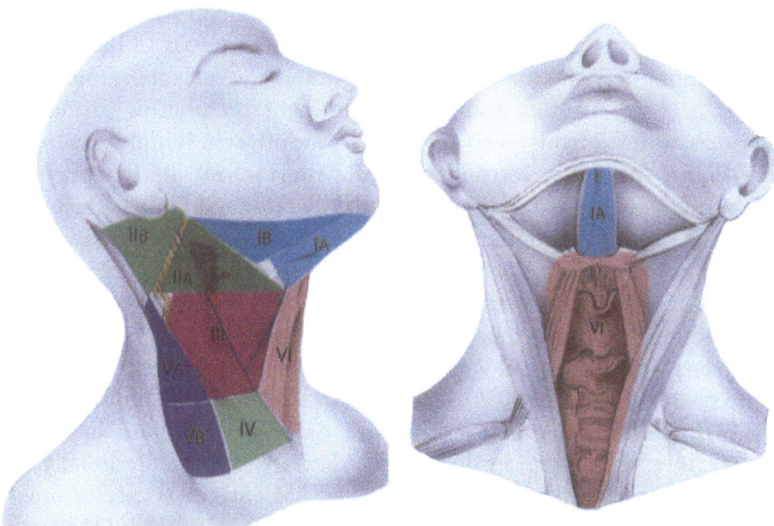

Fig. 3.1. Schematic representation of the various neck node groups: submental (*Ia*) and submandibular (*Ib*); upper jugular (*II*); middle jugular (*III*); lower jugular (*IV*); posterior triangle (*V*); anterior compartment (*VI*)

basilar border of the mandible. Cranially it is limited by the basilar border of the mandible, and caudally by the posterior belly of the digastric muscle. The submandibular nodes receive efferent lymphatics from the submental lymph nodes, the medial canthus, the lower nasal cavity, the hard and soft palate, the maxillary and mandibular alveolar ridges, the cheek, the upper and lower lips, and most of the anterior tongue. Nodes in level Ib are at risk for developing metastases from cancers of the oral cavity, anterior nasal cavity, soft tissue structures of the mid-face and the submandibular gland.

Level II contains the upper jugular lymph nodes located around the upper one-third of the internal jugular vein (IJV) and the upper SAN. It extends from the base of the skull to the carotid bifurcation (surgical landmark) or the caudal border of the body of the hyoid bone (clinical landmark). Previous classifications have used the boundary of the submandibular triangle to separate level Ib from level II, but this separation is not accurate since the posterior belly of the digastric muscle extends across the IJV into level II. Thus Robbins has recently recommended that the stylohyoid muscle be used as a more accurate landmark for separating level Ib from level II (ROBBINS 1999). Level II is limited cranially by the insertion of the posterior belly of the digastric muscle to the mastoid, caudally by the caudal border of the body of the hyoid bone, anteriorly by the stylohyoid muscle, posteriorly by the posterior edge of the sternocleidomastoid (SCM) muscle, medially by the carotid artery and the para-vertebral muscles (levator scapulae and splenius capitis) and laterally by the SCM and the platysma. Level II is further subdivided into two compartments. The lymph nodes located anteriorly to a vertical plane defined by the upper one-third of the SAN are included in level IIa, whereas the lymph nodes located posteriorly to the SAN are included in level IIb. Level II receives efferent lymphatics from the face, the parotid gland, and the submandibular, submental and retropharyngeal nodes. Level II also directly receives the collecting lymphatics from the nasal cavity, the pharynx, the larynx, the external auditory canal, the middle ear, and the sublingual and submandibular glands. The nodes in level II are therefore at greatest risk for harboring metastases from cancers of the nasal cavity, oral cavity, nasopharynx, oropharynx, hypopharynx, larynx, and the major salivary glands. Level IIb is more likely associated with primary tumors of the oropharynx or nasopharynx, and less frequently with tumors of the oral cavity, larynx or hypopharynx.

Level III contains the middle jugular lymph nodes located around the middle third of the IJV. It is the caudal extension of level II. It is limited cranially by the caudal border of the body of the hyoid bone, and caudally by a plane where the omohyoid muscle crosses the IJV (surgical landmark) or by the caudal border of the cricoid cartilage (clinical landmark). The anterior limit is the lateral edge of the sternohyoid muscle, and the posterior limit is the posterior border of the SCM muscle. Laterally, level III is limited by the SCM muscle and medially by the internal carotid artery and the paraspinal muscles. Byers proposed a subdivision of level III into levels IIIa and IIIb (Byers et al. 1997). Level IIIb is far posterior to the IJV. In the case of involvement of level IIIb, there is a higher probability of metastases occurring in level V. Level III contains a highly variable number of lymph nodes and receives efferent lymphatics from levels II and V, and some efferent lymphatics from the retropharyngeal, pretracheal and recurrent laryngeal nodes. It collects the lymphatics from the base of the tongue, tonsils, larynx, hypopharynx and thyroid gland. Nodes in level III are at greatest risk for harboring metastases from cancers of the oral cavity, nasopharynx, oropharynx, hypopharynx and larynx.

Level IV includes the lower jugular lymph nodes located around the inferior third of the IJV from the caudal limit of level III to the clavicle caudally. The anterior and posterior limits are the same as for level III, i.e. the lateral border of the sternohyoid muscle and the posterior edge of the SCM muscle, respectively. Laterally, level IV is limited by the SCM muscle and medially by the internal carotid artery and the paraspinal muscles. As previously proposed by Suen and Goepfert (1987), the American Academy of Otolaryngology-Head and Neck Surgery subdivided level IV into two subgroups to distinguish the anterior jugular (level IVa) from the lateral jugular chain (level IVb). Level IVa includes the nodes located deep in the sternal head of the SCM muscle, whereas level IVb includes those located deep in the clavicular head of the SCM muscle (Robbins 1998). Although involvement of the anterior jugular chain is not generally considered separately from the lateral jugular chain, this subdivision is based on the understanding that in the case of invasion of the latter, there is a higher probability of lymph node metastases in the posterior triangle group. The real clinical implication of such a subdivision, however, needs to be further elucidated. Level IV contains a variable number of nodes and receives efferent lymphatics primarily from levels III and V, some efferent lymphatics from the retropharyngeal, pretracheal and recurrent laryngeal nodes, and collecting lymphatics from the hypopharynx, larynx and thyroid gland (Rouvière 1948). Level IV nodes are at high risk for harboring metastases from cancers of the hypopharynx, larynx and cervical esophagus.

Level V includes the lymph nodes of the posterior triangle group. This group includes the lymph nodes located along the lower part of the SAN and the transverse cervical vessels. Level V is limited cranially by the convergence of the SCM and the trapezius muscles, caudally by the clavicle, anteriorly by the posterior border of the SCM muscle, and posteriorly by the anterior border of the trapezius muscle. Laterally, level V is limited by the platysma muscle and the skin, and medially by the splenius capitis, levator scapulae and scaleni (posterior, medial and anterior) muscles. Level V is currently subdivided into levels Va and Vb. The distinction between the upper posterior triangle (level Va) and the lower posterior triangle (level Vb) allows lymph node involvement of the lower two-thirds of the SAN chain to be differentiated from that of the transverse cervical vessel chain (Robbins 1998, 1999). A horizontal plane defined by the caudal edge of the cricoid cartilage separates these two compartments. During neck dissection, the tendon and posterior belly of the omohyoid muscle serve as landmarks to separate level Va from level Vb.

It should be pointed out that the demarcation between the posterior end of level IIb and the uppermost part of level Va has still not been clearly defined. The American Academy for Otolaryngology-Head and Neck Surgery defined the posterior boundary of level IIb as the posterior border of the SCM muscle, and the apex of the convergence of the SCM and the trapezius muscles as the cranial boundary of level Va. However, the uppermost part of level Va is devoid of any constant lymph node group. In some circumstances, a few lymph nodes lying along the upper third of the SAN may be found, but these nodes are actually included in level IIb (Robbins 1999). The uppermost part of level Va contains superficial occipital lymph node(s) and inconsistently one subfascial lymph node close to the occipital attachment of the SCM muscle (Rouvière 1948). These lymph nodes collect lymphatics from the occipital scalp, and the post-auricular and nuchal regions. They are not involved in the drainage of head and neck cancers except for skin tumors. Consequently, the cranial limit of level Va that is commonly accepted and depicted should be questioned. It appears that defining the lower two-thirds of the SAN as the cranial limit of level Va is more consistent with anatomical reality. This issue should be addressed not only by head and neck surgeons, but also by radiation oncologists in the delineation of lymph node target volumes in head and neck conformal radiotherapy (Grégoire et al. 2000).

Level V receives efferent lymphatics from the occipital and post-auricular nodes as well as those from the occipital and parietal scalp, the skin of the lateral and posterior neck and shoulder, the nasopharynx and the oropharynx (tonsils and base of the tongue). Level V lymph nodes are at high risk for harboring metastases from cancers of the nasopharynx and oropharynx. Nodes in level Va are more often associated with primary cancers of the nasopharynx, oropharynx or the cutaneous structures of the posterior scalp, whereas those in level Vb are more commonly associated with tumors arising in the thyroid gland.

Level VI, also called the anterior compartment group, contains the lymph nodes located in the visceral space: the pre- and paratracheal nodes, the precricoid (Delphian) node and the perithyroid nodes including the lymph nodes along the recurrent laryngeal nerves. It is limited cranially by the hyoid bone, caudally by the suprasternal notch and laterally by the medial border of both carotid sheaths. Level VI receives efferent lymphatics from the thyroid gland, the glottic and subglottic larynx, the hypopharynx and the cervical esophagus. These nodes are at high risk for harboring metastases from cancers of the thyroid gland, the glottic and subglottic larynx, the apex of the piriform sinus and the cervical esophagus.

3.2.2
Neck Node Dissection Procedures

Based on the definition of the neck level, the Committee for Head and Neck Surgery and Oncology of the American Academy for Otolaryngology-Head and Neck Surgery made several recommendations concerning neck dissection terminology. The main objectives of such recommendations were to develop a standardized terminology limited to the use of a few defined procedures in which the lymphatic and non-lymphatic structures removed are unambiguously described. Such recommendations had to correlate with the biology of neck metastases, comply with oncologic principles and meet oncologic standards.

The surgical goal of each type of neck dissection is to remove the lymphatic structures (nodes and vessels) disseminated and non- or poorly individualized in the fatty tissue of the neck with, when oncologically sound, preservation of the non-lymphatic structures, e.g. vessels, nerves, muscles and glands.

The standard procedure is *radical neck dissection* (RND) where levels I–V are removed together with the IJV, the SCM muscle and the SAN. Each procedure which preserves at least one of the non-lymphatic structures (i.e. the IJV, the SCM or the SAN) is called *modified radical neck dissection* (MRND). (Medina and Byers (1989) sub-classified MRND into three types: type I spares the SAN only; type II spares the SAN and the IJV; and type III preserves the SAN, the IJV and the SCM. Type III, as first described by Suarez and popularized by Bocca (Bocca and Pignataro 1967; Bocca et al. 1980; Suarez 1963), is also called by European authors "functional neck dissection". However in their classic description, the submandibular gland was not excised.

A procedure which does not remove all the cervical node levels is called *selective neck dissection* (SND). There are four subtypes of SND: (a) supraomohyoid neck dissection (levels I–III); (b) posterolateral neck dissection (levels II–V); (c) lateral neck dissection (levels II–IV); and (d) anterior compartment neck dissection (level VI).

When additional lymphatic nodes (e.g. the retropharyngeal, upper mediastinal or paratracheal nodes) or non-lymphatic structures (e.g. the parotid gland, the skin, the carotid artery, the hypoglossal nerve) have to be removed, the procedure is called *extended radical neck dissection* (ERND).

3.3 Metastatic Nodal Extension of Squamous Cell Carcinomas of the Oral Cavity, Pharynx or Larynx

3.3.1 Distribution of Clinically Involved Lymph Nodes in the Neck

3.3.1.1 Cervical Lymph Nodes

The metastatic spread of head and neck tumors into the cervical lymph nodes is rather consistent and follows predictable pathways, at least in the neck which has not been violated by previous surgery or radiotherapy. Bataini and Lindberg reviewed the clinical pattern of metastatic neck involvement in patients with head and neck SCC of the larynx, hypopharynx, oropharynx and oral cavity treated between 1948 and 1978 at their respective institutions (Bataini et al. 1985; Lindberg 1972). These data are summarized in Table 3.2. For nasopharyngeal tumors, data from a more recent study have been pooled with those reported by Lindberg (Sham et al. 1990). In their original papers, these authors did not use the Robbins' classification for the neck node levels. Their terminology has been translated into the node levels as shown in Table 3.1. In Table 3.2, the frequency of metastatic lymph nodes is expressed as a percentage of node-positive patients. For example, it can be seen that in patients with oropharyngeal tumors, 64% had clinical lymph node metastases. Among these patients, 13% had nodes in ipsilateral level I, 81% in ipsilateral level II, and so on.

The frequency of neck node metastases as well as the distribution of clinically involved nodes depend to a major extent on the primary tumor site. Typically, nasopharyngeal and hypopharyngeal tumors have the highest propensity for nodal involvement, which occurs in 80% and 70% of cases, respectively. Cranial and anterior tumors (e.g. oral cavity tumors) mainly drain into levels I, II and III, whereas more caudally located tumors (i.e. laryngeal tumors) mainly drain into levels II and III, and to a lesser extent into levels IV and V. Contralateral nodes are very rarely invaded except for midline tumors, or tumors in those sites where bilateral lymphatic drainage has been reported, e.g. the soft palate, base of the tongue and pharyngeal wall. Even in these tumors, the incidence of contralateral involvement is much lower, reaching for example in base of the tongue tumors with clinically positive nodes 31% in contralateral level II compared to 73% in ipsilateral level II (data not shown). Interestingly, node distribution follows the same pattern in the contralateral neck as in the ipsilateral neck. Except for nasopharyngeal tumors, involvement of ipsilateral level V is a rather rare event, occurring in less than 1% of all oral cavity tumors, in less than 10% of all oropharyngeal and laryngeal tumors and in about 15% of all hypopharyngeal tumors. It almost never occurs in contralateral level V. Nasopharyngeal tumors behave differently to other head and neck tumors. These highly lymphophilic tumors carry almost the same risk of nodal involvement in the ipsilateral and contralateral neck, with the preferential involvement of level V in almost one-third of patients.

Metastatic lymph node involvement in the neck depends on the size of the primary tumor, increasing with the T-stage. In the series reported by Bataini, 44% of patients with a T1 tumor had clinical lymph node involvement; this increased to 70% for patients with T4 lesions (Bataini et al. 1985). There are, however, no data suggesting that the relative distribution of involved neck levels varies with the T-stage.

Table 3.2. Distribution of clinical metastatic neck nodes from head and neck SCC

Tumor site	Patients with N+ (%)	Distribution of metastatic lymph nodes per level (percentage of node-positive patients)					
		I	II	III	IV	V	Other[a]
Oral cavity (n=787)	36	42/3.5[b]	79/8	18/3	5/1	1/0	1.4/0.3
Oropharynx (n=1479)	64	13/2	81/24	23/5	9/2.5	13/3	2/1
Hypopharynx (n=847)	70	2/0	80/13	51/4	20/3	24/2	3/1
Supraglottic larynx (n=428)	55	2/0	71/21	48/10	18/7	15/4	2/0
Nasopharynx (n= 440)	80	9/5	71/56	36/32	22/15	32/26	15/10

[a] Parotid, buccal nodes
[b] Ipsilateral/contralateral nodes
Redrawn from Bataini et al. (1985); Lindberg (1972); Sham et al. (1990)

3.3.1.2
Retropharyngeal Lymph Nodes

Retropharyngeal lymph nodes lie within the retropharyngeal space which extends cranially from the base of the skull to the level of C3 caudally. This space is bounded anteriorly by the pharyngeal constrictor muscles and posteriorly by the prevertebral fascia (ROUVIÈRE 1948). Typically, retropharyngeal nodes are divided into medial and lateral groups. The medial group is an inconsistent group which consist of 1–2 lymph nodes intercalated in or near the midline. The lateral group lies medial to the carotid artery. The most superior lymph node of this group is also called the lymph node of Rouvière.

Retropharyngeal lymph nodes represent a special entity inasmuch as they are usually not clinically detectable. The incidence of retropharyngeal lymph node involvement can thus only be estimated from series in which CT or MRI of the retropharynx has been systematically performed as part of the diagnostic procedure. A summary of the available data on the incidence of retropharyngeal lymph node infiltration is presented in Table 3.3 (CHONG et al. 1995; CHUA et al. 1997; MCLAUGHLIN et al. 1995). In all these studies, lymph nodes were investigated by CT and/or MRI and were considered involved when they reached a size of over 10 mm, or showed central necrosis irrespective of their size. Retropharyngeal node involvement occurs in primary tumors arising from (or invading) the mucosa of the occipital and cervical somites, e.g. of the nasopharynx, the pharyngeal wall and the soft palate. Interestingly, the incidence of retropharyngeal lymph nodes is higher in patients in whom involvement of other neck node levels has also been documented. In N0 patients with nasopharyngeal tumors and to a lesser extent in patients with pharyngeal wall tumors the incidence of retropharyngeal nodes is still significant, i.e. between 16 and 40%. Also, as already described for the other lymph node levels, involvement depends on the T-stage, and is typically lower for T1 tumors. Accurate figures are, however, not available.

3.3.2
Distribution of Pathologically Involved Lymph Nodes in the Neck

In previous studies, the pattern of metastatic node involvement was solely established from clinical palpation of the neck. It is likely that the use of modern imaging techniques has slightly altered the reported figures. Indeed, the systematic use of CT scan, MRI or ultrasound has increased both the sensitivity and the specificity of the detection of macroscopic neck node involvement (SOM et al. 1997; VAN DEN BREKEL et al. 1990, 1998). However, even with the use of these modern imaging modalities, there is no reliable diagnostic tool available to detect microscopic neck involvement in patients with clinically or radiologically negative nodes. In this regard, hope has been placed in ultrasound-guided fine needle aspiration. Recent multicentric evaluation, however, has failed to demonstrate a significant added value of this procedure over CT or MRI (TAKES et al. 1998). In order to establish guidelines for the definition of target volumes in the neck of patients with primary tumors of the head and neck, a true estimate of the pattern of macroscopic as well as microscopic metastatic node

Table 3.3. Incidence of retropharyngeal lymph nodes in head and neck primary tumors

Authors	Primary site	Incidence of retropharyngeal lymph nodes (percentage of total number of patients)		
		Overall	N0 neck[a]	N+ neck[b]
MCLAUGHLIN et al. (1995)	Oropharynx			
	Pharyngeal wall	18/93 (19%)	6/37 (16%)	12/56 (21%)
	Soft palate	7/53 (13%)	1/21 (5%)	6/32 (19%)
	Tonsillar fossa	16/176 (9%	2/56 (4%)	14/120 (12%)
	Base of tongue	5/121 (4%)	0/31 (0%)	5/90 (6%)
	Hypopharynx (piriform sinus or post-cricoid area)	7/136 (5%)	0/55 (0%)	7/81 (9%)
	Supraglottic larynx	4/196 (2%)	0/87 (0%)	4/109 (4%)
	Nasopharynx	14/19 (74%)	2/5 (40%)	12/14 (86%)
CHUA et al. (1997)	Nasopharynx	106/364 (29%)	21/134 (16%)	85/230 (37%)
CHONG et al. (1995)	Nasopharynx	Not stated	Not stated	59/91 (65%)

[a] Clinically negative nodes in levels I–V
[b] Clinically positive nodes in levels I–V

distribution is needed. In particular, information on the incidence of microscopic neck involvement in levels contiguous to those with macroscopic node involvement and an estimate of the frequency of microscopic skip metastases are required.

3.3.2.1
Incidence of Pathological Lymph Node Metastases in Levels I–V

The Head and Neck Department at Memorial Sloan-Kettering Cancer Center has established the pattern of cervical lymph node metastases from 1,081 previously untreated patients who underwent 1,119 RND between 1965 and 1986 for tumors of the oral cavity, oropharynx, hypopharynx and larynx (Candela et al. 1990a, b; Shah 1990; Shah et al. 1990). This group was part of the 2,665 patients who underwent RND during the same period for SCC of the upper aerodigestive tract. The remaining 1,584 patients were excluded from the retrospective analysis because of previous surgery, radiotherapy or chemotherapy. Patients with clinically positive nodes at diagnosis were treated by immediate therapeutic RND. Patients with clinically negative nodes were treated either by prophylactic RND at the time of diagnosis, or by subsequent therapeutic RND at the time a node developed during follow-up. The reason for immediate versus delayed RND in N0 patients was not specified. Presumably, the surgeon must have considered that some of these patients were at higher risk of microscopic involvement (e.g. T3–T4 versus T1–T2 tumors, pharyngeal primary). It is likely that during the same period, other patients were referred to the Memorial Sloan-Kettering Cancer Center with the diagnosis of SCC of the upper aerodigestive tract, but were not proposed RND as part of their treatment. Although this retrospective study is thus possibly biased, it represents so far the only large study in which metastatic node distribution in levels I–V of the neck has been established in patients with primaries of the oral cavity, oropharynx, hypopharynx and larynx.

The results of this retrospective study are shown in Tables 3.4–3.7. The data are presented in terms of the number of neck dissections with positive lymph nodes over the total neck dissection procedures and expressed as a percentage. In the 341 patients with a clinically N0 neck, 343 neck dissections were performed, meaning that bilateral dissection was performed only in two patients (<1%). In the

Table 3.4. Incidence of pathological lymph node metastases in SCC of the oral cavity

Tumor site	Distribution of metastatic lymph nodes per level (percentage of neck dissection procedures) Prophylactic RND[a] (192 patients; 192 procedures)						Therapeutic (immediate or subsequent) RND (308 patients; 323 procedures)					
	No. of RND	I (%)	II (%)	III (%)	IV (%)	V (%)	No. of RND	I (%)	II (%)	III (%)	IV (%)	V (%)
Tongue	58	14	19	16	3	0	129	32	50	40	20	0
Floor of mouth	57	16	12	7	2	0	115	53	34	32	12	7
Gum	52	27	21	6	4	2	52	54	46	19	17	4
Retromolar trigone	16	19	12	6	6	0	10	50	60	40	20	0
Cheek	9	44	11	0	0	0	17	82	41	65	65	0
Total	192	20	17	9	3	1	323	46	44	32	16	3

[a] Radical neck dissection
Redrawn from Shah et al. (1990)

Table 3.5. Incidence of pathological lymph node metastases in SCC of the oropharynx

Tumor site	Distribution of metastatic lymph nodes per level (percentage of neck dissection procedures) Prophylactic RND[a] (47 patients; 48 procedures)						Therapeutic (immediate or subsequent) RND (157 patients; 165 procedures)					
	No. of RND	I (%)	II (%)	III (%)	IV (%)	V (%)	No. of RND	I (%)	II (%)	III (%)	IV (%)	V (%)
Base of tongue + vallecula	21	0	19	14	9	5	58	10	72	41	21	9
Tonsillar fossa	27	4	30	22	7	0	107	17	70	42	31	9
Total	48	2	25	19	8	2	165	15	71	42	27	9

[a] Radical neck dissection
Redrawn from Candela et al. (1990a)

Table 3.6. Incidence of pathological lymph node metastases in SCC of the hypopharynx

Tumor site	Distribution of metastatic lymph nodes per level (percentage of neck dissection procedures) Prophylactic RND[a] (24 patients; 24 procedures)						Therapeutic (immediate or subsequent) RND (102 patients; 104 procedures)					
	No. of RND	I (%)	II (%)	III (%)	IV (%)	V (%)	No. of RND	I (%)	II (%)	III (%)	IV (%)	V (%)
Piriform sinus	13	0	15	8	0	0	79	6	72	72	47	8
Pharyngeal wall	11	0	9	18	0	0	25	20	84	72	40	20
Total	24	0	12	12	0	0	104	10	75	72	45	11

[a] Radical neck dissection
Redrawn from Candela et al. (1990a)

Table 3.7. Incidence of pathological lymph node metastases in SCC of the larynx

Tumor site	Distribution of metastatic lymph nodes per level (percentage of neck dissection procedures) Prophylactic RND[a] (78 patients; 79 procedures)						Therapeutic (immediate or subsequent) RND (169 patients; 183 procedures)					
	No. of RND	I (%)	II (%)	III (%)	IV (%)	V (%)	No. of RND	I (%)	II (%)	III (%)	IV (%)	V (%)
Supraglottic larynx	65	6	18	18	9	2	138	6	62	55	32	5
Glottic larynx	14	0	21	29	7	7	45	9	42	71	24	2
Total	79	5	19	20	9	3	183	7	57	59	30	4

[a] Radical neck dissection
Redrawn from Candela et al. (1990b)

736 patients with clinically positive nodes, bilateral neck dissection was performed in 39 patients (5%) with either bilateral nodes at palpation or midline tumors. In both groups, the pathological evaluations of neck dissections were pooled, so that a distinction between the ipsilateral and contralateral neck could not be made.

Overall, metastatic disease was confirmed in 33% of the prophylactic neck dissections and in 82% of the therapeutic neck dissections. In this series, the overall sensitivity and specificity of the clinical examination thus reached 85% and 62%, respectively. As already observed with the pattern of clinical metastatic lymph nodes, the distribution of pathologically confirmed metastatic lymph nodes depended on the primary tumor site. Typically, in clinically N0 patients, metastatic lymph nodes were observed in levels I–III for oral cavity tumors, and in levels II–IV for oropharyngeal, hypopharyngeal and laryngeal tumors. This pattern of node distribution is similar to that determined from the clinical palpation of the neck. It should be noted that the T-stage distribution was different in the various groups. Patients with laryngeal tumors had 54% (42/79) of T3–T4 tumors (mainly supra-glottic) compared to 27% (52/192), 25% (6/24), and 17% (8/47) in patients with oral cavity, hypopharyngeal and oropharyngeal tumors, respectively. Such a difference in T-stage presumably explains the high incidence of node metastases in the larynx group.

When considering the patients who underwent therapeutic neck dissection, the pattern of metastatic node distribution was similar to that observed in N0 patients, with the difference that significant pathological infiltration of an extra level was typically observed, i.e. level IV for oral cavity tumors and levels I and V for oropharyngeal, hypopharyngeal, and to a lesser extent laryngeal tumors. Overall, this observation illustrates the gradual infiltration of node levels in the neck. This concept is well illustrated by the prevalence of metastases in level V. In the Memorial Sloan-Kettering series, the prevalence of pathological infiltration in level V was quite low, averaging 3% in 1,277 neck disssections in patients with oral cavity, oropharyngeal, hypopharyngeal and laryngeal tumors (Davidson et al. 1993). It peaked at 11% for hypopharyngeal tumors with pathologically positive nodes (Table 3.6). A thorough analysis of level V infiltration showed that for all tumor sites pooled together, infiltration of level V without metastases in levels I–IV was only observed in one patient (0.2%). This patient had a hypopharyngeal tumor. Infiltration in level V remained below 1% when a single pathologically confirmed positive node was also observed in levels I–III, but reached 16% when a single pathologically confirmed positive node was also observed in level IV. When more than one level was infiltrated, the probability of level V involvement progressively increased, reaching 40% when levels I–IV were all involved. The pattern of involvement of level I is also a good illustration of the concept of gradual node infiltration. In the Memorial Sloan-Kettering series, pathological involvement of level I was only found in 2% of clinical N0 patients with oropharyngeal tumors (Table 3.5), and was not observed in clinical N0 patients with hypopharyngeal tumors (Table 3.6). On the other hand, in patients with clinically positive nodes, metastases in level I were reported in 15% and 10% of patients with oropharyngeal and hypopharyngeal tumors, respectively. Similar patterns of metastases in levels I and V have been reported by other groups (Andersen et al. 1994; Cole and Hughes 1997; Ferlito and Rinaldo 1998; Schuller et al. 1978; Skolnik et al. 1976).

Anticipating the conclusions that could be drawn from the Memorial Sloan-Kettering Cancer Center data with regard to the extent of neck dissection, several groups have been performing selective neck dissection since the 1950s (Byers 1985; Byers et al. 1988; Chu and Strawitz 1978; Jesse et al. 1978; Kowalski et al. 1993; Lingeman et al. 1977; Medina and Byers 1989; Pellitteri et al. 1997; Pitman et al. 1997; Spiro et al. 1988). Typically, for tumors of the oral cavity, and to a lesser extent for oropharyngeal tumors, dissection of levels I–III (supraomohyoid neck dissection) was performed, whereas for laryngeal and hypopharyngeal tumors, dissection of levels II–IV (lateral neck dissection) or II–V (posterolateral neck dissection) was performed. Such selective neck procedures were initially proposed for clinically node-negative patients, and later extended to clinically node-positive patients. These studies are however biased, as the patients treated by a selective procedure were probably highly selected with regard to the tumor site, tumor stage and nodal status. In addition, in the majority of these patients, post-operative radiotherapy was usually performed in the case of high risk of primary tumor or neck recurrence, e.g. R1 resection, multiple node involvement, large node infiltration, extracapsular spread. It is likely that the irradiated field encompassed those node levels that were not dissected, but that could be at risk for microscopic infiltration.

With these limitations in mind, in some of these studies the level of neck recurrence was reported, allowing an estimate to be made of the failure rate in the neck within and outside the dissected levels (Brazilian Head and Neck Cancer Study Group 1998; Byers 1985; Byers et al. 1988; Chu and Strawitz 1978; Pellitteri et al. 1997; Pitman et al. 1997; Spiro et al. 1988). In five of these studies, neck recurrence was reported only in patients with the primary tumor controlled, thus excluding neck recurrence due to reseeding from the recurrent primary (Byers 1985; Byers et al. 1988; Pellitteri et al. 1997; Pitman et al. 1997; Spiro et al. 1988). In summary, after supraomohyoid or lateral neck dissections, the rate of neck failure in undissected levels was low and typically below 10%. In the study of Chu and Strawitz (1978), a high failure rate of 29% was however reported after a dissection that only removed levels I and II (suprahyoid dissection) for tumors of the oral cavity (Table 3.8).

All these figures can be considered as good estimates of microscopic involvement in the undissected levels at the time of neck dissection. They are in good agreement with the data reported from the Memorial Sloan-Kettering Cancer Center.

Recently, the Brazilian Head and Neck Cancer Study Group reported the results of a randomized trial on modified radical versus supraomohyoid neck dissection for clinically node-negative patients with T2–T4 tumors of the oral cavity (Brazilian Head and Neck Cancer Study Group 1998). Post-operative radiotherapy was indicated in the case of a positive margin at resection of the primary tumor and/or positive lymph nodes. With 64 patients in each group, the 5-year actuarial overall survival reached 63% and 67% in the MRND group and in the supraomohyoid neck dissection group, respectively. A failure rate in the neck of 9% occurred in six patients in each group. In the supraomohyoid neck dissection group, three patients (4.5%) had neck recurrence outside the dissected levels.

In theory, the incidence and distribution of neck node metastases in clinically N0 patients could also be indirectly inferred from neck recurrence outside the irradiated volume in patients treated by radiotherapy. In external radiotherapy, however, typical fields were used to encompass all node levels on both sides of the neck with only few exceptions, e.g. small laryngeal tumors. In addition, in the external radiotherapy series, the pattern of failure usually does not differentiate between in-field and out-field recurrences. Thus adequate sources of data mainly come from patients treated for the sole primary tumor, usually by brachytherapy. In the brachytherapy series, only limited data for oral cavity tumors are available. Pernot et al. (1995) reported a series of 346 carcinomas of the oral cavity (floor of the mouth

Table 3.8. Neck failure after selective neck dissection for SCC of the oral cavity, oropharynx, hypopharynx and larynx

Authors	Site	Clinical stage (AJCC 1980)	Dissected levels	Neck failure (percentage of patients with primary cancer controlled)		
				Total	Dissected levels	Undissected levels
Byers et al. (1997)	Oral cavity, oropharynx, hypopharynx, larynx	T1–T4 N0	I–II, I–III, II–IV, I–V	45/299 (15%)[a]	31/299 (10%)	14/299 (5%)[b]
Byers (1991)	Oral cavity, oropharynx	T1–T4, N0–N3	I–III	21/234 (9%)	16/234 (7%)	5/234 (2%)
Brazilian H&N Cancer Study Group (1998)	Oral cavity	T2–T4, N0	I–III[c]	6/64 (9%)	3/64 (4.5%)	3/64 (4.5%)[d]
Chu and Strawitz (1978)	Oral cavity, oropharynx	Tx–Nx	I–II	10/34 (29%)[e]	0/34 (0%)	10/34 (29%)
Pelliteri et al. (1997)	Oral cavity + oropharynx, hypopharynx + larynx	T1–T4, N0–N3	I–III/I–IV	7/42 (17%)	2/42 (5%)	5/42 (12%)[f]
		T1–T4, N0–N3	II–IV	1/25 (4%)	1/25 (4%)	0/25 (0%)
Pitman et al. (1997)	Oral cavity	T1–T4, N0	I–III/I–IV	5/142 (3.5%)	5/142 (3.5%)	0/142 (0%)
	oro-hypopharynx, larynx	T1–T4, N0	II–IV			
Spiro et al. (1997)	Oral cavity, oropharynx, larynx	T1–T4, N0–N1	I–III	12/107 (11%)	5/107 (4.5%)	7/107 (6.5%)

[a] Patients treated by surgery alone
[b] Six of these patients had failure on the contralateral undissected neck
[c] Part of a randomized study comparing radical modified versus supraomohyoid neck dissection
[d] One of these patients had failure on the contralateral undissected neck
[e] Including N0 patients only
[f] Three of these patients had failure on the contralateral undissected neck

and mobile tongue) treated by brachytherapy in which 227 clinically N0 patients did not have any treatment on the neck. The majority of these patients had T1 tumors. The rate of regional failure alone reached 16% (14% for T1 and 28% for T2), but no information on the distribution of the recurrent node was available. Piedbois et al. (1991) reported similar results in a series of 223 patients with stage I or II carcinoma of the oral cavity (floor of the mouth and mobile tongue) treated by brachytherapy for the primary cancer. Out of the 123 patients who did not have a neck dissection at the time of the primary treatment, 13% (11% for stage I and 25% for stage II) presented neck failure alone. Again, no information on the distribution of the recurrent node was available. The subset of patients from the same institution with floor of the mouth tumors was further analyzed, with similar findings (Mazeron et al. 1990). An old series from Stanford reported a rate of neck failure of 38% in 164 clinically N0 patients treated by radium implants for oral cavity tumors (Goffinet et al. 1975). It should be noted that in the series mentioned above the patients with no neck treatment typically had small T1 or T2 tumors and were highly selected. Besides, because no data were available on the distribution of node failure, these series are of limited value for the assessment of node levels to be treated. However, on average, the reported rates of neck failure are in agreement with the pathological data presented in Table 3.4.

For nasopharyngeal carcinomas, analysis of the pattern of failure in a large series of 5,037 patients treated by external radiotherapy indirectly indicated the incidence of microscopic neck involvement in clinically N0 patients (Lee et al. 1992). In this series, 906 patients did not receive prophylactic irradiation in levels I–V. Among them, 362 (40%) had nodal relapse. It is, however, not known how many of these patients also had local relapse, and the distribution of node failure in the neck was not mentioned.

3.3.2.2 Frequency of "Skip Metastases" in the Neck

"Skip metastases" are those metastases that bypass the orderly progression from one level to a contiguous level, e.g. from level I to level II and from level II to level III. Depending on their frequency, "skip metastases" in patients clinically staged N0 may have a profound implication on the therapeutic management of the neck. In the series from the Memorial Sloan-Kettering Cancer Center, eight out of 343 clinically N0 patients (2.5%) developed "skip metastases" (Shah 1990a). Seven of these patients had oral cavity tumors that metastasized in levels IV or V only. One patient had a laryngeal tumor. These low figures are in good agreement with a rate of neck failure outside the dissected levels of 3% (2/64) observed in pathologically N0 patients treated at the same institution by supraomohyoid neck dissection (SPIRO et al. 1988). The majority of these patients had tumors of the oral cavity. None of them received post-operative radiotherapy, as they were all free of metastases. BYERS et al. (1997) carefully evaluated the frequency of "skip metastases" in 270 patients primarily treated by surgery at the M.D. Anderson Cancer Center from 1970 to 1990 for SCC of the oral tongue. Of these patients, 12 had metastases in level III only, nine had metastases in level IV only and two in level IIb (i.e. nodes that are far enough posterior to the IJV). In addition, in 90 of the patients which were pathologically N0 and did not receive post-operative radiotherapy, nine subsequently developed recurrence in level IV which had not been dissected or irradiated. Altogether (levels IIb, III and IV) the frequency of skip metastases reached 12% (32/270). If one excludes the "skip metastases" in level III, the frequency reached only 7.5% (20/270).

3.3.2.3 Incidence of Pathological Retropharyngeal Lymph Nodes

Retropharyngeal lymph nodes are usually not included in the standard neck dissection procedure, and only limited data are thus available on the incidence of pathological involvement (Table 3.9).

Already in 1964, BALLANTYNE reported a series of 34 patients with pharyngeal wall tumors in whom retropharyngeal node dissection was performed. Pathological involvement of retropharyngeal nodes was observed in 15 patients (44%), 13 of whom also had pathological involvement in other levels in the neck. Ballantyne also reported pathological retropharyngeal node involvement in 11 other patients with oropharyngeal, hypopharyngeal and oral cavity tumors. In this series, no information on the TNM stage was provided, but it is likely that it included selected patients with locally advanced tumors. More recently, two consecutive series from the same Japanese hospital were reported (HASEGAWA and MATSUURA 1994; OKUMURA et al. 1998). These patients were probably highly selected with locally advanced (stages III and IV) oropharyngeal and hypopharyngeal tumors. Pathological retropharyngeal lymph nodes were reported in 12 out of 24 patients (50%), and in six out of 42 patients (14%). Interestingly, comparison of the pathological specimens with the preoperative imaging diagnosis by CT or MRI indicated the high sensitivity (83% for CT and 100% for MRI) and specificity (100% for both CT and MRI) of the radiological examination (OKUMURA et al. 1998). Byers also reported pathological retropharyngeal lymph node involvement in two out of 45 clinically N0 patients with pharyngeal wall tumors (BYERS et al. 1988). Again, these patients were highly selected and the reported figures probably represent an overestimation of pathological involvement in retropharyngeal lymph nodes.

3.3.2.4 Incidence of Anterior Cervical Lymph Nodes

This group of lymph nodes included in level VI comprises the paratracheal, pretracheal, precricoid and perithyroid nodes, and the nodes along the recurrent nerve. These nodes drain the subglottic larynx,

Table 3.9. Incidence of pathological retropharyngeal lymph node metastases in head and neck primary tumors

Authors	Primary site	Incidence of retropharyngeal lymph nodes (percentage of total number of patients)		
		Overall	pN0 neck[a]	pN+ neck[b]
BALLANTYNE (1964)	Oropharynx (pharyngeal wall)	15/34 (44%)	n.a.	n.a.
HASEGAWA and MATSUURA (1994)	Oropharynx	4/11 (36%)	1/2 (50%)	3/9 (33%)
	Hypopharynx	8/13 (62%)	0/3 (0%)	9/10 (90%)
OKUMURA et al. (1998)	Oropharynx + hypopharynx	6/42 (14%)	Not stated	Not stated
BYERS et al. (1988)	Oropharynx (pharyngeal wall)	2/45 (4%)	Not stated	Not stated

[a] Pathologically negative nodes in levels I–V
[b] Pathologically positive nodes in levels I–V

the upper esophagus, the piriform sinus, the thyroid gland and the cervical trachea (VIDIC and SUAREZ-QUIAN 1998; WERNER et al. 1995). The incidence of anterior cervical lymph node metastases is poorly documented in head and neck SCC. In subglottic cancer, it has been reported that paratracheal lymph nodes may be pathologically involved in 50% of cases (HARRISON 1971).

3.3.2.5
Pattern of Node Distribution in the Contralateral Neck

There are very few data available on the pattern of pathological node distribution in the contralateral neck. Bilateral neck dissection was only performed when the surgeon considered that there was a high risk of contralateral node involvement, e.g. tumors of the oral cavity or the oropharynx reaching or extending beyond the midline, or hypopharyngeal and supraglottic tumors. Obviously, in such cases bilateral radical neck dissection was never performed, so that an accurate estimate of the pattern of node involvement in levels I–V of the contralateral neck is not possible. Furthermore, in almost every study, data on both sides of the neck were pooled for presentation. KOWALSKI et al. (1993) presented data on 90 patients who underwent bilateral supraomohyoid neck dissection, and in whom the pattern of node distribution in each side of the neck was reported separately. The majority of these patients had SCC of the lip or the oral cavity. In the ipsilateral neck, pathological infiltration in levels I, II and III reached 20%, 15% and 15%, respectively. In the contralateral neck, corresponding values reached 13%, 11% and 0%, respectively. These figures are in good agreement with data on clinical node distribution showing that both sides of the neck exhibited a similar pattern of node distribution, but with a lower incidence in the contralateral neck. FOOTE et al. (1993) reported the rate of contralateral neck failure in a limited series of 46 clinically N0 patients with base of the tongue tumors treated by some form of glossectomy and ipsilateral neck dissection. None of these patients received post-operative radiotherapy. Ten patients (22%) had contralateral neck recurrence, and the most common sites were in levels II, III and IV. It appears that in two of these patients, recurrence was also observed at the primary site. The development of delayed contralateral neck metastases was not related to the clinical or pathological extent of the base of the tongue tumor.

3.4
Guidelines for the Selection of Target Volumes in the Neck

The data presented in the previous sections indicate that metastatic lymph node involvement of primary SCC of the oral cavity, pharynx, and larynx typically follows a predictive pattern. Both data on clinical and pathological neck node distribution and on neck recurrence after selective dissection procedures support the concept that not all the neck node levels should be treated as part of the initial management strategy of head and neck primaries of squamous cell origin (BYERS 1991; CLAYMAN and FRANK 1998). One should bear in mind, however, that the data on which such a concept is based may include possible bias that could limit its validity.

- First, all the reported series but one are retrospective studies which only included selected patients. As already pointed out, in the large series of the Memorial Sloan-Kettering Cancer Center on pathological node distribution, only 42% of the patients who underwent RND were reviewed (SHAH 1990a). During the period of study, less radical procedures were also performed at the same institution, but the selection criteria were not explicitly described. Similar comments can be made for the series from the M.D. Anderson Cancer Center regarding the selection criteria for selective neck dissection procedures. The T-stage was probably one of the most important selection criteria in these retrospective studies. It should be recalled that at the Memorial Sloan-Kettering Cancer Center, larger tumors were included in the pharyngeal and laryngeal tumor groups in comparison with oral cavity tumors, and the incidence of microscopic metastases is likely to be influenced by the T-stage.
  An unequivocal demonstration of the similitude between RND or MRND and SND procedures (or extended versus localized neck irradiation) would require multicentric randomized trials in which cases are balanced with regards to tumor site, tumor stage and the use of post-operative radiotherapy between treatment groups. The only trial addressing this question failed to demonstrate any difference between the two arms, and its statistical power was not strong enough to demonstrate subtle differences (BRAZILIAN HEAD AND NECK CANCER STUDY GROUP 1998).
- Second, all the figures on pathological involvement of the neck or regional failures after selective treatment are largely based on palpation only,

and the impact of modern imaging techniques on treatment strategy for the neck has not yet been fully investigated. It is likely that the systematic use of imaging will result in up-staging of the neck nodes especially in obese patients, or for deeply located nodes. Whether this will decrease the incidence and modify the distribution of the metastatic neck nodes is still unknown.

- Third, although neck dissection procedures have been well defined, minor variants have been reported by surgical teams. In supraomohyoid neck dissections, Byers reported that lymph nodes located in level IIb were also at risk for microscopic infiltration in SCC of the tongue (Byers 1985; Byers et al. 1988). Apparently, dissection in level IIb is not always performed in supraomohyoid neck dissection. Such practice might thus artificially increase the estimate of the true rate of neck failure outside the dissected levels.
- Fourth, in almost all the series of selective neck dissection, some patients received post-operative radiotherapy on the basis of the characteristics of the primary tumor (e.g. positive margins) or the neck specimen (e.g. extracapsular rupture, more than one infiltrated node). The radiation fields were not described, but it is likely that areas of possible microscopic involvement outside the dissected levels were irradiated. Such management might thus artificially decrease the true estimate of the rate of neck failure outside the dissected levels.
- Fifth, the incidence of retropharyngeal and paratracheal node infiltration cannot be adequately estimated from the literature data. These node areas can only be evaluated by imaging, and such a study has only rarely been performed especially for paratracheal nodes. A few series on pathological infiltration have reported a very high rate of infiltration in these lymph nodes. Unfortunately, the selection criteria for the patients who underwent retropharyngeal or paratracheal node dissection were never mentioned.
- Last, the concept of selective neck treatment in head and neck SCC primaries is mainly based on data collected at large institutions with extensive experience in the management of such cancer patients. The knowledge, experience and technical judgement of the clinicians involved in the treatment of these patients should thus not be underestimated. Great caution should therefore be taken in implementing guidelines for selective neck treatment in smaller institutions, in the best interests of the patients. More than ever, one must emphasize the fact that the management of head and neck cancer patients should be restricted to those institutions with extensive experience, where a multidisciplinary oncologic approach can be offered.

With all these limitations in mind, tentative guidelines for the selection of the appropriate neck node levels to be treated have been proposed. It is assumed that the staging of the neck has been carried out appropriately using clinical and radiological examination including at least CT or MRI. Following the methodology developed by the European "State of the Art in Oncology" (START) project, these recommendations have been based on rational inference, i.e. from available data and knowledge combined, but without indisputable proof resulting from randomized trials or well accepted meta-analysis (see at http://www.cancereurope.net/start/web/methodology.cfm).

In reading these guidelines, the following limitations must be clearly understood.

- These guidelines do not intend to give recommendations on the optimal strategy (observation versus prophylactic treatment) for patients with a clinically N0 neck. Such a decision should be made by the multidisciplinary head and neck tumor board. It has been proposed from decision analysis trees that treatment of the N0 neck is warranted if the probability of occult cervical metastases is higher than 20% (Weiss et al. 1994). It is likely that this very high figure would not be accepted by the majority of European centers, which would probably treat the neck when the probability of occult metastases was higher than 5–10%. Tumor size and depth of infiltration, tumor grade, and tumor site are the most important risk factors for lymph node metastases that should be taken into consideration in making the treatment decision (Shah 1990a).
- These guidelines do not intend to give recommendations on the respective use of radiotherapy or neck dissection in the management of patients with head and neck SCC. The choice between radiotherapy and surgery needs to be considered in the light of the neck stage, the treatment options for the primary tumor, the performance status of the patient, and the local policy agreed upon by a multidisciplinary head and neck tumor board.
- These guidelines do not apply to the treatment of recurrent neck cancer after primary cancer radiotherapy or surgery. In the neck which has been previously treated, lymph node drainage is modified and the pattern of neck node infiltration follows rather unpredictable pathways.

- These guidelines are not inflexible and should be adapted according to the results of forthcoming studies, e.g. a randomized trial of selective versus radical modified treatment of the neck in clinically N0 patients.

For N0 patients with head and neck SCC of the oral cavity, oropharynx, hypopharynx and larynx, selective treatment of the neck is appropriate (Table 3.10) (Byers 1985; Clayman and Frank 1998; Spiro et al. 1988).

Typically, levels I–III should be treated for oral cavity tumors, and levels II–IV for oropharyngeal, hypopharyngeal and laryngeal tumors. Recently, Robbins (1998) has suggested that elective treatment of level IIb is probably not necessary for N0 patients with a primary tumor of the oral cavity, larynx or hypopharynx. On the other hand, Byers et al. (1997) suggested that level IV be included in the treatment of the mobile tongue due to the high incidence (10%) of skip metastases. Retropharyngeal nodes should be treated in tumors of the posterior pharyngeal wall. For subglottic tumors, tumors with subglottic or transglottic extension, or hypopharyngeal tumors with esophageal extension, level VI nodes should also be included in the treatment volume. For nasopharyngeal tumors, levels II–V and retropharyngeal nodes need to be treated even for N0 patients. As proposed by Byers, similar guidelines could also be recommended for N1 patients without evidence of extracapsular infiltration (Table 3.10) (Byers 1985).

For patients with multiple nodes (N2b), the available data suggest that adequate treatment should include levels I–V (Table 3.10). Level I could, however, be omitted for laryngeal tumors, and level V for oral cavity tumors with neck involvement limited to levels I–III. Prophylactic treatment of the retropharyngeal nodes should be systematically performed for oropharyngeal and hypopharyngeal tumors. As for N0 patients, level VI nodes should also be treated for subglottic tumors, tumors with subglottic or transglottic extension, or hypopharyngeal tumors with esophageal extension.

There is no data available on the distribution of pathological metastatic neck nodes in patients presenting with a single ipsilateral large node (N2a or N3) or with bilateral or contralateral nodes (N2c), and thus no recommendation can be made. For N3 patients, the type of treatment of the neck is likely to be dictated by the local extension of the node into the adjacent structures (e.g. paraspinal muscles, parotid gland, blood vessels). For N2c patients, one proposal is to consider each side of the neck separately, e.g. selective treatment in both sides for a small single node in each side, selective treatment for a small single node in one side, and more extensive treatment in the other side in the case of multiple nodes.

Treatment of the contralateral neck is still in the gray zone, and is likely to be based on clinical judgement rather than on strong scientific evidence. Typically, patients with midline tumors or tumors origi-

Table 3.10. Suggested guidelines for the treatment of patients with head and neck SCC

Location of primary tumor	Appropriate node levels to be treated	
	Stage N0–N1 (AJCC 1997)	Stage N2b (AJCC 1997)
Oral cavity	I, II[a], and III (+IV for anterior tongue tumors)	I, II, III, IV and V[c]
Oropharynx	II, III, and IV (+ retropharyngeal nodes for posterior pharyngeal wall tumors)	I, II, III, IV, V and retropharyngeal nodes
Hypopharynx	II[a], III, and IV (+ VI for esophageal extension)	I, II, III, IV, V and retropharyngeal nodes (+ VI for esophageal extension)
Larynx[b]	II[a], III, and IV (+ VI for transglottic and subglottic tumors)	(I), II, III, IV and V (+ VI for transglottic and subglottic tumors)
Nasopharynx	II, III, IV, V and retropharyngeal nodes	II, III, IV, V and retropharyngeal nodes

[a] Nodes in level IIb could be omitted for N0 patients
[b] T1 glottic cancer excluded
[c] May be omitted if only levels I–III are involved

nating from or extending to a site which has bilateral lymphatic drainage (e.g. base of the tongue, vallecula, posterior pharyngeal wall) are thought to benefit from contralateral treatment, whereas well lateralized tumors (e.g. the lateral border of the tongue, retromolar trigone, tonsillar fossa) can be spared contralateral treatment. It has also been reported in tumors of the pharynx and larynx that the risk of contralateral neck metastases increased with involvement of the ipsilateral neck (Marks et al. 1992). One recommendation that can be made regarding treatment of the contralateral neck is that the selection of the node levels to be treated should follow similar rules to those for the ipsilateral neck. Another recommendation is to restrict the treatment to the ipsilateral neck for tumors of the lower gum (not approaching the midline), lateral floor of the mouth, lateral border of the mobile tongue, upper gum, cheek, retromolar trigone, tonsillar fossa (without extension to the base of the tongue, soft palate, posterior pillar) and lateral wall of the piriform sinus.

In principle, a similar approach should apply for the definition of the node levels to be irradiated post-operatively. However, if one agrees on the selection criteria for post-operative radiotherapy (i.e. capsular rupture, patients with a metastatic node over 3 cm in diameter or with more than one metastatic node), irradiation of levels I–V will typically be performed. For laryngeal tumors, level I could be omitted. For oral cavity tumors, post-operative irradiation of level V could be omitted in the case of metastatic nodes located in level I and/or II only. Retropharyngeal and paratracheal nodes should be treated as mentioned above.

3.5 Guidelines for the Delineation of Target Volumes in the Neck

As already discussed in Section 3.2, the Committee for Head and Neck Surgery and Oncology of the American Academy for Otolaryngology-Head and Neck Surgery has recommended the use of a common terminology and procedures for the surgical treatment of the neck (Robbins et al. 1991). We propose that similar recommendations be used for the treatment of the neck by radiotherapy.

Radical neck irradiation would become the reference procedure, with levels I–V included in the target volume along with the IJV, the SAN, and the SCM muscle. Such a procedure is only recommended in the case of infiltration of the SCM muscle and/or infiltration or thrombosis of the IJV as illustrated on CT scan or MRI, or confirmed on pathological examination. *Modified radical neck irradiation* with preservation of the SCM muscle would in fact become the standard procedure. In theory, the IJV and the SAN should also be spared by this procedure. In practice, it will be practically impossible to exclude the IJV and the SAN from the target volume. Similarly, the carotid artery, which is not removed during a neck dissection procedure (unless there is carotid wall infiltration), will always be included in the target volume. On the other hand, the fascia of the SCM muscle on the cutaneous side which is dissected off the muscle during MRND will not be included in the target volume for the obvious reason of skin protection. However, the few lymph nodes included in this fascia will probably be substantially irradiated, irrespective of the technique used. *Selective neck irradiation* would be the procedure of choice when not all levels are included in the target volume. It includes *supraomohyoid neck irradiation* (levels I–III), *lateral neck irradiation* (levels II–IV), and *postero-lateral neck irradiation* (levels II–V). Last, we do not recommend the use of the *extended neck irradiation* terminology. We would prefer to describe separately the irradiation of other lymphatic or non-lymphatic structures. Irradiation of levels II–IV and the retropharyngeal nodes would be called *lateral neck irradiation extended to the retropharyngeal nodes*. Irradiation of levels I–V, the parotid gland and the retropharyngeal nodes would be called *radical modified neck irradiation extended to the parotid and the retropharyngeal nodes*.

The use of such terminology implies that radiation oncologists agree on the use of a standardized procedure for the delineation of the various node levels in the neck. We recommend the use of similar anatomical boundaries to those proposed by Robbins for levels I–VI, and that the concept of node levels be extended to those nodes not covered by the Robbins' classification, i.e. in the retropharyngeal space. The anatomical limits defined by Robbins, however, need to be slightly adapted to take into account the radiological information easily derived from CT or MRI axial sections. In particular, such imaging-based nodal classification needs to address the following specific points. (1) What are the radiological cranial limits of level II and the relationship between these nodes and the retropharyngeal nodes? (2) How can the radiological caudal limits of levels IV and V on axial sections be consistently defined? (3) What are the radiological limits that divide levels IIa and IIb, and levels Va and Vb? (4) What is the upper limit of level V on CT/MRI axial sections?

Table 3.11. Recommendations for the radiological boundaries of neck node levels

Level	Anatomical boundaries					
	Cranial	Caudal	Anterior	Posterior	Lateral	Medial
Ia	Geniohyoid m., plane tangent to basilar edge of mandible	Plane tangent to the body of hyoid bone	Symphysis menti, platysma m.	Body of hyoid bone	Medial edge of ant. belly of digastric m.	n.a.[a]
Ib	Mylohyoid m., cranial edge of submandibular gland	Plane through central part of hyoid bone	Symphysis menti, platysma m.	Posterior edge of sub-mandibular gland	Basilar edge/inner side of mandible, platysma m., skin	Lateral edge of ant. belly of digastric m.
II	Caudal edge of lateral process of C1	Caudal edge of the body of hyoid bone	Post. edge of sub-mandibular gland; ant. edge of int. carotid artery; post. edge of post. belly of digastric m.	Post. border of the sternocleidomastoid m.	Medial edge of sternocleidomastoid	Int. edge of int. carotid artery; paraspinal (levator scapulae) m.
III	Caudal edge of the body of hyoid bone	Caudal edge of the cricoid cartilage	Postero-lateral edge of the sternohyoid m.; ant. edge of the sternocleiomastoid	Post. edge of the sternocleidomastoid m.	Medial edge of sternocleidomastoid	Int. edge of carotid artery, paraspinal (scalenius) m.
IV	Caudal edge of the cricoid cartilage	2 cm cranial to sternoclavicular joint	Anteromedial edge of the sternocleidomastoid m.	Post. edge of the sternocleidomastoid m.	Medial edge of the sternocleidomastoid m.	Medial edge of internal carotid artery, paraspinal (scalenius) m.
V	Cranial edge of body of hyoid bone	CT slice including the transverse cervical vessels[b]	Post. edge of the sternocleidomastoid m.	Ant. border of the trapezius m.	Platysma m., skin	Paraspinal (levator scapulae, splenius capitis) m.
VI	Caudal edge of body of thyroid cartilage[c]	Sternal manubrium	Skin; platysma m.	Separation between trachea and esophagus[d]	Medial edges of thyriod gland, skin and ant.-medial edge of sternocleidomastoid m.	n.a.
Retro-pharyngeal	Base of skull	Cranial edge of the body of hyoid bone	Fascia under the pharyngeal mucosa	Prevertebral m. (longus colli, longus capitis)	Medial edge of the internal carotid artery	Midline

[a] Midline structure lying between the medial border of the anterior bellies of the digastric muscles
[b] For NPC, the reader is referred to the original description of the UICC/AJCC 1977 edition of Ho's triangle – in essence, the fatty planes below and around the clavicle down to the trapezius muscle
[c] For paratracheal and recurrent nodes, the cranial border is the caudal edge of the cricoid cartilage
[d] For paratracheal nodes, trachea and the anterior edge of the cricoid cartilage

Table 3.11 proposes recommendations for the delineation of the various node levels in the neck. These recommendations are based on the imaging classification of cervical nodes proposed by Som and critically reviewed by Robbins (Robbins 1998; Som et al. 1999). They are in good agreement with those proposed by Nowak et al. (1999). Cross-sectional atlases of head and neck nodes have also been recently published (Hayman et al. 1998; Martinez-Monge et al. 1999; Stewart et al. 1998). As far as our demonstration is concerned, they are of limited use, as they do not precisely define the anatomical boundaries of the various nodal spaces. In Table 3.11, the boundaries refer to a patient lying in a supine position with his head in a "neutral" position. This position is different to that adopted during neck dissection. The anatomical landmarks used to define these boundaries may thus be slightly different to those adopted by surgeons (see Section 3.2.1). The terms "cranial" and "caudal" refer to structures close to the cephalic and foot end, respectively. The terms "anterior" and "posterior" were preferred to the terms "ventral" and "dorsal", respectively. Examples of delineated node levels are shown in Figs. 3.2 and 3.3. It should be emphasized that the volumes delineated in these figures correspond to the clinical target volume (CTV), and hence do not include margins for organ motion or set-up inaccuracy.

Regarding the delineation of the upper limit of level II and the relationship of this with the retropharyngeal nodes, a neck dissection of the upper jugular node typically never extends beyond the insertion of the posterior belly of the digastric muscle on the mastoid or beyond the inferior edge of the parotid gland. On CT or MRI, as visualization of the posterior belly of the digastric muscle is not always easy, the caudal edge of the lateral process of C1 is recommended to define the upper limit of level II. This upper limit is slightly more cranial compared to the surgical limit, and thus includes more lymphatic tissue around the IJV and internal carotid artery. Retropharyngeal nodes extend medially to the internal carotid arteries (and thus medially to the level II nodes) from the base of the skull to the upper level of the hypopharynx, which is delineated by an axial plane crossing the cranial edge of the hyoid bone. From there, the retropharyngeal nodes drain into the level II nodes.

The caudal limit of levels IV and V should include the transverse cervical nodal chain which lies along the transverse cervical artery and vein and runs parallel to the clavicle. This nodal chain connects the dorsal cervical nodes to the caudal jugular nodes and drains near the junction between the internal jugular vein and the subclavian vein. For the caudal limit of level IV, an axial section 2 cm above the sternoclavicular joint is recommended. For level V, the axial section encompassing the transverse cervical vessels defines the caudal limit. To limit the inherent variability in delineating the lower limit of levels IV and V, immobilization of the patient on the table coach with a proper fixation device aimed at lowering the shoulders as much as possible is recommended. For the division between levels Va and Vb, the use of the limit between levels III and IV extended posteriorly is recommended.

Regarding the division between levels IIa and IIb the SAN, which is not identified on CT or MRI, cannot be used. Som proposed the use of the posterior edge of the IJV (Som et al. 1999).

The upper limit of level V was originally defined as the base of the skull. As discussed in Section 3.2.1, this limit has been questioned and a better surgical boundary of level V might be the upper two-thirds of the SAN. This nerve is, however, never visualized on either CT or MRI. One proposal is to define the upper limit of level V by an axial plane tangent to the cranial edge of the body of the hyoid bone.

3.6 Conclusions

The increasing use of 3D treatment planning in head and neck radiation oncology has created an urgent need for new guidelines for the selection and delineation of the neck node areas to be included in the CTV. Surgical literature has provided us with valuable information on the extent of pathological nodal involvement in the neck as a function of the primary tumor site. In addition, a few clinical series have also reported data on radiological nodal involvement in those areas not commonly included in RND. Taking all these data together, guidelines for the selection of the node levels to be irradiated for the major head and neck sites could be proposed. To fill the missing link between these guidelines and 3D treatment planning, recommendations for the delineation of these node levels on CT (or MRI) slices have been proposed using the guidelines outlined by the Committee for Head and Neck Surgery and Oncology of the American Academy for Otolaryngology-Head and Neck Surgery. These guidelines have, however, been adapted to take into account specific radiological landmarks more easily identified on CT or MRI slices than in the operating field.

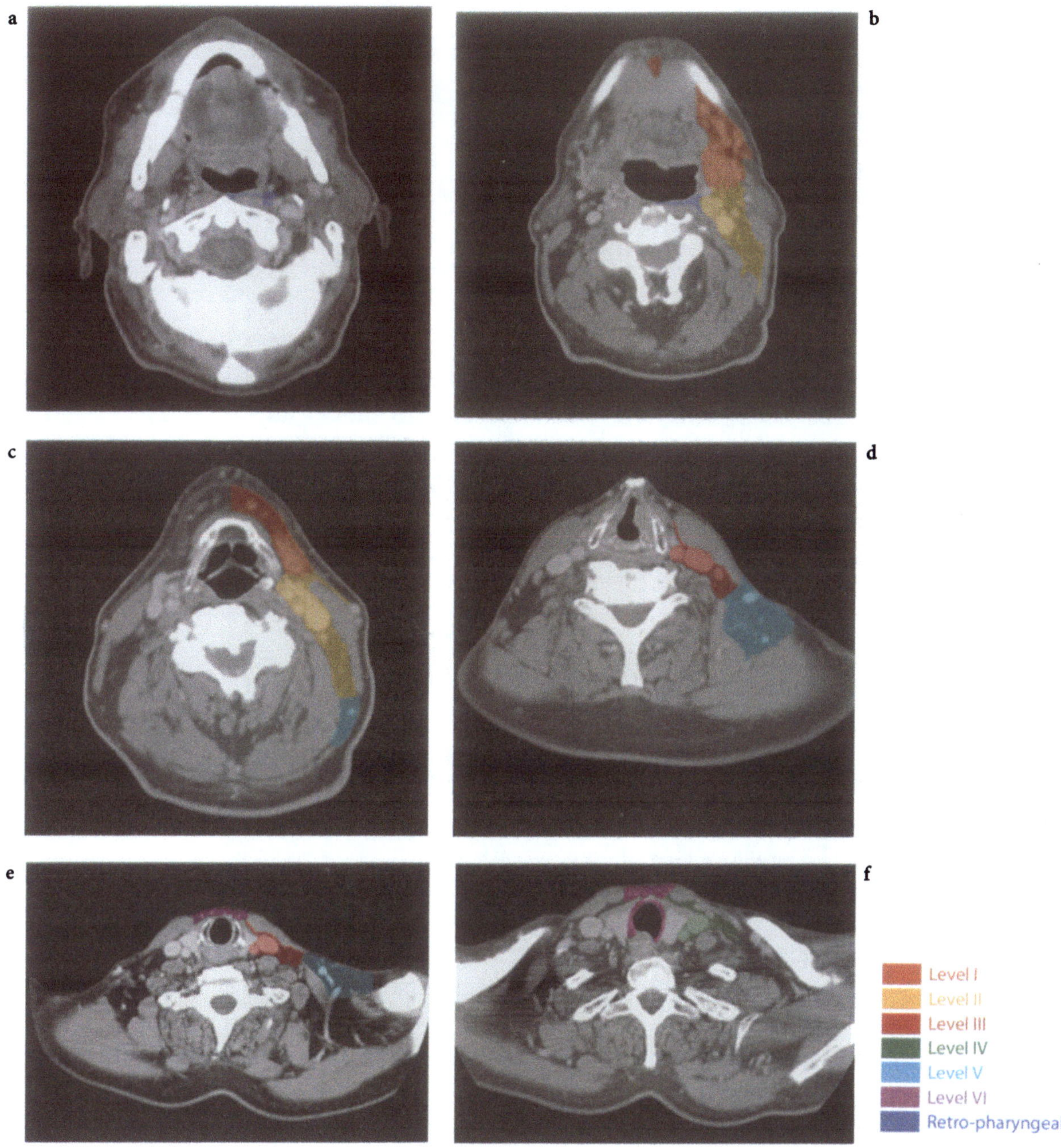

Fig. 3.2. CT imaging of a patient with a T1N0M0 glottic SCC (see tumor in *panel d*). The examination was performed on a dual-detector spiral CT (Elscint Twin, Haifa, Israel) using a slice thickness of 2.7 mm, an interval reconstruction of 2 mm and a pitch of 0.7. Contrast medium was injected intravenously at a rate of 2 ml/s with a total amount of 100 ml. Sections were taken at the level of the bottom edge of C1 (*panel a*), the upper edge of C3 (*panel b*), mid C4 (*panel c*), the bottom edge of C6 (*panel d*), the bottom edge of C7 (*panel e*), and mid D1 (*panel f*). Neck node levels were drawn on each CT slice using the radiological boundaries detailed in Table 3.11. Each node level corresponds to the CTV, and thus does not include a security margin for organ motion or set-up inaccuracy

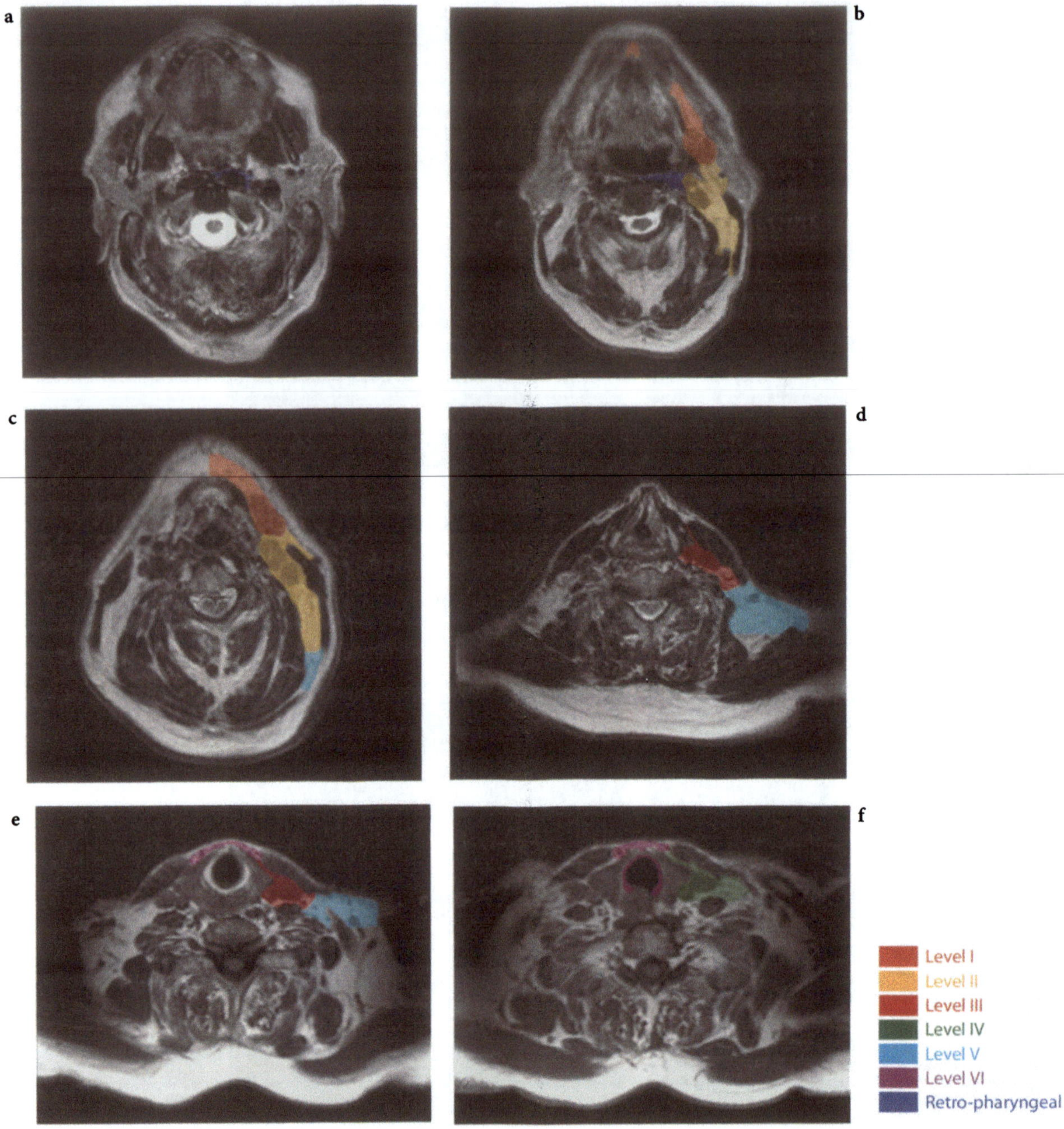

Fig. 3.3. MRI of the same patient with a T1N0M0 glottic SCC (see tumor in *panel d*). The examination was performed on a Gyroscan NT 1.5 T Philips Medical Systems (Eindhoven, the Netherlands) on an axial plane with a slice thickness of 4 mm, a gap of 2 mm, and a field of view of 240 mm. T2-weighted images (TR 7976 ms and TE 90 ms) are displayed in *panels a–d*. *Panels e and f* represent T1-weighted images (TR 500 and TE 12 ms). Sections were taken at the level of the bottom edge of C1 (*panel a*), the upper edge of C3 (*panel b*), mid C4 (*panel c*), the bottom edge of C6 (*panel d*), the bottom edge of C7 (*panel e*), and mid D1 (*panel f*). Neck node levels were drawn on each slice using the radiological boundaries detailed in Table 3.11. The slight difference in the shape of the various levels between Figs. 3.2 and 3.3 is explained by a difference in the positioning of the patient, leading to a slight difference in slice levels. Each node level corresponds to the CTV, and thus does not include a security margin for organ motion or set-up inaccuracy

Implementation of these guidelines in daily radiation oncology practice should assist in reducing treatment variations from patient to patient and in conducting multi-institutional clinical trials or retrospective studies. However, although the guidelines are meant to be applied to the vast majority of patients, there will always be individual cases for whom sound clinical data preclude their use. More than ever, oncologic knowledge and experience are required for the appropriate use of the recommendations proposed in this chapter.

References

Andersen PE, Shah JP, Cambronero E et al (1994) The role of comprehensive neck dissection with preservation of the spinal accessory nerve in the clinically positive neck. Am J Surg 168:499–502

Ballantyne AJ (1964) Significance of retropharyngeal nodes in cancer of the head and neck. Am J Surg 108:500–504

Bataini JP, Bernier J, Brugere J et al (1985) Natural history of neck disease in patients with squamous cell carcinoma of the oropharynx and pharyngolarynx. Radiother Oncol 3: 245–255

Bocca E, Pignataro O (1967) A conservation technique in radical neck dissection. Ann Otol Rhinol Laryngol 76:975–987

Bocca E, Pignataro O, Sasaki CT (1980) Functional neck dissection. A description of operative technique. Arch Otolaryngol Head Neck Surg 106:524–527

Brazilian Head and Neck Cancer Study Group (1998) Results of a prospective trial on elective modified radical classical versus supraomohyoid neck dissection in the management of oral squamous carcinoma. Am J Surg 176:422–427

Byers RM (1985) Modified neck dissection. A study of 967 cases from 1970 to 1980. Am J Surg 150:414–421

Byers RM (1991) Neck dissection: concepts, controversies, and technique. Semin Surg Oncol 7:9–13

Byers RM, Wolf PF, Ballantyne AJ (1988) Rationale for elective modified neck dissection. Head Neck Surg 10:160–167

Byers RM, Weber RS, Andrewa T et al (1997) Frequency and therapeutic implications of "skip metastases" in the neck from squamous carcinoma of the oral tongue. Head Neck 19:14–19

Candela FC, Kothari K, Shah JP (1990a) Patterns of cervical node metastases from squamous carcinoma of the oropharynx and hypopharynx. Head Neck 12:197–203

Candela FC, Shah J, Jaques DP et al (1990b) Patterns of cervical node metastases from squamous carcinoma of the larynx. Arch Otolaryngol Head Neck Surg 116:432–435

Chong VF, Fan YF, Khoo JB (1995) Retropharyngeal lymphadenopathy in nasopharyngeal carcinoma. Eur J Radiol 21:100–105

Chu W, Strawitz JG (1978) Results in suprahyoid, modified radical, and standard radical neck dissections for metastatic squamous cell carcinoma: recurrence and survival. Am J Surg 136:512–515

Chua DTT, Sham JST, Kwong DLW et al (1997) Retropharyngeal lymphadenopathy in patients with nasopharyngeal carcinoma. A computed tomography-based study. Cancer 79:869–877

Clayman GL, Frank DK (1998) Selective neck dissection of anatomically appropriate levels is as efficacious as modified radical neck dissection for elective treatment of the clinically negative neck in patients with squamous cell carcinoma of the upper respiratory and digestive tracts. Arch Otolaryngol Head Neck Surg 124:348–352

Cole I, Hughes L (1997) The relationship of cervical lymph node metastases to primary sites of carcinoma of the upper aerodigestive tract: a pathological study. Aust NZ J Surg 67:860–865

Davidson BJ, Kulkarny V, Delacure MD et al (1993) Posterior triangle metastases of squamous cell carcinoma of the upper aerodigestive tract. Am J Surg 166:395–398

Ferlito A, Rinaldo A (1998) Level I dissection for laryngeal and hypopharyngeal cancer: is it indicated? J Laryngol Otol 112:438–440

Foote RL, Olsen,KD, Davis DL et al (1993) Base of tongue carcinoma: patterns of failure and predictors of recurrence after surgery alone. Head Neck 15:300–307

Goffinet DR, Gilbert EH, Weller SA et al (1975) Irradiation of clinically uninvolved cervical lymph nodes. Can J Otolaryngol 4:927–933

Grégoire V, Coche E, Cosnard G et al (2000) Selection and delineation of lymph node target volumes in head and neck conformal radiotherapy. Proposal for standardizing terminology and procedure based on the surgical experience. Radiother Oncol 56:135–150

Harrison DFN (1971) The pathology and management of subglottic cancer. Ann Otol Rhinol Laryngol 80:6–12

Hasegawa Y, Matsuura H (1994) Retropharyngeal node dissection in cancer of the oropharyngeal and hypopharynx. Head Neck 16:173–180

Hayman LA, Taber KH, Diaz-Marchan PJ et al (1998) Spatial compartments of the neck, part III: axial sections. Int J Neuroradiol 4:393–402

Hermanek P, Henson DE, Hutter RVP, Sobin LH (eds) (1993) TNM supplement 1993. A commentary on uniform use. Springer, Berlin Heidelberg New York

Jesse RH, Ballantyne AJ, Larson D (1978) Radical or modified neck dissection: a therapeutic dilemma. Am J Surg 136: 516–519

Kowalski LP, Magrin J, Waksman G et al (1993) Supraomohyoid neck dissection in the treatment of head and neck tumors. Survival results in 212 cases. Arch Otolaryngol Head Neck Surg 119:958–963

Lee AW, Poon YF, Foo W et al (1992) Retrospective analysis of 5,037 patients with nasopharyngeal carcinoma treated during 1976–1985: overall survival and patterns of failure. Int J Radiat Oncol Biol Phys 23:261–270

Lindberg R (1972) Distribution of cervical lymph node metastases from squamous cell carcinoma of the upper respiratory and digestive tracts. Cancer 29:1446–1449

Lingeman RE, Helmus C, Stephens R et al (1977) Neck dissection: radical or conservative. Ann Otol 86:737–744

Marks JE, Devineni VR, Harvey J et al (1992) The risk of contrategral lymphatic metastases for cancers of the larynx and pharynx. Am J Otolaryngol 13:34–39

Martinez-Monge R, Fernandes PS, Gupta N et al (1999) Cross-sectional nodal atlas: a tool for the definition of clinical target volumes in three-dimensional radiation therapy planning. Radiology 211:815–828

Mazeron JJ, Grimard L, Raynal M et al (1990) Iridium-192 curietherapy for T1 and T2 epidermoid carcinomas of the floor of mouth. Int J Radiat Oncol Biol Phys 18:1299–1306

McLaughlin MP, Mendenhall WM, Mancuso AA et al (1995) Retropharyngeal adenopathy as a predictor of outcome in squamous cell carcinoma of the head and neck. Head Neck 17:190–198
Medina JE, Byers RM (1989) Supraomohyoid neck dissection: rationale, indications, and surgical technique. Head Neck 11:111–122
Nowak PJ, Wijers OB, Lagerwaard FJ et al (1999) A three-dimensional CT-based target definition for elective irradiation of the neck. Int J Radiat Oncol Biol Phys 45:33–39
Okumura K, Fujimoto Y, Hasegawa Y et al (1998) Retropharyngeal node metastasis in cancer of the oropharynx and hypopharynx: analysis of retropharyngeal node dissection regarding preoperative radiographic diagnosis. Nippon Jibiinkoka Gakkai Kaiho 101:573–577
Pellitteri PK, Robbins KT, Neuman T (1997) Expanded application of selective neck dissection with regard to nodal status. Head Neck 19:260–265
Pernot M, Verhaeghe JL, Guillemin F et al (1995) Evaluation de l'importance d'un curage ganglionnaire systématique dans les carcinomes de la cavité buccale traités par curiéthérapie seule pour la lésion primaire (à propos d'une série de 346 patients). Bull Cancer Radiother 82:311–317
Piedbois P, Mazeron JJ, Haddad E et al (1991) Stage I–II squamous cell carcinoma of the oral cavity treated by iridium-192: is elective neck dissection indicated? Radiother Oncol 21:100–106
Pitman KT, Johnson JT, Myers EN (1997) Effectiveness of selective neck dissection for management of the clinically negative neck. Arch Otolaryngol Head Neck Surg 123:917–922
Robbins KT (1998) Classification of neck dissection: current concepts and future considerations. Otolaryngol Clin North Am 31:639–656
Robbins KT (1999) Integrating radiological criteria into the classification of cervical lymph node disease. Arch Otolaryngol Head Neck Surg 125:385–387
Robbins KT, Medina JE, Wolfe GT et al (1991) Standardizing neck dissection terminology. Official report of the Academy's Committee for Head and Neck Surgery and Oncology. Arch Otolaryngol Head Neck Surg 117:601–605
Rouvière H (1948) Anatomie humaine descriptive et topographique, 6th edn. Masson et Cie, Paris
Schuller DE, Platz CE, Krause CJ (1978) Spinal accessory lymph nodes: a prospective study of metastatic involvement. Laryngoscope 88:439–449
Shah JP (1990) Patterns of cervical lymph node metastasis from squamous carcinomas of the upper aerodigestive tract. Am J Surg 160:405–409
Shah JP, Strong E, Spiro RH et al (1981) Surgical grand rounds. Neck dissection: current status and future possibilities. Clin Bull 11:25–33
Shah JP, Candela FC, Poddar AK (1990) The patterns of cervical lymph node metastases from squamous carcinoma of the oral cavity. Cancer 66:109–113
Sham JST, Choy D, Wei WI (1990) Nasopharyngeal carcinoma: orderly neck node spread. Int J Radiat Oncol Biol Phys 19: 929–933
Skolnik EM, Tenta LT, Wineinger DM (1967) Preservation of XI cranial nerve in neck dissection. Laryngoscope 77: 1304–1314
Skolnik EM, Yee KF, Friedman M, et al (1976) The posterior triangle in radical neck surgery. Arch Otolaryngol 102:1–4
Som PM (1997) The present controversy over the imaging method of choice for evaluating the soft tissues of the neck. Am J Neuroradiol 18:1869–1872
Som PM, Curtin HD, Mancuso AA (1999) An imaging-based classification for the cervical nodes designed as an adjunct to recent clinically based nodal classifications. Arch Otolaryngol Head Neck Surg 125:388–396
Spiessl B, Beahrs OH, Hermanek P, Hutter RVP, Scheibe O, Sobin LH, Wagner G (eds) (1992) TNM atlas. Illustrated guide to the TNM/pTNM classification of malignant tumours, 3th edn, 2nd rev. Springer, Berlin Heidelberg New York
Spiro JD, Spiro RH, Shah JP et al (1988) Critical assessment of supraomohyoid neck dissection. Am J Surg 156:286–289
Stewart MG, Hayman LA, Taber KH et al (1998) Clinical pathology of the neck: spatial compartments. Int J Neuroradiol 4:152–158
Suarez O (1963) El problema de las metastasis linfaticas y alejadas del cancer de laringe e hipofaringe. Rev Otorrinolaringol 23:83–89
Suen JY, Goepfert H (1987) Standardization of neck dissection nomenclature. Head Neck 9:75–77
Takes RP, Righi P, Meeuwis CA et al (1998) The value of ultrasound with ultrasound-guided fine-needle aspiration biopsy compared to computed tomography in the detection of regional metastases in the clinically negative neck. Int J Radiat Oncol Biol Phys 40:1027–1032
van den Brekel MWM, Stel HV, Castelijns JA et al (1990) Cervical lymph node metastasis: assessment of radiologic criteria. Radiology 177:379–384
van den Brekel MWM, Castelijns JA, Snow GB (1998) The size of lymph nodes in the neck on sonograms as a radiologic criterion for metastasis: how reliable is it? Am J Neuroradiol 19:695–700
Vidic B, Suarez-Quian C (1998) Anatomy of the head and neck. In: Harrison LB, Sessions RB, Ki Hong W (eds) Head and neck cancer. A multidisciplinary approach, 1st edn. Lippincott-Raven, Philadelphia, pp 79–114
Weiss MH, Harrison LB, Isaacs RS (1994) Use of decision analysis in planning a management strategy for the stage N0 neck. Arch Otolaryngol Head Neck Surg 120:699–702
Werner JA, Schünke M, Lippert BM et al (1995) Das laryngeale Lymphgefäbsystem des Menschen. HNO 43:525–531

4 Lung Cancer

P. Van Houtte, F. Mornex, P. Rocmans, P. Loubeyre, F. Vaylet

CONTENTS

4.1 Introduction

Radiation still plays an important role in the management of lung cancer either alone or combined with surgery and/or chemotherapy, not only with the intent to cure the patient but also to improve his quality of life. During the last decades, several prognostic factors have been clearly identified regarding tumor extent (e.g. size, nodal invasion), the host response (e.g. performance status, weight loss) or radiation treatment (total dose, fractionation and technique). Nevertheless, local control remains a major challenge: figures as low as 20% have been reported following doses of 60 Gy or more with or without induction chemotherapy (Arriagada et al. 1991; Saunders et al. 1999). One means of improving treatment efficacy is to increase the physical or biological doses (conformal 3D radiotherapy, accelerated hyperfractionated schedule, concurrent chemotherapy). The main limitation remains that of the tolerance of normal tissue, the spinal cord, the heart, the esophagus, and the lung. The volume of irradiated normal tissue also has a direct influence on the risk of occurrence of subsequent late effects. Reducing this volume implies a precise knowledge of tumor extent and the clinical target volume (CTV) to be treated. In the present chapter, we will attempt to examine the nodal spread of lung cancer and review the data available from surgical and radiotherapeutic series.

4.2 The Lymphatic Drainage of the Lung: Anatomy and Classification

4.2.1 Normal Lymphatic Drainage

Rouvière divided the visceral nodes of the thorax into four different groups: the anterior mediastinal nodes, the posterior mediastinal nodes, the peritracheobronchial nodes and the intrapulmonary nodes (Rouvière 1967).

4.2.1.1 The Intrapulmonary Nodes

The first lymph nodes are situated within the lung: the subsegmental nodes, the segmental nodes, and the lobar or interlobar nodes. They are located either at the bifurcation of the bronchi or close to the angle

P. Van Houtte, MD, PhD
Department of Radiotherapy, Institut Jules Bordet, Brussels, Belgium
F. Mornex, MD
Department of Radiotherapy, Centre Hospitalier Lyon Sud, Pierre Bénite, France
P. Loubeyre, MD
Service de Radiologie, Hopital Cantonal Universitaire de Geneve, Geneve, Swizerland
P. Rocmans, MD
Department of Thoracic Surgery, Hôpital Erasme, Brussels, Belgium
F. Vaylet, MD
Department of Respiratory Diseases, Hôpital d'Instruction des Armées Percy, Clamart, France

formed by the division of the arteries and veins. Some small nodes are located under the visceral pleura. Hilar nodes are located at the pulmonary hilum, outside the reflection of the pleura.

4.2.1.2
The Peritracheobronchial Nodes

The most important group of nodes is located around the trachea and the main bronchi. They are divided into the following:

- The nodes of the pulmonary pedicles: these lie between the different structures of the pulmonary pedicle from the origin of the bronchus to the mediastinal reflection of the pleura. They are divided into the anterior, posterior, superior and inferior nodes according to their position in relation to the bronchus.
- the subcarinal nodes: these lie within the bifurcation of the trachea.
- the peritracheal nodes:
  a) the right laterotracheal group is located along the anterior and right lateral plane of the trachea within the Barety space: this space is delineated anteriorly by the superior vena cava and the right brachiocephalic trunk, inside by the trachea, the aortic arch, at the top by the subclavian artery and at the bottom by the azygos arch.
  b) the left laterotracheal or recurrent nodes directly follow the recurrent nerve.
  c) the posterior tracheal nodes are small and infrequent, and follow the lymphatic channels connecting the subcarinal nodes to the right laterotracheal nodes.

4.2.1.3
Anterior Mediastinal Groups

These are located in the upper part of the mediastinum in front of the main vessels. They are divided into three groups:

a) the right anterior mediastinal group, which follows the upper diaphragmatic vessels, the superior vena cava and the right brachiocephalic veins from the diaphragm to the base of the neck.
b) the left anterior mediastinal group, which extends from the left pulmonary pedicle to the neck in front of the aortic arch and the left carotid artery.
c) the anterior and transverse group, which follows the left brachiocephalic trunk and connects the left and right anterior groups.

4.2.1.4
The Posterior Mediastinal Nodes

These lie along the esophagus and the thoracic aorta.

In essence, lymph from the right upper lobe drains to the right tracheobronchial lymph nodes, and lymph from the right middle and lower lobes drains to the lobar, interlobar and finally to the hilar, subcarinal, ipsilateral and mediastinal nodes. On the left, lymph from the upper lobe drains not only to the angle of the confluence between the subclavian and internal jugular veins at the same site, but also crosses over to the right lower and upper mediastinum. Lymphatic drainage from both lower lobes can also reach the pulmonary ligament and paraesophageal nodes (Nohl-Oser 1981). The different lymph channels drain the lymph to the jugulosubclavicular vein on the right, or to the thoracic canal. In the case of chest wall involvement, there is a risk of spread to the intercostal nodes located close to the intercostal vessels and nerves; the different lymph vessels reach the thoracic canal except for those of the first space which extend to the supraclavicular region and the subclavian veins. Paravertebral nodes situated either laterally or in front of the vertebral bodies may be located along the pathway of the intercostal lymph collector.

Hata et al. performed an interesting analysis of the different lymphatic pathways by carrying out lymphoscintigraphy in 179 patients without known nodal invasion. For the right lobes, most of the lymph flowed into the right scalene nodes through the subcarinal or right tracheobronchial nodes, but there was some drainage to the left scalene lymph nodes through the subcarinal nodes. In contrast, the lymphatic drainage from the left lung was more variable: the lymph flowed both to the left and right scalene lymph nodes especially in the case of the lower lobe (Fig. 4.1) (Hata et al. 1990).

4.2.2
Classification

The TNM classification divides the nodal stations into three broad categories:

- N1 metastases in the ipsilateral peribronchial and/or ipsilateral hilar lymph nodes.
- N2 metastases in the ipsilateral mediastinal and/or subcarinal lymph nodes.
- N3 metastases in the contralateral mediastinal, contralateral hilar, ipsilateral or contralateral scalene or supraclavicular lymph nodes.

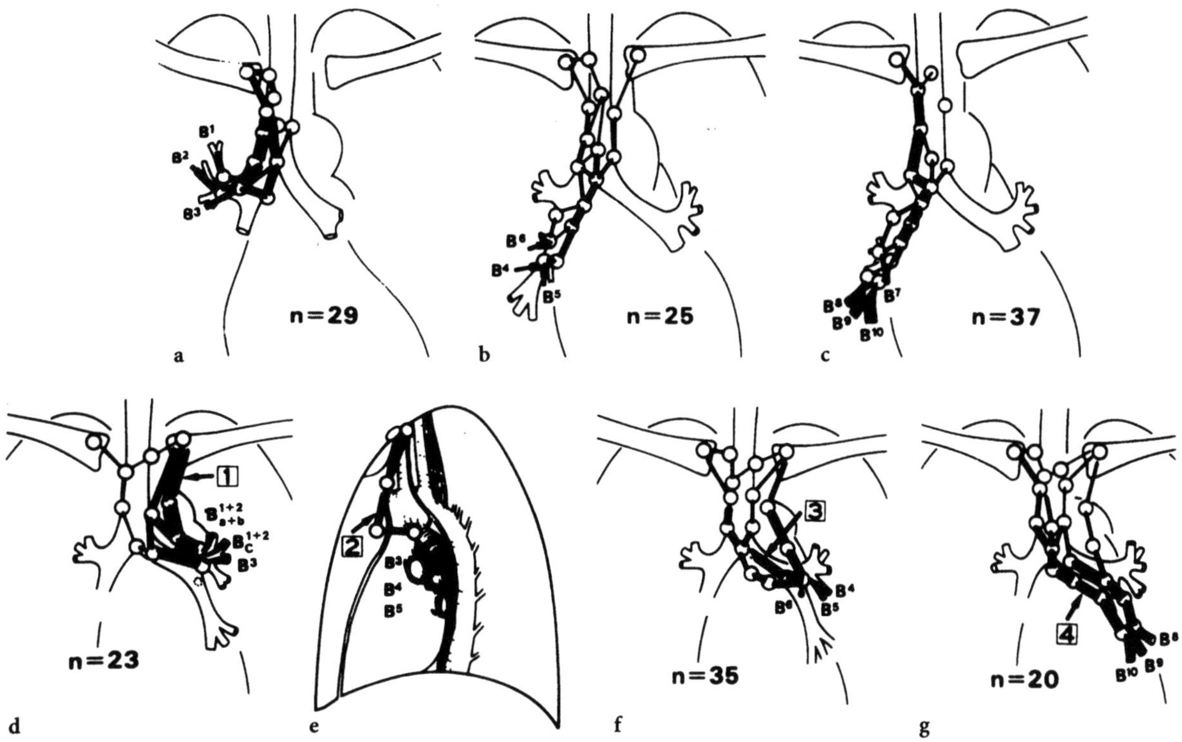

Fig. 4.1. Standard pattern of lymphatic drainage based on 192 lymphoscintigraphies carried out in 179 patients without known nodal dissemination (from HATA et al. 1990)

The location of the lymph nodes within the mediastinum has been described according to the American Thoracic Society's definition (ATS map) modified in 1997 which defines the nodal stations in relation to fixed anatomical structures, allowing a correlation between CT and MRI imaging procedures and surgical findings (MOUNTAIN and DRESLER 1997). The anatomical structures concerned are the trachea, bronchi, aortic arch and other vascular structures (Figs. 4.2, 4.3). This map classifies the lymph nodes into 11 different stations:

- 2R: right upper paratracheal nodes: at the intersection of the caudal margin of the innominate artery with the trachea and the apex of the lung.
- 2L: upper left paratracheal nodes: between the top of the aortic arch and the apex of the lung (supra-aortic nodes).
- 4R: right lower paratracheal nodes: between the intersection of the caudal margin of the innominate artery with the trachea and the cephalic border of the azygos vein.
- 4L: left lower paratracheal nodes: between the top of the aortic arch and the carina (medial to the ligamentum arteriosum).
- 5: aortopulmonary nodes: subaortic and para-aortic nodes lateral to the ligamentum arteriosum (proximal to the first branch of the left pulmonary artery).
- 6: anterior mediastinal nodes: anterior to the ligamentum arteriosum.
- 7: subcarinal nodes: caudal to the carina of the trachea.
- 8: paraesophageal nodes: dorsal to the posterior wall of the trachea and to the right or left of the midline of the esophagus.
- 9: pulmonary ligament nodes: nodes within the inferior pulmonary ligament.
- 10R: right tracheobronchial angle nodes: from the cephalic border of the azygos to the origin of the right upper lobe bronchus.
- 10L: left tracheobronchial angle nodes: between the carina and the left upper lobe of the bronchus (medial to the ligamentum arteriosum).
- 11: interlobar nodes.
- 12: lobar nodes.
- 13: segmental nodes.
- 14: subsegmental nodes.

This lymph node map was developed from that proposed by NARUKE and the Japanese Lung Cancer Society. There are still a number of small differences between both maps: in the NARUKE map, station 1

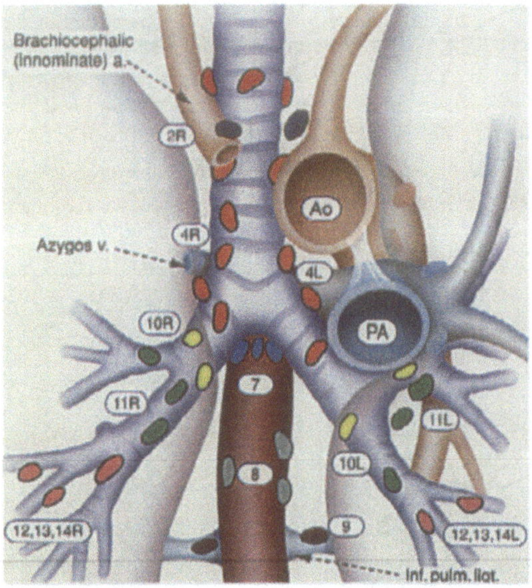

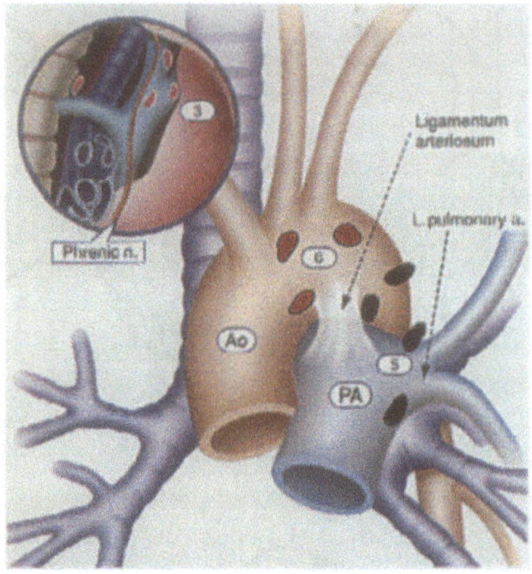

Fig. 4.2. Regional nodal stations for lung cancer: reproduced from MOUNTAIN and DRESLER (with permission of the American College of Chest Physicians)

includes the superior or highest mediastinal nodes, station 3 the anterior or posterior mediastinal nodes, while station 10 represents the hilar nodes. In an interesting study, 20 consecutive patients were subjected to systematic nodal dissection and all nodal stations were separately designated in a blind fashion by one of two European surgeons and one Japanese surgeon. The total concordance was only 60% (WATANABE et al. 2002).

4.3 Detection of Lymph Node Metastasis

4.3.1 Surgical Staging Procedures

Mediastinoscopy is a useful tool for assessing mediastinal lymph node involvement. This procedure should be carried out by an expert thoracic surgeon, capable of performing an emergency thoracotomy or sternotomy in the event of mediastinal damage. It usually requires general anesthesia. A 4-cm incision is made above the sternal notch. After division of the pretracheal fascia, the trachea is exposed and serves as a guide for further finger dissection and endoscopic exploration. Different nodal stations are explored and samples obtained: the superior mediastinal lymph node (station 2), the upper paratracheal (station 2) and the lower paratracheal node (station 4), and the anterior portion of the subcarinal nodes (station 7). In capable hands, this is a very safe procedure without risk of mortality and with very low morbidity: LUKE et al., in a series of 1,000 patients reported 3 cases of severe complications requiring additional surgery and 20 cases of minor problems including pneumothorax, wound infections, and left recurrent nerve damage (LUKE et al. 1986).

For left upper lobe lesions, the subaortic and para-aortic mediastinal nodes may require an anterior mediastinotomy or an extended cervical mediastinoscopy. Video-assisted thoracoscopic surgery (VATS) is a minimally invasive technique which facilitates assessment of the subaortic and para-aortic nodes (stations 5 and 6) as well as the para-esophageal (station 8) and the pulmonary ligament (station 9) nodes. In a selected group of patients, the Memorial Team performed ipsilateral scalene lymph node biopsy at the time of mediastinoscopy using a reversed mediastinoscope. The rate of unexpected scalene node dissemination was 0%, 30% and 80% for pN0, pN2 and mediastinal pN3 respectively (LEE and GINSBERG 1996).

In his series, GOLDSTRAW discovered at thoracotomy unexpected N2 disease in 25% of cases even after a careful staging procedure including CT, mediastinoscopy and even mediastinostomy for enlarged nodes (GOLDSTRAW 1997).

4.3.2 Chest Imaging: CT and MR

The radiological detection of lymph node metastases is based mainly on the demonstration of nodal enlargement. Therefore microscopic metastases cannot be

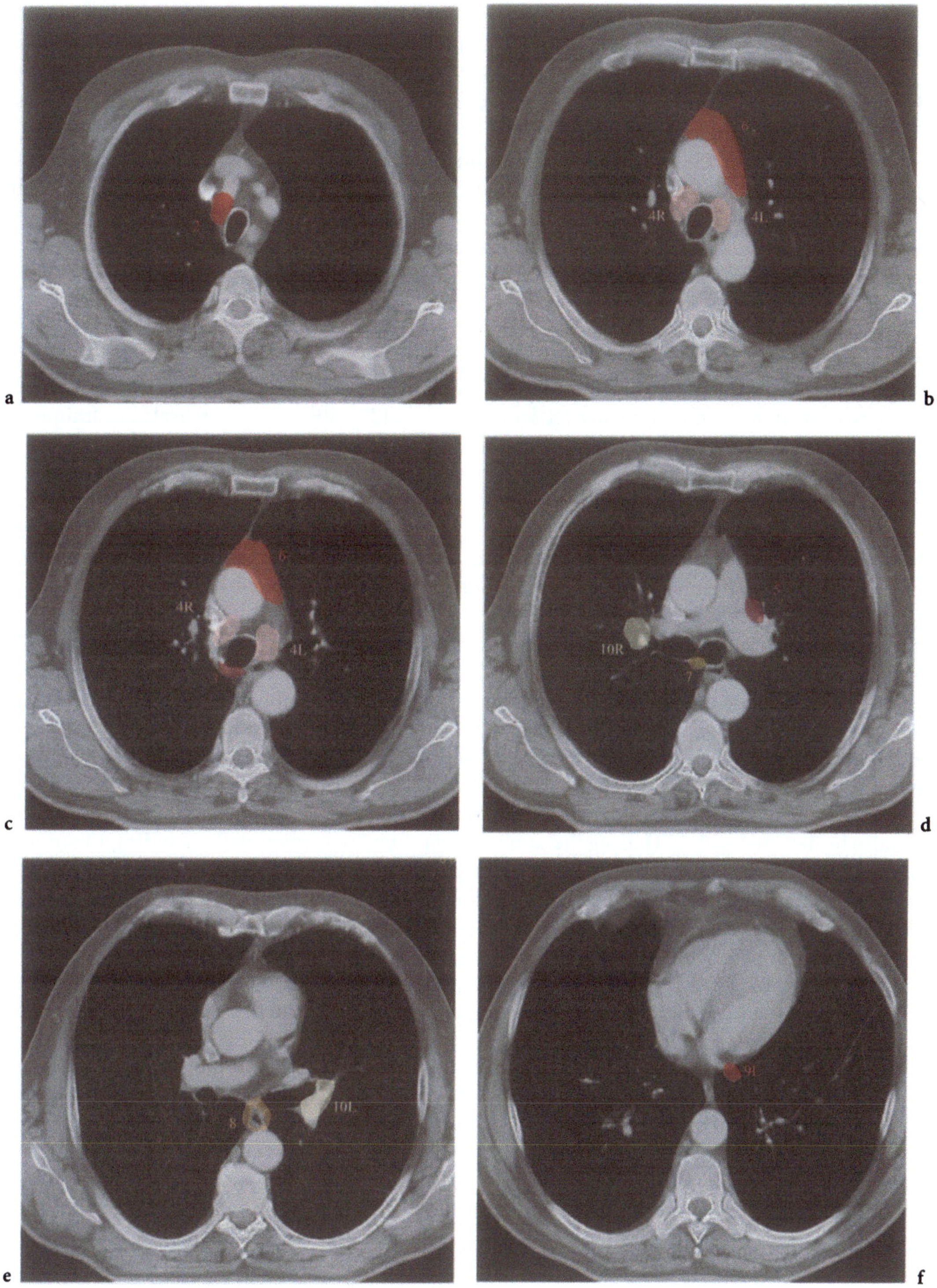

Fig. 4.3. Chest CT with the different regional nodal stations according to MOUNTAIN and DRESLER (with permission of the American College of Chest Physicians)

detected, or major nodal enlargement may be due to benign disease, e.g. infection or to coincidental occupational or granulomatous lung disorders. The choice of the upper limit for normal nodal size is a complex issue, and may vary with nodal position: from 11 mm in the paratracheal to 3 mm in the hilar regions (Hanson and Armstrong 1999). Short axis diameter measurements are widely used to avoid the variation due to node orientation in cross-sectional imaging: a convenient and reasonably easy approach is to use the landmark of 10 mm in the short axis diameter (Glazer et al. 1985). In the study of MacLoud et al., the rate of positive mediastinal lymph node involvement increased from 13% when the node measured less than 1 cm to 62% for nodes of 2 to 2.9 cm (MacLoud et al. 1992). Furthermore, CT specificity according to mediastinal nodal site varied from 72% for station 10R (right hilar) to 94% for station 10L (left hilar) when the criteria for positivity were 10 mm or over (MacLoud et al. 1992). In the presence of obstructive pneumonitis, the rate of false positive lymph node involvement increased to 45%. One way to improve the accuracy of CT is to take into account natural lymphatic drainage: if nodes in the draining territory of the tumor are enlarged (over 10 mm in the short axis) and at least 5 mm larger than nodes in the non-draining territories, CT specificity improves with a positive predictive value of 95% (Buy et al. 1988). Mediastinal node enlargement can also be detected with MRI using the same criteria as for CT scan. Comparative studies have shown little difference between CT and MR imaging techniques.

Nevertheless, the discrepancy between clinical staging including CT with or without mediastinoscopy and pathologically confirmed classification including surgical resection is well known. In a series of 305 patients with clinical N0 disease and tumors smaller than or equal to 3 cm, Asamura et al. observed 24 cases of pN1 disease, 43 cases of ipsilateral mediastinal involvement (pN2) and 1 case of pN3 disease: in fact, 22% of cases showed nodal involvement (Asamura et al. 1996). In the study of Greedo et al., patients underwent thoracotomy only after a negative cervical mediastinoscopy: the nodal status was correctly assessed by CT scan in 35%, overstaged in 44% and understaged in 20% of the patients (Greedo et al. 1997). In the large Heidelberg database, the agreement between clinical and pathological staging regarding nodal status was only 56% (Bulzebruck et al. 1992).

Last but not least, the technique used to obtain good mapping via CT scan implies the use of a helical CT with contiguous slices 5-mm thick or less and a bolus injection of contrast medium to better differentiate the vascular structures. Furthermore, in subjects with atelectasia, the contrast medium may help to delineate the tumor, which in these cases will be less dense. Concerning the mapping of the different nodal stations, CT cannot differentiate between a hilar node and a tracheobronchial angle node (station 10L or R), the limit being the pleural reflection.

4.3.3 PET Scan

Fluorodeoxyglucose-positron emission tomography (FDG-PET) is a very useful technique for evaluating tumor extent in non-small cell lung cancer (NSCLC): the staging appears to be more accurate than that obtained with conventional imaging procedures, including CT scan (Fig. 4.4). Furthermore, without the use of anesthesia, PET allows not only a good staging of lymphatic spread but also that of distant metastases to be obtained. This is not only an anatomical imaging procedure, but it also provides a functional evaluation. In a review of 991 cases from different published series, Vaylet et al. reported the following values: a sensitivity of 86% for PET vs. 59.9% for CT and a specificity of 89.6% vs. 74.6% respectively (Vaylet et al. 2000). These figures are very close to the results of the meta-analysis made by Dwamena et al. including 14 studies of PET (514 patients) and 29 studies of CT performance (2,226 patients): the sensitivity increased from 60% for CT to 79% for PET, and the specificity from 77% to 91% (Dwamena et al. 1999). In a series of 102 patients with resectable non-small cell lung cancer, the staging procedure included CT, liver echography, bone scan and FDG-PET; if indicated, additional imaging procedures and biopsy were performed. The use of PET changed the disease stage in 62 out of 102 patients: the stage was lower in 20 and increased in 42 (Pieterman et al. 2000). In a randomized trial including 188 patients, the addition of PET to a classical staging procedure reduced by 51% the risk of unnecessary thoracotomy due to the presence of more extensive disease, exploratory thoracotomy or early relapse (van Tinteren et al. 2002).

We should, however, be aware of the limits of PET: false-positive or false-negative results may be observed. False-positive lymph node uptake may be seen due to inflammatory processes, anatomical factors or inaccurate localization of uptake: Roberts et al. in a series of 100 patients reported 7 cases of false-positive results for mediastinal uptake, due in 6

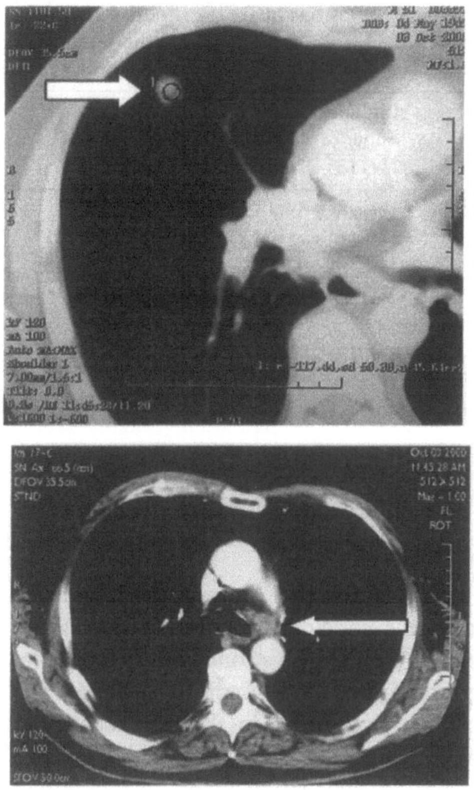

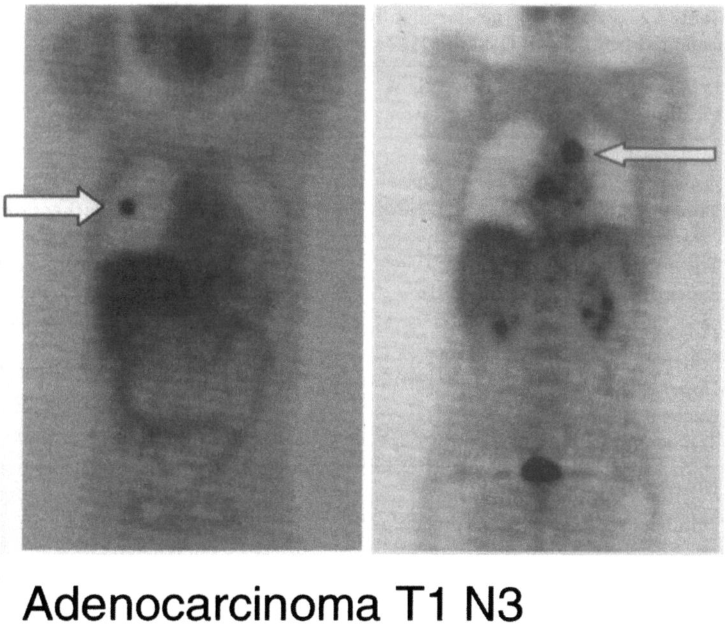

Fig. 4.4. Chest CT of small right lower adenocarcinoma with a positive node in the subaortic window. This is well illustrated by PET showing two hot spots in the right lung and in the mediastinum

cases to inflammatory disease (ROBERTS et al. 2000). False-negative results may be due to minimal tumor involvement of the lymph node. In the large series of VANUYTSEL et al, PET showed no nodal uptake only for 20 out of 859 nodes of normal size on CT, which were resected with confirmed metastatic disease (VANUYTSEL et al. 2000).

4.4 Probability and Pattern of Nodal Involvement

The probability of nodal involvement is directly related to tumor extent or size. In the series of OGATA and NARUKE, the probability of mediastinal nodal involvement increased from 24% for tumors under 2 cm in size to more than 40% for tumors larger than 5 cm (Table 4.1). In a series of 157 patients with small peripheral adenocarcinomas (between 1 and 2 cm in size), 27 patients displayed either hilar or mediastinal metastases (TAKIZAWA et al. 1998).

NOHL-OSER examined the location of nodal involvement in 749 patients based on data obtained via mediastinoscopy, scalene lymph node biopsy and surgical specimens. The right upper lobe tumors spread to the right upper and lower paratracheal and scalene nodes and rarely to the subcarinal nodes or to the contralateral nodes. In contrast, right lower lobe tumors spread to the right tracheobronchial and subcarinal nodes. Left lobe tumors might cross the midline, and the right mediastinal nodes might be invaded (Table 4.2) (NOHL-OSER 1981). OGATA and NARUKE reported similar figures in a surgical series of 434 patients (Table 4.3) (OGATA and NARUKE 1986): the subcarinal nodes were rarely invaded for upper lobe tumors either on the right or on the left side. In contrast to these figures, WATANABE et al. reported a higher number of positive subcarinal nodes when investigating only N2 disease: 36% in a series of 124 patients with upper right lobe tumors (WATANABE et al. 1990).

Table 4.1. Probability of lymph node metastasis in relation to tumor size (adapted from OGATA and NARUKE)

Tumor size (cm)	pN0 (%)	pN1 (%)	pN2 (%)
0–2	57.4	18	24.6
2.1–3	51.9	20.1	27.9
3.1–5	35.4	19.9	44.7
>5	37.3	18.9	43.8
Total no. of patients	277	129	256

Table 4.2. Pattern of mediastinal lymph node metastases (adapted from NOHL-OSER 1981)

Lymph node location	Right upper	Right lower	Left upper	Left lower
Ipsilateral				
Scalene	27	10	13	5
Upper and lower tracheal	78	21	4	0
Tracheobronchial	36	9	46	15
Subcarinal	2	13	9	5
Contralateral				
Scalene	6	3	10	6
Upper and lower tracheal	1	1	10	6
Tracheobronchial	0	0	3	5
No. of patients	230	108	202	68

Numbers are expressed in percentages

Table 4.3. Percentage of positive mediastinal nodes according to tumor location in a series of 434 patients who underwent surgical resection (modified from OGATA and NARUKE 1986)

Nodes	Right upper N=113	Right lower N=108	Left upper N=113	Left lower N=68
Tracheobronchial	16	14.3		11.8
Pretracheal	13.8		6.7	14.3
Paratracheal	15.9	11.1		
Subcarinal	6.3	22.2	2.4	18.5
Para-aortic			16.7	
Subaortic			15.1	19.1

Another issue is the problem of skip metastasis: if a nodal station is negative, what is the probability of discovering positive nodes in another nodal area? GAER and GOLDSTRAW reported 14 cases of positive mediastinal lymph nodes without hilar involvement in a series of 227 patients (GAER and GOLDSTRAW 1990). In contrast to this very low figure, BONNER et al. reviewed the experience of the Mayo Clinic in a series of 336 subjects treated by surgery only: 52 patients (15%) showed involvement of N2 lymph nodes only (BONNER et al. 1999). Risk factors included enlarged mediastinal nodes at CT scan, or T1–T2 lesions. An extensive review of surgical data on skip metastases (pN2 with disease-free hilar lymph nodes following complete mediastinal dissection) has been presented in Table 4.4. Among cases without hilar node dissemination, routine mediastinal dissection revealed 6% unexpected mediastinal lymph node involvement (pN2): each pN2 case would have been missed if mediastinal exploration had not been performed. An average of 34% of pN2 cases have mediastinal dissemination without hilar lymph node involvement. So the sentinel lymph node concept is not an accurate indicator for lung cancer peroperative staging. However, the main drainage pathways are determined for each lobe, and priority should be given to their exploration at the time of thoracotomy, followed by routine mediastinal radical lymphadenectomy (NARUKE 1993).

In contrast to these surgical series, little information is available on patients treated by radiation only. KIRICUTA et al. carried out a retrospective study on pretreatment CT scans of 512 patients who were candidates for radiotherapy (KIRICUTA et al. 1994). On the basis of CT criteria (lymph node larger than 10 mm in the short axis or 15 mm in the long axis), 266 subjects were considered to be node-positive. They correlated their observations with tumor location using a modified ATS mapping scheme. The incidence of positive nodes in the supraclavicular area or in the contralateral hilum was less than 10% (Table 4.5). In their study, using an irradiation volume modified according to nodal extent based on CT observations, none of the patients with positive supraclavicular or contralateral hilar nodes survived more than 2 years post-treatment.

Table 4.4. Skip metastases from mediastinal lymph nodes in surgical series (patients without any pathologically determined N1 nodes)

Authors	All patient groups (%)	Only the pN2 group (%)
MARTINI et al. (1983)		27
ISHIDA et al. (1990)	10	41
NARUKE et al. (1993)		31.5
ARITA et al. (1995)		21
ASAMURA et al. (1996)	5.3	25
YOSHINO et al. (1996)		30
TAKIZAWA et al. (1997)	5.5	33
TAKIZAWA et al. (1998)	2.2	
ODA et al. (1998)	5	70
OKADA et al. (1998)		37.6
SAGAWA et al. (1999)		43
BONNER et al. (1999)		41
GRAHAM et al. (1999)	9.3	34
ASAMURA et al. (1999)		25
Mean	6.2%	34%

Results are expressed in percentage of all groups of patients without pathologically determined N1 disease or only for pathologically determined N2 disease

Table 4.5. Incidence of positive lymph nodes for NSCLC based on CT data (Adapted from KIRICUTA et al. 1994)

	Tumor location	
	Right	Left
No. of patients	161	105
Supraclavicular		
Right	8.6	9.5
Left	1.8	3.8
Upper mediastinal	0.6	0
Paratracheal		
Right	19.9	5.7
Left	2.5	6.7
Lower tracheobronchial		
Right	77	43.8
Left	30.4	76.2
Hilar		
Right	34.2	4.8
Left	3.7	41.9
Anterior tracheal	27.3	25.7
Subcarinal	50.9	44.8

Numbers are expressed in percentages

4.5 What Have We Learnt from Surgical Series?

The probability of locoregional relapse is directly correlated with tumor stage. It varies from less than 10% for pathologically determined stage I disease to 20% or more for stage III disease after complete resection (Table 4.6). The study of SAWYER et al. is intriguing: in a series of 370 patients operated on for pathologically determined stage I disease, the actuarial risk at 5 years of local recurrence was only 15%, but three factors had a significant association with local failure: the number of lymph nodes dissected and pathologically evaluated (at least 15); more limited resection than lobectomy; and T2 tumors (SAWYER et al. 1999). The first two factors concern the issue of skip metastases, the quality of the surgical procedure and the Lung Cancer Study Group trial. Indeed, the Lung Cancer Study Group conducted a randomized trial on T1N0 tumors to compare lobectomy to more limited resection (segmentectomy or wedge resection): 247 patients were included in this study, which demonstrated a clear benefit in terms of locoregional recurrence and survival in favor of patients randomized to lobectomy. The locoregional recurrence rate of 17% after limited resection dropped to 5% after lobectomy (GINSBERG and RUBINSTEIN 1995).

Table 4.6. Pattern of failure after surgery for lung cancer

Authors	Tumor stage	No. of patients	Local failure (%)
MARTINI (1977)	T1–T2 N0	110	0
PAIROLERO et al. (1984)	T1 N0	170	6
	T2 N0	158	6
FELD et al. (1984)	T1 N0	162	9
	T2 N0	196	11
LAFFITE et al. (1996)	T2 N0	70	14
LUNG CANCER STUDY GROUP (1986)	N1–N2	108	20
IMMERMAN et al. (1981)	T1–T2 N0	77	12
	T1–T2 N1	22	41
SAWYER (1999)	T1–T2 N0	370	15
STEPHENS et al. (1996)	T1–T2 N1	91	49
	T1–T2 N2	54	41

Another question is that of the impact of mediastinal clearance by surgery. Is it useful or not to perform a complete dissection of the different mediastinal lymph nodes? This question may be of interest to the radiation oncologist in regard to the extent of the CTV, which should include all microscopic tumor extension. In the study of SAWYER et al., the number of lymph nodes removed had a direct influence on survival (SAWYER et al. 1999). Furthermore, an interesting observation was made in the ECOG trial which included patients with completely resected stage II and IIIa disease who were randomized to treatment by mediastinal irradiation with or without chemotherapy. Stratification factors included radical mediastinal lymph node dissection versus systematic sampling. The latter included the removal of at least one lymph node at levels 4, 7 and 10 during right thoracotomy; and at levels 5 and/or 6 and 7 during left thoracotomy, whereas the former approach required the complete removal of all lymph nodes at those levels. Among the 222 patients with N2 disease, multiple levels of N2 were documented in 30% of patients with complete mediastinal dissection compared to 12% in the systematic sampling patient group. In this nonrandomized comparison between a radical mediastinal lymph node dissection and a simple sampling, the radical dissection led to a survival benefit for patients with right side lung tumors (KELLER et al. 2000). Three trials investigated the question of the usefulness of radical systemic mediastinal lymphadenectomy. One hundred and sixty-nine patients were randomized between lymph node sampling and systematic mediastinal dissection. No difference in overall survival was found, although the number of local recurrences was reduced after mediastinal dissection. Nevertheless, mediastinal dissection resulted in better local control and improved survival for patients with pathologically determined N1 or limited N2 disease: the local recurrence rate of 44.8% after systematic sampling dropped to 29% after radical dissection (Izbicki et al. 1998). In the trial of Yi-Long et al., 471 patients were randomized between systematic nodal dissection and mediastinal lymph node sampling: the median survival of 34 months following mediastinal lymph node sampling increased to 59 months after systematic nodal dissection. This was mainly observed for stage I and IIIa disease (Yi-Long et al. 2002). A similar trend was observed in a small trial including 94 patients (Passlick et al. 2002).

4.6 Clinical Target Volume for Non-small Cell Lung Cancer

The optimal CTV remains a controversial issue in lung cancer treatment, especially as regards the extent of prophylactic nodal irradiation. In the 1970s and 1980s, there was a trend in favor of "large" radiation fields covering all the mediastinal nodes, the contralateral hilum and both supraclavicular areas. This approach was based on a double assumption, i.e. that some patients with nodal involvement might be cured due to the high efficacy of radiation treatment in controlling microscopic disease; and that the spread of disease to the lymph nodes occurred in an orderly fashion. The retrospective study of Choi and Doucette and the radiation quality audit of the RTOG protocol 73–01 supported this hypothesis (Choi and Doucette 1981; Perez et al. 1982). In the latter study, the survival of patients with a normal contralateral hilum was improved when the hilar regions were well included in the radiation fields: median survival increased from 22 weeks to 50 weeks (Perez et al. 1982). We should recall that this trial was largely conducted during a period when CT scan was not routinely performed.

Several surveys of radiation practice have outlined a wide variation in the CTV used by radiation oncologists but also in that reported between studies. There was a general trend to limit prophylactic nodal irradiation by omitting either the contralateral hilum and/or the supraclavicular areas except for upper lobe tumors (Van Houtte et al. 1994, 1998, 1999). In a recent review of different RTOG protocols including more than 1,700 patients, Emami et al. made the following observations: a worse prognosis was only observed if the margins around the ipsilateral hilum were inadequate; and if the doses delivered to the ipsilateral hilar or to the mediastinal lymph nodes were below those specified by the protocol (Emami et al. 1996). Last but not least, a careful pattern of failure analysis has clearly demonstrated that the main issue remains the local control of gross disease: in several randomized studies, local control has been reported to remain below 20% (Arriagada et al. 1991; Saunders et al. 1999).

The practice of radiation oncology is governed by the existence of a dose-response, and more particularly of a tumor-size dose-response relationship. From the original findings of G. Fletcher, it is generally accepted that for most epithelial tumors, the dose required to eradicate microscopic disease is around 50 Gy, and that for a tumor measuring 1 to 3 cm between 65 and 75 Gy. So it is clear that a T2 bronchogenic carcinoma is already greater than 3 cm; the standard radiation doses are far too low to be able to adequately treat a large number of patients suffering from this dreadful disease.

Several avenues were explored in the 1990s to improve these poor results, either by increasing the physical or the biological dose. The question arises of whether we are certain that more aggressive treatment is better than the conventional radiotherapeutic approach. The best illustration certainly is that of the results obtained in a randomized trial testing the accelerated radiation schedule, i.e. continuous hyperfractionated accelerated radiotherapy (CHART): the use of this technique statistically improved survival compared to the 60 Gy schedule. The 2- and 3-year survival rates were 21% and 13% after 60 Gy and 30 and 20% after CHART therapy respectively; the 3-year local control rate increased from 12% to 17%. This improvement in local control also led to a lesser incidence of distant metastases: the 3-year metastasis-free survival rates increased from 33% for the standard 60 Gy schedule to 40% for CHART (Saunders et al. 1999). Therapeutic benefit was mainly observed for cases of squamous cell carcinoma.

Thoracic irradiation represents a challenge to the radiation oncologist due to the limited tolerance of many major organs including the lungs, heart, spinal cord and even the esophagus. Any extension of margin or volume of elective nodal irradiation increases the amount of normal tissue, especially the esophagus and the lungs, that is exposed to radiation. Dose-volume histogram analysis (DVH) has shown a relation between the volume of normal lung receiving doses in excess of 20 Gy and the risk of subsequent radiation-induced pneumonitis. In the study made by Graham et al., no case of grade 3 pneumonitis was observed when less than 25% of the lung received more than 20 Gy; this rate amounted to 23%

when the volume was greater than 40% (GRAHAM et al. 1999). In contrast, by limiting the CTV to the gross tumor volume (GTV), the amount of normal lung spared allows a dose escalation to be included of about 30% without an increase in the probability of radiation-induced pneumonitis (BELDERBOS et al. 1997). Another problem is certainly that of acute esophagitis, a dose-limiting factor, especially in the case of an accelerated radiation procedure or in a situation involving drugs combined with radiation. Grade 3 esophageal toxicity implies a state of severe dysphagia with a weight loss of over 15% that requires artificial alimentation. In the BALL et al. trial, in which 60 Gy were delivered over 3 weeks at two fractions per day, either without or with one injection of carboplatin, 30% of the patients experienced grade 3 esophagitis (BALL et al. 1995).

The current trend is to design more aggressive radiation treatment using accelerated schedules, increasing the total dose with a 3D conformal approach, or combining radiation with concurrent chemotherapy. The extent of elective nodal irradiation tends to be increasingly reduced. During the First International Workshop on Prognostic and Predictive Factors in Lung Cancer, the following guidelines were proposed:

- CTV for involved nodes consists of a 1-cm margin of normal tissue around the involved hilar lymph nodes, a 2-cm circumferential and a 2.5-cm craniocaudal margin for the coverage of one sentinel node station beyond the involved mediastinal lymph nodes.
- An additional margin of 0.7 is added to the CTV to take into account setup error and patient motion.

Thus, for example, the nodal CTV for involved mediastinal nodes at stations 7 and 4R should include stations 4L, 5, 6 2R and 2L (CHOI et al. 2001). Another approach is to use software that evaluates the risk of mediastinal node involvement according to individual parameters; GIRAUD et al. have developed a program that includes the following parameters: primary tumor location, histology, T and N stage (GIRAUD et al. 2001).

Current 3-D conformal radiotherapy studies using doses in excess of 70 Gy have suggested the feasibility of this approach. Pattern of failure analysis has outlined that most relapses occur within the initial GTV, and nodal failures are rarely observed (ARMSTRONG et al. 1997; GRAHAM et al. 1999; ROZENSWEIG et al. 1999; SIBLEY et al. 1998). Nevertheless, in these studies the intended CTV was usually strictly limited to the initial GTV, but incidental doses to the adjacent uninvolved nodal stations within the mediastinum are also relevant. In a series of 10 patients with stage IIIa or b disease, irradiated to doses above 69 Gy, MARTEL et al. reported the percentage for the different nodal stations receiving at least 50 Gy as follows: ipsilateral hilum 100%; contralateral hilum 40%; subcarinal 96%; inferior paratracheal 68%; superior paratracheal 0%, the aortopulmonary nodes 57% (MARTEL et al. 1999). ROZENSWEIG et al. reported their own experience in a series of 132 patients treated with 3D conformal radiotherapy: the 2-year rates for elective nodal control and local control were 92% and 40% respectively. Only 8 patients showed elective nodal failure, underlining that local control of the GTV remains the main issue (ROZENSWEIG et al. 1999) (Table 4.7). In his series, 6 cases of failure were observed in supraclavicular areas, a figure very close to the 3% observed in a prospective trial by PIGGOT and SAUNDERS (1993). In the past, the inclusion of a supraclavicular field was justified as a measure of preventing relapse without additional toxicity: in the RTOG trial 73–01, the failure rate of 8% in the absence of irradiation dropped to 2% for doses in excess of 45 Gy (PEREZ et al. 1987). Tide margins may expose the subject to the risk of geographical error and possibly with improved gross tumor control, the issue of limited versus widespread nodal irradiation may provide a new subject of investigation.

Table 4.7. Pattern of failure after 3D conformal radiotherapy limited to the GTV (adapted from ROZENSWEIG et al. 1999)

Elective nodal region	No. of patients	Median dose (Gy)	Patients receiving >40 Gy (%)	No. of failures
Ipsilateral Supraclavicular	125	0	8	2
Contralateral Supraclavicular	132	0	0	4
Ipsilateral sup. Mediastinum	115	18	34	0
Contralateral sup. Mediastinum	129	5	8	1
Subcarinal	91	33	41	2
Ipsilateral inf. Mediastinum	59	60	63	2
Contralateral inf. Mediastinum	121	18	21	2

Stage I disease often represents a challenge for radiation oncologists. The patients involved are frequently referred for further treatment as a result of medical contraindications regarding classical treatment, i.e. surgery. Poor lung function is a common reason for avoiding surgical resection. The issue in these cases is whether the CTV should be limited to the primary tumor in the absence of CT evidence of nodal involvement, or whether the hilar and mediastinal nodes should be treated prophylactically. Table 4.8 summarizes data from the literature showing 5-year survival rates ranging from 5% to 31% without the major influence of elective nodal irradiation. When irradiation was restricted to the primary tumor, the incidence of relapse in the regional nodes as the first and only site of failure was low: in the series of Slotman et al., including 31 patients, three locoregional recurrences were observed; in the study of Krol et al., 50 patients achieved complete remission at the primary site and 4 developed loco-regional failure including 2 nodal relapses; and in the study of Cheung et al., which included 102 patients, 4 patients experienced regional failure (Cheung et al. 2000; Krol et al. 1996; Slotman et al. 1996). In a series of 132 patients treated in different European centers, 6 patients displayed mediastinal relapse: one of them only had isolated mediastinal relapse (Gouders et al. 2000). These figures are very close to the data reported in surgical series: locoregional relapse has been reported in the range of 0% to 14% for T1 and T2 N0 tumors (Table 4.8). In contrast, Morita et al. reported improved results following elective hilar/mediastinal irradiation: the 5-year survival rate amounted to 31.3% with elective irradiation vs. 14.9% after limited irradiation (Morita et al. 1997). However, patients with untreated nodes were more likely to have adenocarcinomas and tumors located in the lower lobe (in these instances, treatment was often limited to the primary tumor to avoid excessive toxicity to the large field). In the Sibley et al. study, prophylactic mediastinal irradiation resulted in improved local control at 2 years follow-up, but not in a statistically better overall survival (Sibley et al. 1998). Therefore, the inclusion of at-risk nodal regions may be useful in treating a subset of patients, but should be weighed against the possible drawbacks. The treatment should therefore be adapted to patient needs (lung function) and to tumor location. A small tumor located close to the mediastinum may be a suitable candidate for nodal irradiation, whereas this is certainly not the case for a peripheral lesion: a large amount of normal lung will be destroyed. The main question regarding these patients remains our ability to improve local control by more aggressive treatment. This is well illustrated by a subset analysis of the CHART trial: amongst 169 patients with stage I or II disease, the 4-year survival rate increased from 12% after 60 Gy in 6 weeks to 18% after a CHART schedule (Bentzen et al. 2000).

In any case, PET is being increasingly used in daily practice, including our treatment plan especially as regards the differentiation of normal or abnormal nodes. Several interesting studies have been reported during recent years. PET scan is a useful tool for treatment planning, especially in the case of atelectasia; it is often not an easy task to differentiate diseased tissue from normal tissue. In the retrospective evaluation made by Kiffer et al., the impact of PET on the anterior-posterior radiation volumes was reviewed in a series of 15 patients: in 3 patients with a poorly demarcated tumor mass, PET defined primary lesions

Table 4.8. Irradiation for early NSCLC: influence of an elective mediastinal irradiation

Authors	No. of pts	Radiation scheme Gy	Radiation scheme weeks	Elective nodal irradiation	Survival rate (%) 3 years	Survival rate (%) 5 years
Burt et al. (1989)	133	50–55	3	No		20
Cheung et al. (2000)	102	48	4	No	35	16
Coy and Kennely (1980)	141	50–57	4	Yes	18	10
Dosoretz et al. (1992)	152	50–70	5–7	Yes		10
Gauden et al. (1995)	347	50	4	Yes		27
Gouders et al. (2000)	123	40–70		Yes (59%)	18	5
Graham et al. (1995)	150	60	6	Yes		14
Krol et al. (1996)	108	60–65	6–7s	No	31	15
Morita et al. (1997)	66	55–74	6–7	Yes		31
	83			No		15
Noordijk et al. (1988)	50	60	6–7s	No	16	
Sandler et al. (1990)	77	60	6	Yes	21	17
Sibley et al. (1998)	141	64	5–7	Yes (73%)		13
Zhang et al. (1989)	44	55–70	6–7	Yes		16

s: Split course

that extended beyond the radiation margins, whereas a good agreement was found for 12 well-defined tumors (Kiffer et al. 1998). In a study involving 34 patients, Nestle et al. reported that in 12 cases the treated volume was modified after PET exploration; this was more marked in the presence of atelectasia: 8 out of 17 patients vs. 3 out of 17 subjects without atelectasia (Nestle et al. 1999). An interesting study was also conducted by Vanuytsel et al: in a series of 105 patients operated on for NSCLC; they were able to obtain imaging studies including PET and CT scans, as well as a precise surgical mapping. For 73 patients with positive lymph nodes, a theoretical GTV was defined based on CT and PET scans. A total of 988 lymph node stations were available for review. When the nodes were not enlarged on CT scan (equal to or more than 1.5 cm at maximal cross-sectional diameter), PET findings displayed 20 false-negative findings amongst 859 nodes and 6 false-positive results amongst 33 nodes. The figures for enlarged nodes on CT scan were respectively: 5 false-negative out of 45 nodes, and 14 false positive for 51 nodes. Based on these data, the CT defined volume was identical to that of the PET-CT defined volume in 28 patients. Additional PET altered the treatment volumes in the remaining 45 patients. In 16 patients the PET-CT volume was larger, and this was proven to be correct by surgical investigation in 11 patients, whereas it was found to be insufficient in four patients, and unnecessary in one patient. In 29 patients, the PET-CT volume was smaller, and in 25 cases this modified volume was proven to be correct, whereas the coverage was still insufficient for 3 patients. Therefore, GTV defined via PET-CT was found to be incorrect for 8 patients; this was due to findings in 3 patients with only minimal lymph node metastases, and 5 cases of misinterpretation of the exact localization of the positive nodes (Vanuytsel et al. 2000).

To conclude this review, we would like to re-examine the consensus meeting held in Annecy in 1998. The group of experts made the following 3 recommendations regarding the issue of target volume definition:

1. GTV identification requires the injection of contrast medium. Therefore, contrast i.v. (bolus) injection should be used during dosimetric CT acquisition if a diagnostic CT scan with contrast is not available for proper identification of mediastinal opacities. This issue is certainly well illustrated by a study conducted in Australia and New Zealand; 14 radiation oncologists were asked to draw their GTV and CTV on 12 sample cases. In 25% of cases, normal structure was considered as tumor-associated; there was a frequent misinterpretation by the clinician of normal structures such as the superior vena cava or the pulmonary artery, but the CT images were taken with a variable amount of contrast (Denham et al. 1993).
2. Because tumor metastases can be present in the primary tumor itself as well as in the lymph nodes, it might be helpful to distinguish between a GTV(t) for the primary and GTV(n) for enlarged and therefore supposedly involved nodes.
3. "Prophylactic" nodal irradiation, i.e., inclusion of mediastinal nodes in CTV, is a desirable and probably useful approach, particularly in cases of centrally located tumors, but should be weighed against NTCP, patient performance status, and other factors relevant to survival and quality of life (Scalliet et al. 1998).

4.7 Conclusions

The optimal target volume for NSCLC remains a controversial issue, but there is a general trend toward reducing the target volume, in contrast to the recommendations made in the 1970s and 1980s. Further reports on patterns of failure are necessary to clarify this problem. Furthermore, the introduction of PET in treatment planning may prove to be a very helpful tool, and may be able to assist us in determining an optimal solution. Until now, the main concern has been that of the local control of the GTV. Elective nodal irradiation has now become a secondary issue. The main issue remains that of providing more aggressive treatment approaches (i.e., 3D conformal radiotherapy, accelerated hyperfractionated schedules; concurrent chemotherapy, surgery) for well-selected patients based on different prognostic factors; this may help to improve both the survival and the quality of life in this patient population.

References

Arita T, Kuramitsu T, Kawamura M, Matsumoto T, Matsunaga N, Sugi K, Esato K (1995) Bronchogenic carcinoma: incidence of metastases to normal size lymph nodes. Thorax 50:1267

Armstrong J, Raben A, Zelefsky M, Burt M, Leibel S, Burman C, Kutcher G, Harrison L, Hahn C, Ginsberg R, Rusch V, Kris M, Fuks Z (1997) Promising survival with three-dimensional conformal radiation therapy for non-small cell lung cancer. Radiother Oncol 44:17

Arriagada R, Le Chevalier T, Quoix E, Ruffie P, De Cremoux H, Douillard JY, Tarayre M, Pignon JP, Laplanche A (1991) Effect of chemotherapy on locally advanced non-small lung carcinoma: a randomized study of 353 patients. Int J Radiat Oncol Biol Phys 20:1183

Asamura H, Nakayama H, Kondo H, Tsuchiya R, Shimosato Y, Naruke T (1996) Lymph node involvement, recurrence and prognosis in resected small, peripheral non-small-cell lung carcinomas: are these carcinomas candidates for video-assisted lobectomy? J Thorac Cardiovasc Surg 111:1125

Asamura H, Nakayama H, Kondo H, Tsuchiya R, Naruke T (1999) Lobe-specific extent of systematic lymph node dissection for non-small cell carcinomas according to a retrospective study of metastasis and prognosis. j Thorac Cardiovasc Surg 117:1102

Ball D, Bishop J, Smith J, Crennan E, O'Brien P, Davis S, Ryan G, Joseph D, Walker Q (1995) A phase III study of accelerated radiotherapy with and without carboplatin in non-small cell lung cancer: an interim toxicity analysis of the first 100 patients. Int J Radiat Oncol Biol Phys 31:267

Belderbos JSA, Lebesque JV, Barillot I (1997) Normal tissue complication probabilities for irradiation of NSCLC patients with and without elective nodal irradiation. Lung Cancer 18:126

Bentzen SM, Saunders MI, Dische S, Parmar MK (2000) Updated data for CHART in NSCLC: further analyses. Radiother Oncol 55:86

Bonner JA, Garces YI, Gould PM, Foote RL, Deschamps C, Lange CM, Li H (1999) Frequency of noncontiguous lymph node involvement in patients with resectable non-small cell lung carcinoma. Cancer 86:1159

Bulzebruck H, Bopp P, Drings R, Bauer E, Krysa S, Probst G, van Kaick G, Muller KM, Vogt-Moykopf I (1992) New aspects in the staging of lung cancer. Prospective validation of the International Union Against Cancer TNM classification. Cancer 70:1102

Burt PA, Hancock BM, Stout R (1989) Radical radiotherapy for carcinoma of the bronchus: an equal alternative to radical surgery? Clin Oncol 1:86

Buy JN, Ghossain MA, Poirson F (1988) Computed tomography of mediastinal lymph nodes in non-small cell lung cancer: a new approach based on the lymphatic pathway of tumor spread. J Comput Assist Tomogr 12:545

Cheung PC, Mackillop WJ, Dixon P, Brundage MD, Youssef YM, Zhou S (2000) Involved-field radiotherapy alone for early stage non-small cell lung cancer. Int J Radiat Oncol Biol Phys 48:703

Choi NC, Doucette JA (1981) Improved survival of patients with resectable non-small cell bronchogenic carcinoma by an innovative high dose en bloc radiotherapeutic approach. Cancer 48:101

Choi N, Baumann M, Flentjie M, Kellokumpu-Lehtinen P, Senan S, Zamboglou N, Kosmidis P (2001) Predictive factors in radiotherapy for non-small cell lung cancer: present status. Lung Cancer 31:43

Coy P, Kennelly GM (1980) The role of curative radiotherapy in the treatment of lung cancer. Cancer 45:698

Denham JW, Hamilton CS, Joseph DJ, Lamb DS, Spry NA, Gray AJ, Atkinson CH, Wynne CJ, Abdelaal A, Bydder PV, Chapman PJ, Matthews JHL, Stevens G, Ball DL, Kearsley J, Ashcroft JB, Janke P, Gutmann A (1993) The use of simulator and CT information in the planning of radiotherapy for non-small cell lung cancer: an Australian patterns of practice study. Lung Cancer 8:275

Dosoretz DE, Katin MJ, Blitzer PH, Rubenstein JH, Salenius S, Rashid M, Dosani RA, Mestas G, Siegel AD, Chadha TT, Chandrahasa T, Hannan SE, Bhat SB, Metke M (1992) Radiation therapy in the management of medically inoperable carcinoma of the lung: results and implications for future treatment strategies. Int J Radiat Oncol Biol Phys 24:3

Dwamena BA, Sonnad SS, Angobaldo JO, Wahl RL (1999) Metastases from non-small cell lung cancer: mediastinal staging in the 1990s – metaanalytic comparison of PET and CT. Radiology 213:530

Emami B, Scitt C, Byhardt R, Graham MV, Andras EJ, John M, Herskovic A, Urtasun RC, Asbell SO, Perez CA, Cox J (1996) The value of regional nodal radiotherapy (dose/volume) in the treatment of unresectable non-small cell lung cancer: an RTOG analysis. Int J Radiat Oncol Biol Phys 36 [Suppl 1]:209

Feld R, Rubinstein LV, Weisenberger TH, the Lung Cancer Study Group (1984) Sites of recurrence in resected stage I non small cell lung cancer: a guide for future studies. J Clin Oncol 2:1352

Gaer JA, Goldstraw P (1990) Intraoperative asssessment of nodal staging at thoracotomy for carcinoma of the bronchus. Eur J Cardio Thorac Surg 4:207

Gauden S, Ramsay J, Tripciony L (1995) The curative treatment by radiotherapy alone of stage I non-small cell lung cancer. Chest 108:1278

Ginsberg RJ, Rubinstein LV (1995) Lung Cancer Study Group Randomized trial of lobectomy versus limited resection for T1N0 non-small cell lung cancer. Ann Thorac Surg 60:615

Giraud P, De Rycke Y, Minet P, Danhier S, Dubray B, Helfre S, Dauphinot C, Rosenwald JC, Cosset JM (2001) Estimation de la probabilité d'envahissement tumoral médiastinal: une définition statistique du volume-cible anatomoclinique pour la radiothérapie conformationnelle des cancers bronchiques non à petites cellules? Cancer Radiother 5:725

Glazer GM, Gross BH, Quint LE, Francis IR, Bookstein FL, Orringer MB (1985) Normal mediastinal lymph nodes: number and size according to the American Thoracic Society mapping. Am J Roentgenol 144:261

Goldstraw P (1997) Report on the International workshop on intrathoracic staging London October 1996. Lung Cancer 18:107

Gouders D, Maingon P, Rodrigus P, Hahn B, Arnaiz M.D, Nguyen T, Landmann C, Bosset J.F, Danhier S, Van Houtte P (2000) Exclusive radiotherapy for inoperable stage I non-small cell lung cancer (NSCLC): a multicentric study. Lung Cancer 29 [Suppl 1]:166

Graham AN, Chan KJ, Pastorino U, Goldstraw P (1999) Systematic nodal dissection in the intrathoracic staging of patients with non-small cell lung cancer. J Thorac Cardiovasc Surg 117:246

Graham PH, Gebski VJ, Langlands AO (1995) Radical radiotherapy for early non-small cell lung cancer. Int J Radiat Oncol Biol Phys 31:261–266

Graham MV, Purdy JA, Emami B, Harms W, Bosch W, Lockett MA, Perez CA (1999) Clinical dose-volume histogram analysis for pneumonitis after 3D treatment of non-small cell lung cancer. Int J Radiat Oncol Biol Phys 45:323

Greedo A, Van Schil P, Corthouts B, Van Miegheme F, Van Meerbeeck J, Van Marck E (1997) Comparison of imaging TNM (iTNM) and pathological TNM (pTNM) in staging of bronchogenic carcinoma. Eur J Cardiothorac Surg 12:224

Hanson JA, Armstrong P (1999) Radiological evaluation of intrathoracic extension and resectability of non-small cell lung cancer. In: Van Houtte P, Klastersky J, Rocmans P (eds) Progress and perspectives in lung cancer. Springer, Berlin Heidelberg New York, pp 23–38
Hata E, Hayakawa K, Miyamoto H, Hayashida R (1990) Rationale for extended lymphadenectomy for lung cancer. Theor Surg 5:19
Immerman SC, Vanecko RM, Fry WA, Shields TW (1981) Site of recurrence in patients with stages I and II carcinoma of the lung resected for cure. Ann Thorac Surg 32:23
Ishida T, Yano T, Maeda K, Kaneko S, Tateishi M, Sugimachi K (1990) Strategy for lymphadenectomy in lung cancer three centimeters or less in diameter. Ann Thorac Surg 50:708
Izbicki JR, Passlick B, Pantel K, Pitchmeier U, Hosch SB, Karg O, Thetter O (1998) Effectiveness of radical systematic mediastinal lymphadenectomy in patients with resectable non-small cell lung cancer. Results of a prospective randomized trial. Ann Surg 227:138
Keller SM, Adak S, Wagner H, Johnson DH (2000) Mediastinal lymph node dissection improves survival in patients with stages II and IIIa non-small cell lung cancer. Eastern Cooperative Oncology Group. Ann Thorac Surg 70:358
Kiffer JD, Berlangieri SU, Scott AM, Quong G, Feigen M, Schumer W, Clarke P, Knight SR, Daniel FJ (1998)The contribution of 18F-fluoro-2-deoxy-glucose positron emission tomographic imaging to radiotherapy planning in lung cancer. Lung Cancer 19:167
Kiricuta IC, Mueller G, Stiess J, Bohndorf W (1994) The lymphatic pathways of non-small cell lung cancer and their implication in curative irradiation treatment. Lung Cancer 11:71
Krol ADG, Aussems P, Noordijk EM, Hermans J, Leer JWH (1996) Local irradiation alone for peripheral stage I lung cancer: could we omit the elective regional nodal irradiation? Int J Radiat Oncol Biol Phys 34:297
Lafitte J, Ribert ME, Prévost BM, Gosselin BH, Copin MC, Brichet AH (1996) Postresection irradiation for T2NOMO non-small cell carcinoma: a prospective, randomized study. Ann Thorac Surg 62:830
Lee JD, Ginsberg RJ (1996) Lung cancer staging – the value of ipsilateral scalene lymph node biopsy obtained at mediastinoscopy. Ann Thorac Surg 62:338
Luke WP, Pearson FG, Todd TRJ, Patterson GA, Cooper JD (1986) Prospective evaluation of mediastinoscopy for assessment of carcinoma of the lung. J Thorac Cardiovasc Surg 91:53
Lung Cancer Study Group (1986) Effects of postoperative mediastinal radiation on completely resected stage II and stage III epidermoid cancer of the lung. N Engl J Med 315:1377
MacLoud TC, Bourgouin PM, Greenberg RW, Kosiuk JP, Templeton PA, Shepard JA, Moore EH, Wain JC, Mathisen DJ, Grillo HC (1992) Bronchogenic carcinoma: analysis of staging in the mediastinum with CT by correlative lymph node mapping and sampling. Radiology 182:319
Martel MK, Strawderman M, Hazuka MB, Turrisi AT, Fraass BA, Lichter AS (1997) Volume and dose parameters for survival of non-small cell lung cancer patients. Radiother Oncol 44:23
Martel MK, Sahijdak WM, Hayman JA, Ball D (1999) Incidental dose to clinically negative nodes from conformal treatment fields for non-small cell lung cancer. Int J Radiat Oncol Biol Phys 45:244
Martini N, Beattie EJ (1977) Results of surgical treatment in stage I lung cancer. J Thorac Cardiovasc Surg 74:499
Martini N, Flehinger BJ, Zaman MB, Beattie EJ (1983) Results of resection in non-oat cell carcinoma of the lung with mediastinal lymph node metastases. Ann Surg 198:386
Morita K, Fuwa N, Suzuki Y, Nishio M, Sakai K, Tamaki Y, Niibe H, Chujo M, Wada S, Sugawara T, Kita M (1997) Radical radiotherapy for medically inoperable non-small cell lung cancer in clinical stage I: a retrospective analysis of 149 patients. Radiother Oncol 42:31
Mountain CF, Dresler CM (1997) Regional lymph node classification for lung cancer staging. Chest 111:1718
Naruke T (1993) Signifcance of lymph node metastases in lung cancer. Semin Thorac Cardiovasc Surg 5:210
Nestle U, Walter K, Schmidt S, Licht N, Nieder C, Motaref B, Hellwig D, Niewald M, Ukena D, Kirsch CM, Sybrecht GW, Schnabel K (1999) 18F-Deoxyglucose positron emission tomography (FDG-PET) for the planning of radiotherapy in lung cancer: high impact in patients with atelectasis. Int J Radiat Biol Phys 44:593
Nohl-Oser HC (1981) Surgery of the lung. In: Nohl-Oser HC, Nissen R, Schreiber HW (eds) Surgery of the lung. Thieme, Stuttgart, pp 37–184
Noordijk EM, Van Poest-Clement E, Hermans J, Wever AMJ, Leer JWH (1988) Radiotherapy as an alternative to surgery in elderly patients with resectable lung cancer. Radiother Oncol 13:83
Oda M, Watanabe Y, Shimizu J, Murakami S, Onta Y, Sekido N, Watanabe S, Ishikawa N, Nonomura A (1998) Extent of mediastinal node metastasis in clinical stage I non-small-cell lung cancer: the role of systematic nodal dissection. Lung Cancer 22:233
Ogata T, Naruke T (1986) Twenty year's experience with lymph node dissection in patients with lung cancer. The mode of lymph node metastases and the effect of dissection of nodes on the prognosis. In: Motta G (ed) Cancer of the lung and pleura: surgical considerations. Masson, Paris, pp 35–46
Okada M, Tsubota N, Yoshimura M, Miyamoto Y (1998) Proposal for reasonable mediastinal lymphadenectomy in bronchogenic carcinomas: role of subcarinal nodes in selective dissection. J Thorac Cardiovasc Surg 116:949
Paiorolero PC, Williams DE, Bergstrahl MS, Piehlen JM, Bernartz PE, Payne WJ (1984) Post-surgical stage I bronchogenic carcinoma: morbid implications of recurrent disease. Ann Thorac Surg 38:331
Passlick B, Kubuschock B, Sienel W, Thetter O, Pantel K, Izbicki J.R. (2002) Mediastinal lymphadenectomy in non-small cell lung cancer: effectiveness in patients with or without nodal micrometastases – results of a preliminary study. Eur J Cardiothorac Surg 21:520
Perez CA, Stanley K, Grundy G, Hanson W, Rubin P, Kramer S, Brady L, Marks JE, Perez-Tamayo R, Brown GS, Concannon JP, Rotman M (1982) Impact of irradiation technique and tumor extent in tumor control and survival of patients with unresectable non-oat cell carcinoma of the lung. Report by the Radiation Therapy Oncology Group. Cancer 50:1091
Perez CA, Pajak TF, Rubin P, Simpson JR, Mohiuddin M, Brady LW, Perez-Tamayo R, Rotman M (1987) Long-term observations of the patterns of failure in patients with unresectable non-oat cell carcinoma of the lung treated with definitive radiotherapy. Cancer 59:1874

Pieterman RM, van Putten JW, Meuzelaar JJ, Mooyaart EL, Vaalburg W, Koeter GH, Fidler V, Pruim J, Groen HJ (2000) Preoperative staging in non-small cell lung cancer with positron-emission tomography. N Engl J Med 343
Pigott KH, Saunders MI (1993) The long-term outcome after radical radiotherapy for advanced localized non-small cell carcinoma of the lung. Clin Oncol 5:360
Roberts PF, Follette DM, von Haag D, Park JA, Valk PE, Pounds TR, Hopkins DM (2000) Factors associated with false-positive staging of lung cancer by positron-emission tomography. Ann Thorac Surg 70:1154
Rouvière H (1967) Anatomie humaine: descriptive et topographique. Masson, Paris
Rozensweig KE, Sim S, Mychalczak B, Schindelheim R, Fuks SZ, Leibel SA (1999) Elective nodal irradiation in the treatment of non-small cell lung cancer with three-dimensional conformal radiation therapy (3D-CRT). Int J Radiat Oncol Biol Phys 45:243
Sagawa M, Sakurada A, Fujimura S, Sato M, Takahashi S, Usuda K, Endo C, Aikawa H, Kondo T, Saito Y (1999) Five-year survivors with resected pN2 non-small cell lung carcinoma. Cancer 85:864
Sandler HM, Curran WJ, Turrisi AT (1990) The influence of tumor size and pre-treatment staging on outcome following radiation therapy alone for stage I non-small cell lung cancer. Int J Radiat Oncol Biol Phys 19:9
Saunders M, Dische S, Barrett A, Harvey A, Griffiths G, Parmar M (1999) Continuous, hyperfractionated, accelerated radiotherapy (CHART) versus conventional radiotherapy in non-small cell lung cancer: mature data from the randomised multicentre trial. Radiother Oncol 52:137
Sawyer TE, Bonner JA, Gould PM, Deschamps C, Lange CM, Li H (1999) Patients with stage I non-small cell lung carcinoma at postoperative risk for local recurrence, distant metastasis and death: implications related to the design of clinical trials. Int J Radiat Oncol Biol Phys 45:315
Scalliet P, Saunders M, Van Houtte P, Mornex F (1998) Target volume definition: a practical CT contouring exercise by a panel of experts and derived recommendations. In: Mornex F, Van Houtte P (eds) Treatment optimization for lung cancer: from classical to innovative procedures. Elsevier, New York, pp 49–58
Sibley GS, Mundt AJ, Shapiro C, Jacobs R, Chen G, Weichselbaum R, Vijayakumar S (1995) The treatment of stage III non-small cell lung cancer using high-dose conformal radiotherapy. Int J Radiat Oncol Biol Phys 33:1001
Sibley GS, Jamieson TA, Marks LB, Anscher MS, Prosnitz LR (1998) Radiotherapy alone for medically inoperable stage I non-small cell lung cancer: the Duke experience. Int J Radiat Oncol Biol Phys 40:149
Slotman BJ, Antonisse IE, Njo KH (1996) Limited field irradiation in early stage (T1–2, N0) non-small cell lung cancer. Radiother Oncol 41:41
Stephens RJ, Girling DJ, Bleehen NM, Moghissi K, Yosef HMA, Machin D, Medical Research Council Lung Cancer Working Party (1996) The role of post-operative radiotherapy in non-small cell lung cancer: a multicentre randomised trial in patients with stage T1–2, N1–2 M0 disease. Br J Cancer 74:632
Takizawa T, Terashima M, Koike T, Akamura H, Kurita Y, Yokoyama A (1997) Mediastinal lymph node metastasis in patients with clinical stage I peripheral non-small cell lung cancer. J Thorac Cardiovasc Surg 113:248
Takizawa T, Terashima M, Koike T, Watanabe T, Kurita Y, Yokoyama Y, Honma K (1998) Lymph node metastasis in small peripheral adenocarcinoma of the lung. J Thorac Cardiovasc Surg 116:276
Talton BM, Constable WC, Kersh CR (1990) Curative radiotherapy in non-small cell carcinoma of the lung. Int J Radiat Oncol Biol Phys 19:15
Van Houtte P, Gregor A, Philips P (1994) An international survey of radiotherapy practice for radical treatment of non-small cell lung cancer. Lung Cancer 11:S129
Van Houtte P, Mornex F, Acharki A (1998) Survey of treatment indications and radiotherapy practice for lung cancer. In: Mornex F, Van Houtte P (eds) Treatment optimization for lung cancer: from classical to innovative procedures. Elsevier, New York, pp 71–80
Van Houtte P, Ball D, Danhier S, Scalliet P (1999) Treatment indications and clinical target volume. In: Van Houtte P, Klastersky J, Rocmans P (eds) Progress and perspectives in lung cancer. Springer, Berlin Heidelberg New York, pp 225–239
Vansteenkiste JF, Stroobants SG, De Leyn PR et al (1998) Lymph node staging in non-small cell lung cancer with FDG-PET scan: a prospective study on 690 lymph node stations from 68 patients. J Clin Oncol 16:2141
van Tinteren H, Hoekstra OS, Smit EF, van den Bergh JH, Schreurs AJ, Stallaert RA, van Velthoven PC, Comans EF, Diepenhorst FW, Verboom P, van Mourik JC, Postmus PE, Boers M, Teule GJ (2002) Effectiveness of positron emission tomography in the preoperative assessment of patients with suspected non-small cell lung cancer: the PLUS multicentre randomised trial. Lancet 359:1388
Vanuytsel LJ, Vansteenkiste JF, Stroobants SG, De Leyn PR, De Wever W, Verbeken E, Gatti GG, Huyskens DP, Kutcher GJ (2000) The impact of 18 F-fluoro-2-deoxy-D-glucose positron emission tomography (FDG-PET) lymph node staging on the radiation treatment volumes in patients with non-small cell lung cancer. Radiother Oncol 55:317
Vaylet F, Foëhrenbach H, Guigay J, de Dreuille O, Maszelin P, Grassin F, Margery J, Dot JM, Gaillard JF, L'Her P (2000) Apport de la tomographie par émission de positons à la radiothérapie thoracique. Cancer Radiother 4 [Suppl 1]: 13s
Watanabe Y, Shimizu J, Tsubota M, Iwa T (1990) Mediastinal spread of metastatic lymph nodes in bronchogenic carcinoma. Chest 97:1059
Watanabe S, Ladas G, Goldstraw P (2002) Inter-observer variability in systematic nodal dissection: a comparison of European and Japanese nodal designation. Ann Thorac Surg 73:245
Yi-Long W, Zhi-Fan H, Si-Yu W, Wei O (2002) A randomized trial of systematic nodal dissection in resectable non-small cell lung cancer. Lung Cancer 36:1
Yoshuno I, Yokoyama H, Yano T, Ueda T, Takai E, Mizutani K, Asoh H, Ichinose Y (1996) Skip metastasis to the mediastinal lymph nodes in non-small cell lung cancer. Ann Thorac Surg 62:1021
Zhang HX, Yin WB, Yang ZY, Zang ZX, Wang M, Chen DF, Gu XZ (1989) Curative radiotherapy of early operable non-small cell lung cancer. Radiother Oncol 14:89

5 Esophageal Tumors

K. Haustermans and A. Lerut

CONTENTS

5.1 Introduction

When radiation is used with curative intent in the treatment of esophageal cancer, either alone or in combination with surgery and/or chemotherapy, the radiation volume should encompass the detectable tumor and the anatomic areas at risk for metastatic spread. In esophageal cancer it is hard to determine these areas for the individual tumor. Moreover, the areas at risk are very large and this implies that if all areas at risk need to be covered, large radiation fields are also necessary. This chapter describes the anatomy of the esophagus and its draining lymph node regions as a basic requirement when delineating the clinical target volume (CTV) to irradiate these cancers.

K. Haustermans, MD, PhD
Professor, UZ Gasthuisberg, Radiation Oncology, Herestraat 49, 3000 Leuven, Belgium
A. Lerut, MD
Professor, UZ Gasthuisberg, Thoracic Surgery, Herestraat 49, 3000 Leuven, Belgium

5.2 Definition of the Different Anatomical Regions of the Esophagus

The esophagus has been artificially subdivided into regions to facilitate analysis and comparison of results based on an accurate definition of tumor site. The different parts according to the UICC TNM classification are described below (Hermanek et al. 1997).

The cervical esophagus begins at the lower border of the cricoid cartilage and terminates at the level of the thoracic inlet or suprasternal notch.

The thoracic esophagus is subdivided into three parts, namely the upper, middle and lower esophagus. The upper thoracic esophagus begins at the suprasternal notch and ends at the carina. The segment of the esophagus between the levels of the tracheal bifurcation and the esophagogastric junction is divided into two equal parts, the proximal of which is known as the middle thoracic esophagus. The lower esophagus compromises both the lower thoracic esophagus and the hiatal segment of the esophagus. The latter is also termed the abdominal esophagus or gastroesophageal junction (GEJ) (Fig. 5.1).

Most carcinomas that develop in the cervical and thoracic esophagus are squamous cell carcinomas. Tumors arising in the lower esophagus and cardia are almost always adenocarcinomas.

5.3 Classification of Node Levels – Anatomy

Lymphatic drainage of the esophagus is complex. Nodes draining the organ are widely distributed, and are located anywhere between the neck and the upper

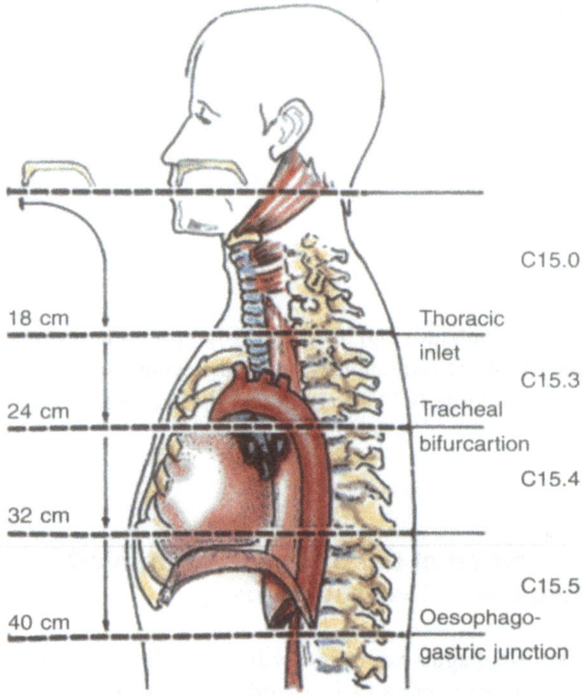

Fig. 5.1. The different anatomical regions of the hypopharynx, esophagus and gastric cardia

abdomen. SAKATA (1903) stated that the submucosal lymphatics drain mainly longitudinally. He showed that, in the midportion of the esophagus, the lymphatics drain upward through the submucosa and, on reaching the neck, they pass through muscle toward the nodes in that area. The lymph of the lower thoracic esophagus drains distally toward the cardiac nodes.

Lymphatic drainage was extensively studied by HAAGENSEN (1972) by injecting blue dye directly into both the mucosal and submucosal layers of the esophagus during resection for carcinomas. By examining the extent of spread of dye in the lymphatics of the resected specimen, he noted that lymph flows more freely in the longitudinal than in the circumferential direction. Haagensen also observed that the inferior esophageal segment empties its lymph mostly into several subdiaphragmatic nodes in the region of the celiac trunk and nodes around the left gastric artery and left infradiaphragmatic artery.

TANABE et al. (1986) injected technetium labeled rhenium colloid into the esophageal wall of 42 patients with carcinoma using endoscopic techniques. After surgery, the radioactive uptake of each lymph node dissected was measured using a scintillation counter. He concluded that:

1. The lymphatic flow of the upper and middle third of thoracic esophagus was mainly in the direction of the neck and upper mediastinum although there was drainage also to the abdomen; and that
2. Lymph from the lower third drained mainly into the abdomen and, in some cases, to the tracheal bifurcation and nodes around the left renal vein.

AKIYAMA (1990) integrated the various published classifications and nomenclatures for lymph nodes into one practical classification. These groups of nodes and their corresponding regions are a modification of the guidelines drawn up by the JAPANESE SOCIETY FOR ESOPHAGEAL DISEASES (1976) combined with the descriptions of HAAGENSEN (1972). The lymph nodes are usually classified into seven groups, as shown in Fig. 5.2.

5.3.1 Cervical Nodes

Carcinoma of the esophagus inevitably spreads to the deep cervical lymph nodes, but the superficial cervical nodes are frequently spared until the advanced stages. Three groups of cervical lymph nodes are distinguished (Fig. 5.3):

1. The deep lateral nodes (spinal accessory lymphatic chain or level Vb).
2. The deep external lymph nodes (lateral to the internal jugular vein including inferiorly the supraclavicular nodes or level IV).
3. The deep internal nodes (recurrent laryngeal nerve lymphatic chain medial to the internal jugular vein or level VI). These deep internal nodes medial to the internal jugular vein are associated with a high incidence of metastatic spread.

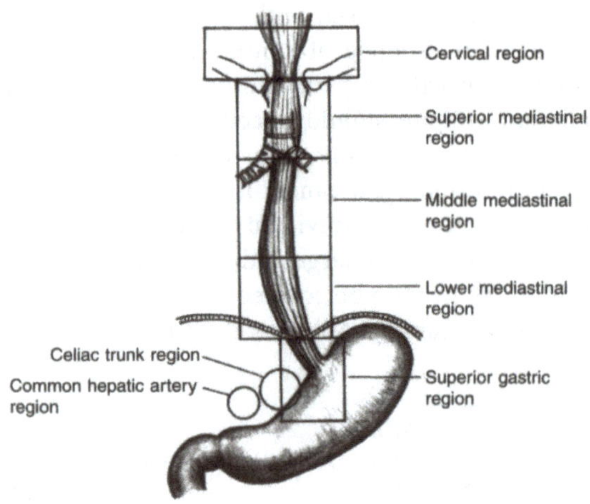

Fig. 5.2. The seven different regions of lymph nodes of the thoracic esophagus

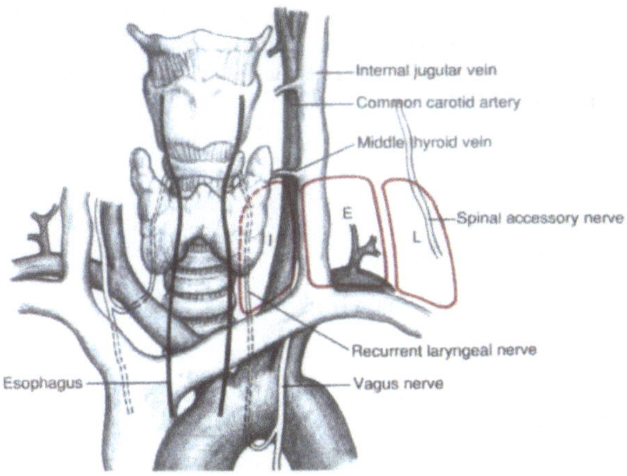

Fig. 5.3. The different groups of cervical lymph nodes. I is the deep internal cervical region or level VI, E is the deep external cervical region or level IV and L is the deep lateral cervical region or level Vb

5.3.2 Superior Mediastinal Group of Lymph Nodes

These are divided into five subgroups (Fig. 5.4):

1. The recurrent laryngeal nerve chain nodes. To the right of the superior mediastinum, several nodes are found along the right recurrent laryngeal nerve where it hooks around the subclavian artery. To the left of the superior mediastinum, smaller lymph nodes are found in line with the left recurrent laryngeal nerve.
2. The paratracheal nodes. These are the counterparts of the recurrent laryngeal nerve chain nodes on the left side. The right paratracheal nodes are located on the right main trunk of the vagus nerve, between the trachea and the superior vena cava. The latter are less frequently invaded.
3. The brachiocephalic nodes. These are located anterior and medial to the vagus nerve where it crosses the brachiocephalic artery.
4. The paraesophageal nodes. Only nodes in close proximity to the esophageal wall may be classified as paraesophageal. These nodes are located dorsal to the posterior wall of the trachea and to the right or left of the midline of the esophagus.
5. The infraaortic arch nodes. Several nodes are found beneath the aortic arch. These nodes are occasionally involved by tumor infiltration.

5.3.3 Middle Mediastinal Group of Lymph Nodes

These are divided into three groups (Fig. 5.4):

1. The tracheal bifurcation nodes. These are also known as carinal nodes and are closely related to the mid-esophagus.
2. The pulmonary hilar nodes. These are found in the right and the left terminal parts of the main bronchi.
3. The paraesophageal nodes. The posterior mediastinal nodes, paraaortic nodes, and nodes along the thoracic duct are all included in this category. Normally these nodes are freely scattered within the sparse mid-mediastinal tissue and are not easily identifiable within a particular group.

5.3.4 Lower Mediastinal Group of Lymph Nodes

The lower mediastinal group of lymph nodes includes the paraesophageal nodes and the diaphragmatic nodes. The latter group forms part of the retrocardiac and infracardiac group of nodes (Fig. 5.4).

5.3.5 Superior Gastric Group of Lymph Nodes

These are divided into three groups (Fig. 5.4):

1. The cardiac nodes. These are frequently involved. They are found along the most superior branch of the left gastric artery. Although cardiac nodes are located separately to the right and the left of the cardia, they are considered as one group since they are closely related to one vascular branch of the left gastric artery.
2. The lesser curvature nodes. It is by this route that tumor spread occurs from the esophagus to the celiac nodes.
3. The left gastric artery nodes.

5.3.6 Celiac Trunk Nodes

These comprise the nodes around the short celiac trunk and those at the root of the common hepatic, and splenic arteries. Metastases beyond this point represent systemic disease.

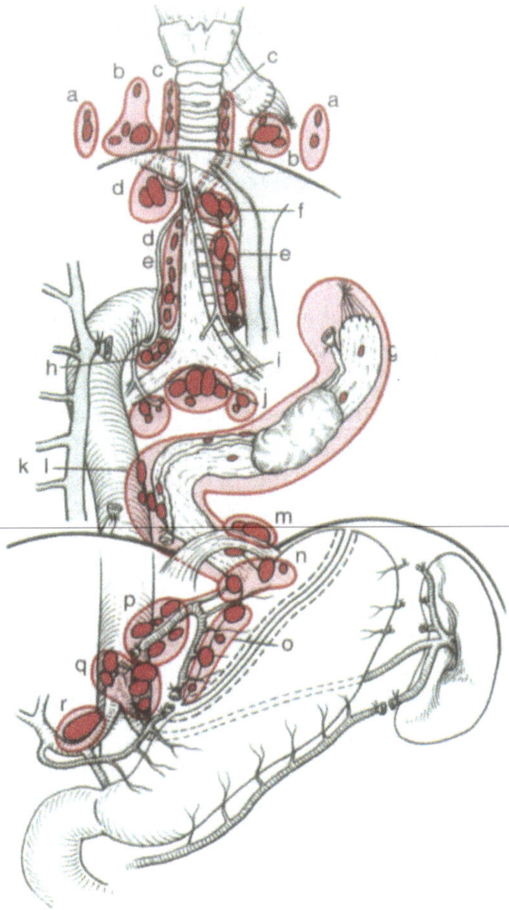

Fig. 5.4. Classification of lymph nodes according to Akiyama (1990). The mediastinal part is the lateral view from the right. The right main bronchus is retracted anteriorly. The cervical and abdominal part are seen from the front

Cervical lymph nodes
Deep lateral nodes Vb (a)
Deep external nodes IV (b)
Deep internal nodes VI (c)
Superior mediastinal nodes
Recurrent nerve lymphatic chain (d)
Paratracheal nodes (e)
Brachiocephalic artery nodes (f)
Paraesophageal nodes (g)
Infraaortic arch nodes (h)
Middle mediastinal nodes
Tracheal bifurcation nodes (i)
Pulmonary hilar nodes (j)
Paraesophageal nodes (k)
Lower mediastinal nodes
Paraesophageal nodes (l)
Diaphragmatic nodes (hiatal part, m)
Superior gastric lymph nodes
Paracardiac nodes (n)
Lesser curvature nodes (o)
Left gastric artery nodes (p)
Celiac trunk nodes (q)
Common hepatic artery nodes (r)

5.3.7 Common Hepatic Artery Nodes

The presence of metastases in the common hepatic artery nodes again represents systemic disease. In squamous cell carcinoma of the esophagus, lymph node involvement is rarely found in the hepatoduodenal ligament, around the greater curvature of the stomach, the distal portion of the splenic artery, the splenic hilum or the left renal vein. These nodes are therefore not included in the list.

5.3.8 RTOG classification of node levels

To facilitate and standardize regional lymph node staging of esophageal cancer, the RTOG has developed a lymph node map that simply adds nodal stations to the widely used lung cancer lymph node map originally reported by Naruke et al. (see chapter on Lung Cancer). The additional nodal stations include the posterior crural nodes (station 15, lying posterior to the diaphragm), paracardial nodes (station 16, immediately adjacent to the GEJ), left gastric nodes (station 17, along the course of the left gastric artery), common hepatic nodes (station 18, along the course of the common hepatic artery), splenic nodes (station 19, along the course of the splenic artery), and celiac nodes (station 20, at the base of the celiac artery). Paraesophageal nodes are described by 3P above the tracheal bifurcation and by 8 below. The latter may be further subdivided into 8M (between the tracheal bifurcation and the caudal margin of the inferior pulmonary vein) and 8L (from the inferior pulmonary vein to the GEJ). The inferior border of the phrenoesophageal ligament serves as the anatomic landmark separating lower paraesophageal nodes (8L) from paracardial nodes (Baba et al. 1997; Casson 1994; Korst et al. 1998) (Fig. 5.5). As most extensive data on lymph node involvement come from the Japanese surgical series, the classification of Akiyama (1990) has been used throughout this chapter.

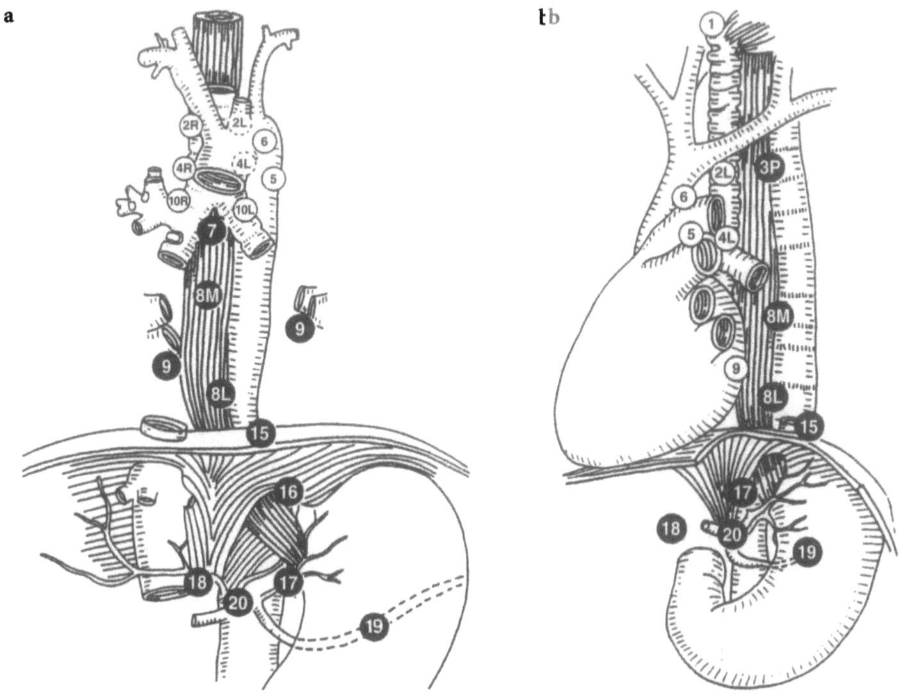

Fig. 5.5a, b. Regional lymph node stations from front (A) and side (B) according to the NARUKE map (see chapter on lung cancer) and adding station 15 (posterior crural nodes), station 16 (paracardial nodes), station 17 (left gastric artery), station 18 (common hepatic nodes), station 19 (splenic nodes) and station 20 (celiac axis) (KORST et al. 1998; CASSON 1994)

Station/description	Location
1 Supraclavicular nodes	Above suprasternal notch and clavicles
2R Right upper paratracheal nodes	Between intersection of caudal margin of innominate artery with trachea and apex of lung
2L Left upper paratracheal nodes	Between top of aortic arch and apex of lung
• 3P Posterior mediastinal nodes	Upper paraesophageal nodes, above tracheal bifurcation
4R Right lower paratracheal nodes	Between intersection of caudal margin of innominate artery with trachea and cephalic border of azygos vein
4L Left lower paratracheal nodes	Between top of aortic arch and carina
5 Aortopulmonary nodes	Subaortic and paraaortic nodes lateral to the ligamentum arteriosum
6 Anterior mediastinal nodes	Anterior to ascending aorta or innominate artery
• 7 Subcarinal nodes	Caudal to carina of trachea
• 8M Middle paraesophageal lymph nodes	From tracheal bifurcation to caudal margin of interior pulmonary vein
• 8L Lower paraesophageal lymph nodes	From caudal margin of inferior pulmonary vein to esophagogastric junction
• 9 Pulmonary ligament nodes	Within inferior pulmonary ligament
10R Right tracheobronchial nodes	From cephalic border of azygos vein to origin of RUL bronchus
10L Left tracheobronchial nodes	Between carina and LUL bronchus
• 15 Diaphragmatic nodes	Lying on dome of diaphragm, and adjacent to or behind its crura
• 16 Paracardial nodes	Immediately adjacent to gastroesophageal junction
• 17 Left gastric nodes	Along course of left gastric artery
• 18 Common hepatic nodes	Along course of common hepatic artery
• 19 Splenic nodes	Along course of splenic artery
• 20 Celiac nodes	At base of celiac artery

5.4 Patterns of Esophageal Cancer Spread

Esophageal cancer can spread longitudinally and radially. The esophagus is marked by a rich network of submucosal lymphatics, which allows easy tumor spread along the esophagus to lymph nodes far from the primary tumor. Longitudinal spread occurs in both distal and proximal directions along the intramural lymphatic network and perineural spaces, with intramural localizations up to 5 to 6 cm from the primary tumor. Intramural localizations are defined as being clearly separated from the primary tumor, located in the esophageal or gastric wall, not surrounded by endothelium and not accompanied by intraepithelial cancerous extension. Thus they are presumably metastatic deposits which have extravasated from the submucosal lymphatics. Of 393 patients with squamous cell carcinoma in the thoracic esophagus, 60 were found by histological examination to have intramural metastasis (Kato et al. 1992). Fifty of these were identified by gross inspection. A strong correlation was found between intramural metastasis and lymph node involvement.

Because the esophagus has no serosa, radial spread and direct invasion into the adjacent anatomical structures such as the pleura, tracheobronchial tree, lung and recurrent laryngeal nerves, occurs at an early stage.

The esophagus has a dual longitudinal interconnecting system of lymphatics, in the lamina propria and in the muscularis mucosae. This is in contrast with other parts of the gastrointestinal tract, where lymphatics are located below the submucosa. As a result of this system, lymph fluid can pass through the entire length of the esophagus before draining into the lymph nodes. Lymphatics enter the mucosa to lie just below the basement membrane of the epithelium and drain the lamina propria and muscularis mucosae. Lymphatics pierce the muscularis propria and drain into regional lymph nodes or directly into the thoracic duct (see Fig. 5.6).

5.5 Distribution and Incidence of Regional Nodes

Periesophageal lymph node involvement is an early process (Table 5.1).

The percentage possibility for positive locoregional nodes is close to 0% for intra-epithelial tumors (Nishimaki et al. 1993), 31% to 56% for T1b tumors (Nishimaki et al. 1994), 58% to 78% for T2, 74% to 81% for T3, and 83% to 100% for T4 tumors (Akiyama 1990; Lerut et al. 1993, 1999; Natsugoe et al. 1995; Nishimaki et al. 1993, 1994, 1995, 1999).

Because of the early and wide spread of lymphatic metastasis, Kato et al. (Kato et al. 1992) recommend esophagectomy with three-field lymph node dissection even for patients with lesions diagnosed as submucosal cancer. In a series of 43 patients with early stage tumors they found that 46.5% had positive nodes. The lymph nodes around the right recurrent nerve and the right paracardiac nodes were the most frequent sites of metastasis, whereas no metastases were found in the right paratracheal, infracarinal, infraaortic arch, common hepatic, and celiac nodes.

Nodal metastases occur in about 70% of patients with thoracic esophageal tumors. The most commonly affected node groups are the lesser curvature, parahiatal and the right recurrent nodes. Cervical node metastases occur in about 35% of patients, irrespective of tumor location or T-stage. The metastatic

Table 5.1. The relationship between depth of tumor infiltration and incidence of lymph node metastases; *M* represents the mucosa, and *Sm* the submucosa, both divided into three sublayers (Kodama and Kakegawa 1998).

Depth of infiltration	% of *N*+ (*N*+/Total)
M1	0 (0/199)
M2	3.3 (5/153)
M3	12.2 (28/230)
Sm1	26.5 (58/219)
Sm2	35.8 (133/372)
Sm3	45.9 (260/567)

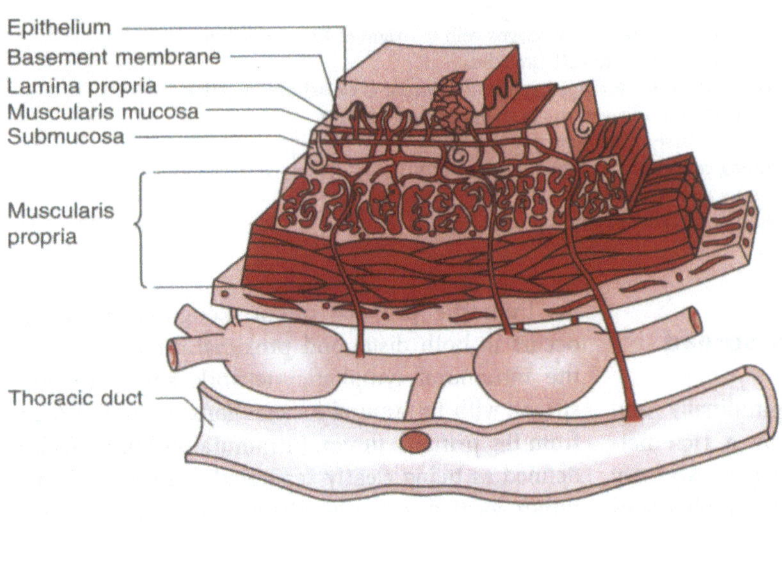

Fig. 5.6. Lymphatic anatomy of the esophagus (Rice et al. 1998)

rate to mediastinal and abdominal nodes is around 45%. In the mediastinum most positive nodes are found in the bilateral recurrent lymph nodes, the bifurcation nodes and the paraesophageal nodes, while in the abdomen the highest rate of positive nodes is found in the bilateral cardial nodes.

Table 5.2 and Fig. 5.7 demonstrate the frequency of cases with positive lymph nodes per number of lymph nodes resected according to the location of the primary tumor (Table 2) or per number of cases resected (Fig. 5.7) (Akiyama 1990). Although there is a clear correlation between the anatomical location of the tumor and the frequency of positive lymph nodes in the various anatomical drainage sites, it is also clear that metastases occur frequently at long distances from the primary tumor through longitudinal lymphatic pathways (Fig. 5.7). It is surprising to find that 28.6% of patients have lymph node involvement in the superior gastric area when the tumor is located high up in the upper esophagus. Similarly, when the tumor is located in the lower esophagus, positive nodes in the superior mediastinum are found in as many as 33.3% of patients.

Adenocarcinoma has replaced squamous cell carcinoma as the most common esophageal tumor in the Western world. Less extensive series have been reported on the prevalence and location of lymph node metastases (Hagen et al. 2001; Steup et al. 1996). However, there is no reason to assume that there is a different mode of spread for adenocarcinomas compared to squamous cell carcinomas (Law et al. 1992). An en bloc esophagectomy was performed in 44 patients with transmural adenocarcinoma of the distal esophagus or GEJ (Nigro et al. 1999b). The incidence of positive lymph nodes is represented in Table 5.3. An upper mediastinal and neck dissection was not performed in these patients, so no data are available on the incidence of positive nodes in these regions.

Table 5.2. Frequency of metastases per number of dissected lymph nodes according to location of the primary tumor (Akiyama 1990)

Group of lymph nodes	Location of primary tumor		
	Upper esophagus	Middle esophagus	Lower esophagus
Mediastinum			
Superior	51/401 (12.7%)	115/2092 (5.5%)	28/1002 (2.8%)
Middle	16/385 (4.2%)	121/2201 (5.5%)	51/1048 (4.9%)
Lower	12/256 (4.7%)	53/1082 (4.9%)	59/ 711 (8.3%)
Abdomen			
Superior gastric	21/754 (2.8%)	17/ 631 (2.7%)	253/2035 (12.4%)
Celiac trunk	1/145 (0.7%)	204/3660 (5.6%)	30/ 354 (8.5%)
Common hepatic	0/102 (0%)	27/ 681 (4.0%)	8/ 310 (2.6%)

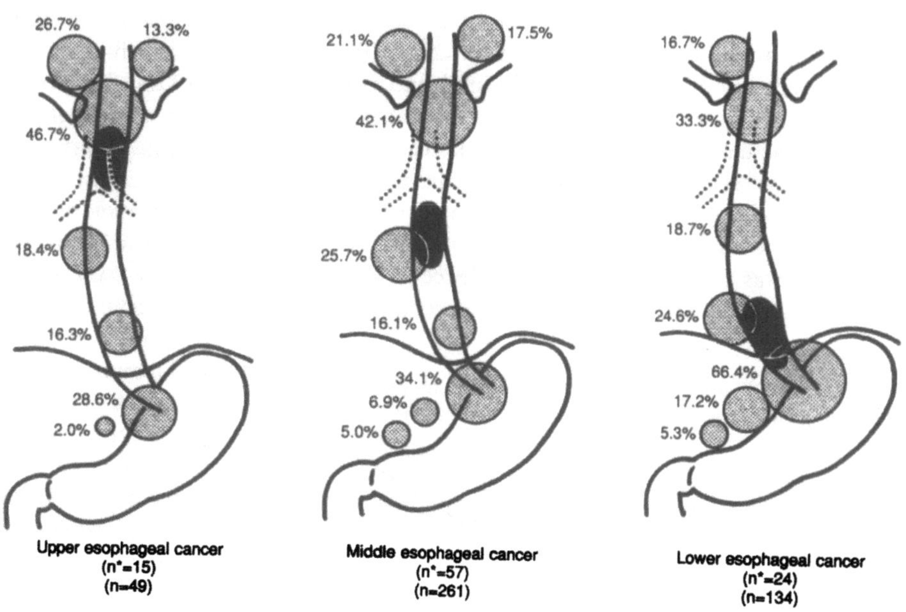

Fig. 5.7. Frequency of lymph node metastases per number of cases resected according to tumor location. N^* represents the number of cases for analysis of cervical nodes

Table 5.3. Frequency of lymph node metastases by nodal location for patients with transmural adenocarcinoma located in the distal esophagus (n=36) or GEJ (n=8)

Group of lymph nodes	Distal esophagus (%)	GEJ (%)
Mediastinum		
Middle	8.3	13
Lower	33	50
Abdomen		
Superior gastric	78	50
Splenic artery and hilum	6	13
Celiac trunk	14	25
Common hepatic	3	0

The prevalence of positive lymph nodes in adenocarcinoma of the esophagus and GEJ is also related to the T-stage of the primary tumor (see Table 5.4). The prevalence of regional node involvement increased progressively with the depth of tumor invasion, with involved lymph nodes identified in 80% of patients with muscular invasion. Lymph node metastases are also more common at distant node stations in intramuscular tumors (Nigro et al. 1999a).

Esophageal cancer also has a high propensity to invade distant lymph nodes without involving local nodes (skip metastases), e.g. 24% of "early" submucosal tumors may have skip metastases to distant cervical or abdominal nodes without local lymph node involvement (Nishimaki et al. 1999). Skipping of one or more than one level of lymph node groups was reported in 34% of patients in a study by Hosch et al. (2001), who studied 86 patients with resected esophageal cancer. A total of 1,584 resected lymph nodes were obtained and evaluated by routine histopathology and immunohistochemistry with Ber-EP4, an anti-epithelial cell monoclonal antibody. Forty-six percent (n=23) of the patients with supracarinal esophageal cancer had skip metastases compared to 47% (n=17) of the patients with supracarinal tumors (not significant). Regarding tumor type, 31% (n=18) of patients with squamous cell carcinoma and 41% (n=11) of patients with adenocarcinoma showed skip metastases (not significant). No correlation was found between the incidence of skip metastases and tumor type, grade of differentiation, T stage or N stage of the primary tumor. The presence of skip metastases was associated with a significantly decreased disease-free survival. In a group of 37 patients with T3 adenocarcinoma of the distal esophagus or GE-junction, unforeseen cervical lymph node involvement was observed in 20% of the GEJ tumors and in 35.3% of the distal esophageal tumors. Especially in tumors of the GEJ there is an important skip phenomenon (Van de Ven et al. 1999). However, in this group of tumors, skip metastases had no independent prognostic impact on disease-free or overall survival. It seems that this phenomenon may not necessarily reflect more aggressive or advanced disease in tumors of the GEJ, but is an indicator that limited lymph node sampling in the context of a complex lymphatic anatomy might lead to false-negative histopathological staging.

Table 5.4. Lymph node prevalence and number in patients undergoing en bloc esophagectomy (Nigro et al. 1999a)

Tumor location	Prevalence of involved nodes	No. of involved nodes (median, range)
Intramucosal (n=10)	1/ 5 (7%)	0 (0–1)
Submucosal (n=12)	6/12 (50%)	0.5 (0–9)
Intramuscular (n=10)	8/10 (80%)	1.0 (0–6)

5.6 Diagnosis of Local and Regional Lymph Node Involvement

Nishimaki et al. (1999) studied the accuracy of preoperative tumor staging by using esophagography, esophagoscopy, percutaneous and endoscopic ultrasonography, and CT scan in 224 patients with resectable esophageal cancer. For T-staging, the overall accuracy was 80%. For N-staging, the overall accuracy was 72% with a sensitivity of 78%, a specificity of 60% and a positive predictive value of 78%. Overall, the accuracy of stage grouping was only 56%.

The study of Flamen et al. confirmed that endoscopic ultrasound (EUS) is the preferred method for the assessment of local lymph node involvement with a superior sensitivity of 81% compared to CT (0%) or FDG-PET (33%) (Flamen et al. 2000). EUS, however, suffers from a lack of specificity (67%), resulting in overstaging. Botet et al. (1991) found a similar rate of overstaging with EUS. The use of trans-EUS-guided lymph node biopsies offers new possibilities for more specific minimally invasive staging (Mallery and Van-Dam 1999). For the assessment of regional and distant lymph node involvement, FDG-PET has a higher specificity (98%) and a similar sensitivity (43%) compared to the combined use of EUS and CT scan. Most false-negative FDG-PET scans have involved lymph nodes with only microscopic involvement. So clinical staging remains deficient in regard to lymph node metastases. This probably reflects the impossibility of detecting microscopic metastases and the wide distribution of lymph node metastases as well as other technical factors.

5.7 Patterns of Locoregional Recurrence After Surgery

The differential diagnosis of local recurrence, regional recurrence and anastomotic recurrence in these cases is difficult. Only very few papers report on their results in such detail (Fujita et al. 1994). Tumor recurrences evaluated by CT scan are most commonly diagnosed as some combination of locoregional disease, distal metastasis and abdominal lymph node enlargement. CT findings isolated to one region are only occasionally reported (Carlisle et al. 1993).

A study of the patterns of tumor recurrence was performed in 112 consecutive patients after resection and reconstruction for esophageal carcinoma (Akiyama 1990). Blood-borne metastases were most frequent (52%) followed by lymphatic recurrence (40%). Recurrence in the cervical lymph nodes was most frequently seen with primary carcinoma of the upper thoracic esophagus (33%). Of all other lymphatic drainage sites, abdominal recurrence was most infrequent (6%). Local recurrence at the anastomotic site was confirmed in only 3% of cases. This low number of local recurrences was confirmed in a study by Law et al. (1992). He examined a series of 500 patients undergoing surgery and found a local recurrence rate of 6.1% in patients with squamous cell carcinomas compared to 7.6% among patients with adenocarcinomas. In a recent series (Altorki and Skinner 2001), 111 patients with esophageal cancer underwent an en bloc esophagectomy with radical lymph node dissection. Recurrence occurred in 39% of the patients and was local in only 8% of cases. Other reports suggest a higher locoregional failure rate ranging from 25% to 35% for patients with pT3N1 tumors (Fok et al. 1993; Law et al. 1996). Locoregional recurrence is mainly found in the region around the recurrent nerves and the main bronchi (Matsubara et al. 1996). In a series of 90 patients who underwent extensive radical esophagectomy with three-field dissection for squamous cell carcinoma of the thoracic esophagus, 21% developed locoregional recurrence. All lymph node recurrences were clinically diagnosed via US, CT and MRI. Lymph nodes larger than 1 cm, round in shape and with enlargement at follow-up were scored as being malignant. The locoregional recurrence was clearly correlated with the number of metastatic nodes at the time of surgery (see Table 5.5) (Bhansali et al. 1997).

In contrast to these results, Whittington et al. (1990) reported a locoregional recurrence rate of 77% in patients treated with surgery alone, the most common site of recurrence being the anastomosis. A possible explanation for this big difference in locoregional recurrence rate is related to the difference in surgical technique used (transhiatal esophagectomy yielding a high rate compared with en bloc esophagectomy with three-field lymph node dissection).

The rate of locoregional failure following chemoradiation varies from 17% to 47% (al-Sarraf et al. 1997; Coia et al. 1991; Herskovic et al. 1992; John et al. 1989; Urga et al. 2001; Walsh et al. 1996). An intergroup study (RTOG 9405, INT 0123) compared concurrent chemotherapy with 50.4 Gy to concurrent chemotherapy with 64.8 Gy. The higher radiation dose did not lead to an improved survival or locoregional control. The trial was closed because of increased toxicity and treatment-related mortality (Minsky et al. 2002). The failure to find a dose-response quite likely reflects geographic underdosage to subclinical lymphatic metastases because treatment fields extended only 5 cm from the primary detectable tumor volume. Defining whether locoregional recurrences were situated within the radiation fields would address this question, but was not reported in these studies. A combined approach using preoperative chemoradiation followed by surgery led to the lowest percentage of locoregional recurrences varying between 2% and 36% (Bosset et al. 1997). This may reflect more complete elimination of widespread lymphatic metastasis.

5.8 Guidelines for Selection of Target Volumes and Radiation Field Design

When delineating the CTV for esophageal cancer the radiation oncologist should make sure that the volume treated adequately encompasses the tumor and lymph nodes at risk. Due to the anatomy of the esophagus, this will lead to large radiation fields. The use of shrinking fields is a logical approach to eliminate distant microscopically invaded nodes while limiting toxicity. However, many of these nodes are only microscopically invaded and the total dose given to these regions at risk does not need to be as high as the dose needed to treat macroscopic disease. Nevertheless, the toxicity and morbidity of such treatment is substantial as radiation needs to be combined with chemotherapy.

Esophageal cancer is notorious for its ability to spread intramurally to locations distant from the

Table 5.5. Lymph node metastases and recurrence in 90 patients with squamous cell carcinoma of the thoracic esophagus who underwent extended radical esophagectomy with three-field dissection (Bhansali et al. 1997)

Nodes	Extent of lymphadenectomy (%)	Metastases at operation (%)	First site of recurrence (%)
Cervical nodes			
Submandibular			
Right	0	0	1(1)
Left	0	0	0
Internal jugular			
Right	6(7)	1(1)	3(3)
Left	10(11)	0	3(3)
Supraclavicular			
Right	90(100)	10(11)	3(3)
Left	90(100)	6(7)	3(3)
Cervical paraesophageal			
Right[a]	87(97)	3(3)	1(1)
Left	86(96)	6(7)	6(7)
Thoracic nodes			
Right recurrent nerve	90(100)	29(32)	0
Left paratracheal	86(96)	13(14)	2(2)
Right paratracheal	45(50)	3(3)	1(1)
Infraaortic arch	53(59)	3(3)	1(1)
Periesophageal	90(100)	18(20)	0
Infracarinal	90(100)	10(11)	0
Lower posterior mediastinal	90(100)	8(9)	0
Abdominal nodes			
Paracardiac			
Right	90(100)	23(26)	0
Left	90(100)	10(11)	0
Lesser curvature	90(100)	14(16)	0
Left gastric	90(100)	12(13)	0
Celiac[b]	44(49)	2(2)	2(2)
Abdominal paraaortic	0	0	2(2)
Other nodes			
Axillary	–		
Right	0	0	0
Left	0	0	1(1)

[a]Includes the cervical paraesophageal and paratracheal nodes
[b]Includes the common hepatic, splenic, and celiac nodes

main lesion (Kato et al. 1992). Some surgeons advocate the removal of at least 5 cm of normal esophagus to ensure a safe surgical margin. Not infrequently, primary tumors with multicentric lesions and tumor spread are encountered and a 5 cm margin may not be sufficient. However, with new advances in endoscopic and radiological techniques, the tumor extent and spread, together with synchronous lesions, are frequently accurately detected.

In a series of 154 patients treated with radical esophagectomy for invasive carcinoma of the thoracic esophagus it has been shown that cervical lymphadenectomy should only be performed routinely as part of a radical esophagectomy when the tumor is in the upper or middle esophagus. Survival did not differ in these patients according to whether they had regional or distant lymph node metastases. In a study of lower esophageal cancer however, none of the 10 patients with distant node metastases survived for more than 4 years. However, this subgroup of patients is too small to draw such firm conclusions. The inclusion of cervical lymphadenectomy in these patients is to be considered as investigational (Nishimaki et al. 1997).

Less than a three-field lymph node dissection may be appropriate in selected cases; for instance, in patients considered to be poor risk, or too old and frail. Those lymph nodes to be removed need to be selected from the viewpoint of frequency of metastases (Fig. 5.7).

These surgical guidelines can also be used to delineate the CTV. We have adapted the different lymph node regions described from surgical experience so that it is possible to delineate them on a CT scan in the treatment position. We have added the supraclavicular lymph node regions as separate regions. The paraesophageal nodes are divided into two groups: above or below the carina. The superior gastric lymph nodes are not subdivided intosubgroups (Fig. 5.8).

It is generally accepted that lymph node regions with a probability of 10% or more of being microscopically invaded should be included in the CTV. This would mean that the celiac trunk nodes do not need to be included in the CTV for tumors of the upper and middle esophagus. However, most cases referred for radiation are at an advanced stage at diagnosis and are referred for preoperative neoadjuvant treatment. So the estimated percentage of involved nodes deduced from the surgical series is probably a low estimate of the probability among those patients referred for radiotherapy.

In order to optimize the delineation of the CTV, we studied the additional value of performing FDG-PET scans to delineate the CTV. Thirty patients with advanced esophageal cancer were studied prospectively. All patients underwent a CT scan of the chest and the abdomen, EUS and FDG-PET before the start of the preoperative chemoradiotherapy. Fourteen different lymph nodes regions were defined on the basis of surgical series. All these regions (n=1260) were scored individually for lymph node involvement with the help of an experienced radiologist and nuclear medicine physician.

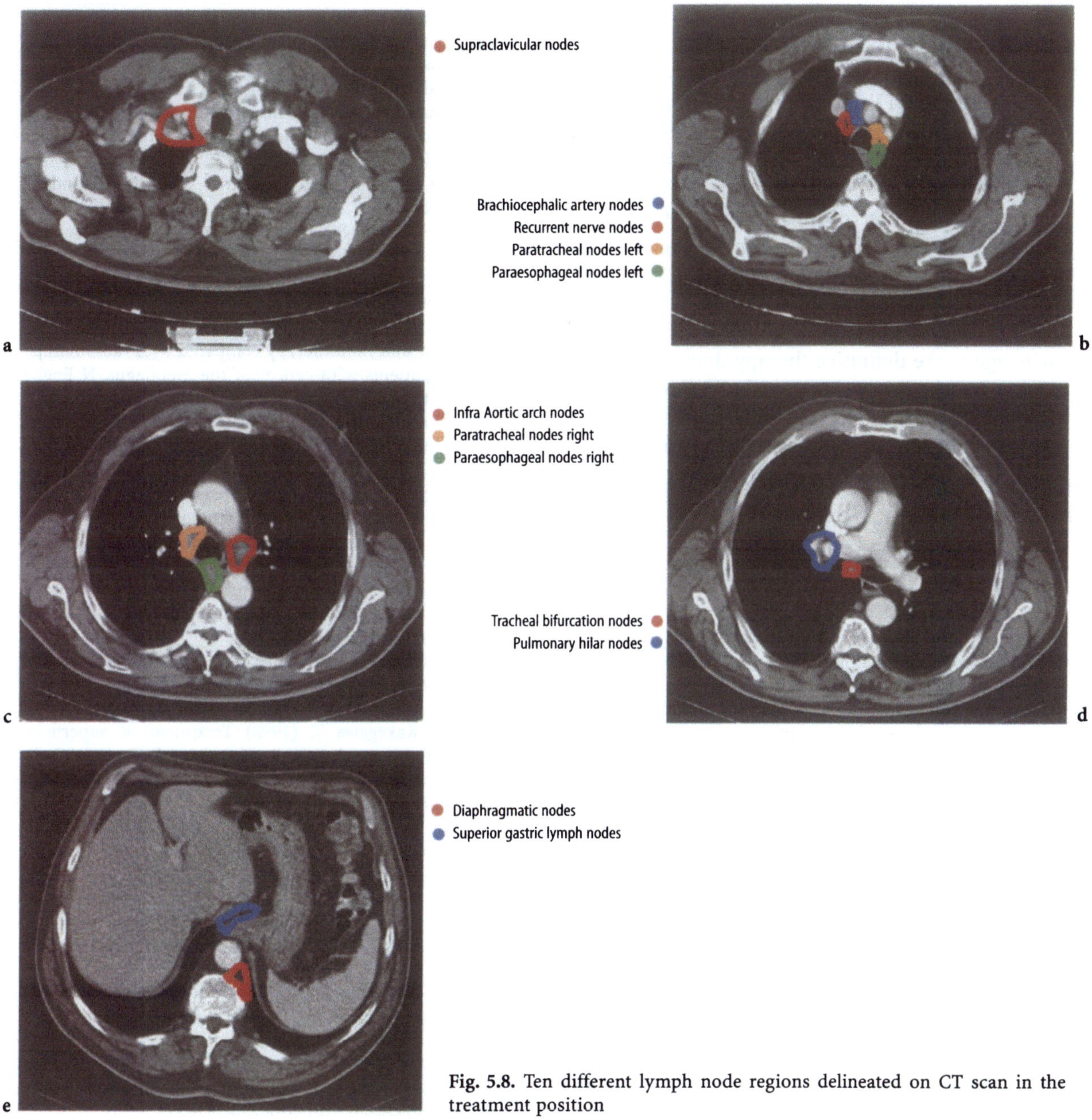

Fig. 5.8. Ten different lymph node regions delineated on CT scan in the treatment position

Radiation fields were defined on the basis of conventional imaging modalities. The supraclavicular nodes were included in the treatment fields for primary tumors located above the carina. When FDG uptake was found in a lymph node region without pathological nodes determined on CT and/or EUS, the influence of this finding on the radiation fields was assessed. In 14 of the 30 patients (47%), there were discordant findings for the regional lymph nodes between CT/EUS and FDG-PET. Nine positive lymph nodes (larger than 1 cm) in 8 patients were detected on CT/EUS, but these nodes did not show FDG uptake. However, due to the low sensitivity of FDG-PET, the fields were not reduced on the basis of these findings. Six patients had a positive PET scan in a CT/EUS negative lymph node region. In three of these cases, the radiation fields had to be enlarged on the basis of the PET scan, including the supraclavicular region for infracarinal tumors or including the celiac trunk for tumors located above the carina. In this study, 10% of the radiation fields were altered on the basis of the FDG-PET scan, indicating a potential role for PET in radiotherapy treatment planning for esophageal cancer.

5.9 Conclusion

Delineating the CTV for esophageal cancer remains a challenging task. Lymphatic spread is more extensive along the length of the esophagus than in other organs. All efforts should be made to adapt and delineate the CTV according to the location of the primary tumor and the relative incidence of lymph node involvement in the different regions. In general, subclinical lymphatic deposits should be treated by appropriate doses to large volumes with subsequent shrinkage if the definitive therapy does not include surgery. In selecting a chemo-radiotherapy regimen, the benefit of including the different lymph node regions should be weighed against the risk of morbidity and complications during surgery.

References

Akiyama H (1990) Surgery for cancer of the esophagus. Williams and Wilkins, Baltimore

al-Sarraf M, Martz K, Herskovic A et al (1997) Progress report of combined chemoradiotherapy versus radiotherapy alone in patients with esophageal cancer: an intergroup study. J Clin Oncol 15:277

Altorki N, Skinner D (2001) Should en bloc esophagectomy be the standard of care for esophageal carcinoma? Ann Surg 234:581–587

Baba M, Aikou T, Natsugoe S et al (1997) Lymph node and perinodal tissue tumor involvement in patients with esophagectomy and three-field lymphadenectomy for carcinoma of the esophagus. J Surg Oncol 64:12–16

Bhansali MS, Fujita H, Kakegawa T et al (1997) Pattern of recurrence after extended radical esophagectomy with three-field lymph node dissection for squamous cell carcinoma in the thoracic esophagus. World J Surg 21:275–281

Bosset JF, Gignoux M, Triboulet JP et al (1997) Chemoradiotherapy followed by surgery compared with surgery alone in squamous cell cancer of the esophagus. N Engl J Med 337:161

Botet JF, Lightdale CJ, Zauber AG et al (1991) Preoperative staging of esophageal cancer: comparison of endoscopic US and dynamic CT. Radiology 181:419–425

Carlisle JG, Quint LE, Francis IR et al (1993) Recurrent esophageal carcinoma: CT evaluation after esophagectomy. Radiology 189:271–275

Casson AG (1994) Lymph node mapping of esophageal cancer. Ann Thorac Surg 58:1569–1570

Coia L, Engstrom P, Paul A et al (1991) Long-term results of infusional 5-FU, mitomycin-C and radiation as primary management of esophageal cancer. Int J Radiat Oncol Biol Phys 20:29

Flamen P, Lerut A, Van Cutsem E et al (2000) Utility of positron emission tomography for the staging of patients with potentially operable esophageal carcinoma. J Clin Oncol 18:3202–3210

Fok M, Sham JS, Choy D et al (1993) Postoperative radiotherapy for carcinoma of the esophagus: a prospective, randomized controlled study. Surgery 113:138–147

Fujita H, Kakegawa T, Yamana H et al (1994) Lymph node metastasis and recurrence in patients with a carcinoma of the thoracic esophagus who underwent three-field dissection. World J Surg 18:266–272

Haagensen CD (1972) The lymphatics in cancer. Saunders, Philadelphia

Hagen JA, De Meester SR, Peters JH (2001) Curative resection for esophageal adenocarcinoma. Ann Surg 234:520–531

Hermanek P, Hutter RVP, Sobin LH et al (1997) TNM atlas, 4th edn. Springer, Berlin Heidelberg New York

Herskovic A, Martz K, al-Sarraf M et al (1992) Combined chemotherapy and radiotherapy compared with radiotherapy alone in patients with cancer of the esophagus. N Engl J Med 326:1593

Hosh SB, Stoecklein NH, Pichlmeier U et al (2001) Esophageal cancer: the mode of lymphatic tumor cell spread and its prognostic significance. J Clin Oncol 19:1970–1975

Japanese Society for Esophageal Diseases (1976) Guidelines for the clinical and pathologic studies on carcinoma of the esophagus, part I. Clinical classification. Jpn J Surg 6: 69–78

John MJ, Marshall SF, Mowry PG et al (1989) Radiotherapy alone and chemoradiation for nonmetastatic esophageal carcinoma. Cancer 63:2397

Kato H, Tachimori Y, Watanabe H et al (1992) Intramural metastasis of thoracic esophageal carcinoma. Int J Cancer 50:49–52

Kodama M, Kakegawa T. (1998) Treatment of superficial cancer of the esophagus: a summary of responses to a questionnaire on superficial cancer of the esophagus in Japan. Surgery 123:432–439

Korst RJ, Rush VW, Venkatraman E et al (1998) Proposed revision of the staging classification for esophageal cancer. J Thorac Cardiovasc Surg 3:660–670

Law SY, Fok M, Cheng SW et al (1992) A comparison of outcome after resection for squamous cell carcinomas and adenocarcinomas of the esophagus and cardia. Surg Gynecol Obstet 172:107–112

Law SY, Fok M, Wong J (1996) Pattern of recurrence after oesphageal resection for cancer: clinical implications. Br J Surg 83 :107–111

Lerut T, De Leyn P, Coosemans W et al (1993) Surgical strategies in esophageal carcinoma with emphasis on radical lymphadenectomy. Ann Surg 216:583–590

Lerut T, Coosemans W, De Leyn P et al (1999) Is there a role for radical esophagectomy. Eur J Cardiothorac Surg 16 [Suppl 1]:44–47

Mallery S, Van-Dam J (1999) Increased rate of complete EUS staging of patients with esophageal cancer using the non-optical, wire-guided echoendoscopy. Gastrointest Endosc 50:53–57

Matsubara T, Ueda M, Takahashi T et al (1996) Localization of recurrent disease after extended lymph node dissection for carcinoma of the thoracic esophagus. J Am Coll Surg 182:340–346

Minsky BD, Pajak TF, Ginsberg RJ et al (2002) INT 0123 (Radiation Therapy Oncology Group 94-05) Phase III trial of combined-modality therapy for esophageal cancer: high-dose versus standard-dose radiation therapy. J Clin Oncol 20:1167–1174

Natsugoe S, Aikou T, Yoshinaka H et al (1995) Lymph node metastasis of early stage carcinoma of the esophagus and of the stomach. J Clin Gastroenterol 20:325–328
Nigro JJ, Hagen JA, Demeester TR et al (1999a) Prevalence and location of nodal metastases in distal esophageal adenocarcinoma confined to the wall: implications for therapy. J Thorac Cardiovasc Surg 117:16–25
Nigro JJ, De Meester SR, Hagen JA et al (1999b) Node status in transmural esophageal adenocarcinoma and outcome after en bloc esophagectomy. J Thorac Cardiovasc 117:960–968
Nishihira T, Sayama J, Ueda H et al (1995) Lymph flow and lymph node metastasis in esophageal cancer. Jpn J Surg 25:307–317
Niskimaki T, Tanaka O, Suzuki T et al (1993) Tumor spread in superficial esophageal cancer: histopathologic basis for retional surgical treatment. World J Surg 17:766–771; discussion 771–772
Nishimaki T, Tanaka O, Suzuki T et al (1994) Patterns of lymphatic spread in thoracic esophageal cancer. Cancer 74:4–11
Nishimaki T, Suzuki T, Tanaka Y et al (1997) Evaluating the rational extent of dissection in radical esophagectomy for invasive carcinoma of the thoracic esophagus. Surg Today 27:3–8
Nishimaki T, Suzuki T, Kanda T et al (1999) Extended radical esophagectomy for superficially invasive carcinoma of the esophagus. Surgery 125:142–147
Rice TW, Zuccaro G, Adelstein DJ et al (1998) Esophageal carcinoma: depth of tumor invasion is predictive of regional lymph node status. Ann Thorac Surg 65:787–792
Sakata K (1903) Über die Lymphgafässe des Oesophagus und über seine regionären Lymphdrüsen mit Berücksichtigung der Verbreitung des Karcinoms. Mitt Grenzgeb Med Chir 11:634–656
Steup WH, De Leyn P, Deneffe G et al (1996) Tumors of the esophagogastric junction. Long-term survival in relation to the pattern of lymph node metastasis and a critical analysis of the accuracy or inaccuracy of pTNM classification. J Thorac Cardiovasc Surg 111:85–94; discussion 94–95
Tanabe G, Baba M, Kuroshima K et al (1986) Clinical evaluation of esophageal lymph flow system based on the RI uptake of removed regiocal lymph nodes following lymphoscintigraphy [in Japanese]. J Jpn Surg Soc 87:315–323
Urga SG, Orringer MD, Turrisi A et al (2001) Randomized trial of preoperative chemoradiation versus surgery alone in patients with locoregional esophageal carcinoma. J Clin Oncol 19:305
Van de Ven C, De Leyn P, Coosemans W et al (1999) Three-field lymphadenectomy and pattern of lymph node spread in T3 adenocarcinoma of the distal esophagus and the gastro-esophageal junction. Eur J Cardiothorac Surg 15:769–773
Walsh TN, Noonan N, Hollywood D et al (1996) A comparison of multimodality therapy and surgery for esophageal adenocarcinoma. N Engl J Med 335:462
Whittington R, Coia LR, Haller DG et al (1990) Adenocarcinoma of the esophagus and esophago-gastric junction: the effect of single and combined modalities on the survival and patterns of failure. Int J Radiat Oncol Biol Phys 19: 593–603

6 Target Volume Selection and Delineation in Breast Cancer Conformal Radiotherapy

I. C. Kiricuta

CONTENTS

I. C. Kiricuta, MD, PhD
Associate Professor, Institute for Radiation Oncology, St. Vincenz-Hospital, Auf dem Schafsberg, 65549 Limburg/Lahn, Germany

6.1 Introduction

The selection and delineation of target volumes in computed tomography (CT) axial slices is of paramount importance for the transition from standard radiation therapy (RT) to conformal or intensity modulated RT. A CT based nodal classification for standard target volume selection is necessary. Clinical and pathological data from large studies exist, enabling individual target volume selection and delineation.

In daily clinical practice the integration of postmastectomy radiation therapy (PMRT) varies from accepted to very controversial indications, whereas postoperative irradiation is with very few exceptions well established in breast conserving strategy. Indications for the irradiation of locoregional lymphatics like the internal mammary lymph chain (IMC) and/or the axillary and supraclavicular lymph nodes are a subject of controversy (Morrow 1999; Perez et al. 1992). A lack of consensus on whether or not to irradiate the internal mammary lymph nodes exists worldwide, as reported by Kuske (1998). The French and the Scandinavian radiation oncologists tend to treat the IMC, whereas the English and the Italians do not. In the United States, some radiation oncologists such those from the University of Michigan, Duke University and Ochsner Clinic/Tulane Cancer Center do so routinely whereas others, including radiation oncologists from the Harvard Joint Center, Fox Chase Cancer Center and Memorial Sloan-Kettering Cancer Center, tend not to irradiate these lymphatics.

In recent years, a new concept and procedure has been introduced and validated to indicate the negativity or positivity of the axillary nodal status. The sentinel node concept (SNC) will quite likely revolutionize the treatment of early-stage breast cancer in the near future.

The SNC is fundamentally based on the orderly progression of tumor cells within the lymphatic system. It is the most important new concept in surgical and radiation oncology. A high rate of success in the identification of the sentinel node (SN) for breast cancer has been reported. The presence or absence of metastases in this node is a very accurate predictor of overall nodal status.

The implications of the TNM classification (TNM ATLAS 1998; TNM SUPPLEMENT 1993) and the ICRU 62 recommendations (ICRU 62 1999) for target volume selection and delineation have been considered. Guidelines for the selection of clinical target volumes (CTV) based on consensus statements and on the results of the sentinel node procedure (SNP) have been proposed. Guidelines for clinical target volume delineation have been adapted to take into account specific radiological landmarks more readily identified on CT slices.

6.2 Hypotheses on Tumor Spread in Breast Cancer

The debate concerning tumor spread, ongoing since the last century, has centered on two basic and interrelated views. The first involves the anatomical extent of surgical dissection based on the orderly pattern of tumor spread. The second considers the blood and lymphatic system as inseparable insofar as tumor spread is concerned, implying that there can be no orderly pattern of tumor cell dissemination based on mechanical considerations, hence the systemic nature of the cancer. In breast cancer these two contradictory opinions are known as the Halstedian (HALSTED 1907) and the Fisher theory, proposed in 1968 (FISHER 1998; FISHER and SLACK 1970; FISHER et al. 1985). In Fisher's theory, patterns of tumor spread are not solely dictated by anatomical considerations but are influenced by intrinsic factors in tumor cells and in the organs they invade. The Halstedian theory of orderly progression considers the involvement of the axillary nodes as local and the supraclavicular nodes as regional disease. Fisher's theory views breast cancer as a systemic disease; thus locoregional disease does not exist. Clinical practice shows that despite nodal involvement, long-term survivors who received only local treatment exist. The involvement of the axillary nodes is considered as local disease, whereas the involvement of the supraclavicular nodes must be considered as systemic disease (KIRICUTA 1993; KIRICUTA et al. 1994).

The evolution of breast cancer therapy was influenced by the above-mentioned hypotheses. From aggressive surgery in the early years, the treatment approach evolved to more conservative surgery followed by adjuvant RT, systemic chemotherapy and hormonal therapy. The recent introduction of the SNC and SNP can be expected to influence the treatment strategy in the direction of more conservative surgery and well-defined indications for adjuvant RT.

The randomized Danish Breast Cancer Group study (OVERGAARD et al. 1997) on 1,708 high-risk premenopausal breast cancer patients supported the hypothesis of Halsted, and succeeded in demonstrating that postoperative RT improved distant disease-free survival, and reported an improved overall survival of 9% and a reduced incidence of locoregional disease. The Fisher point of view was sustained by the randomized NSABP study (FISHER et al. 1985), which failed to demonstrate that postoperative RT improved distant disease-free survival even when it reduced the incidence of locoregional disease.

According to the Halstedian theory, radical local treatment should improve survival. Adjuvant irradiation of the breast/chest wall and the regional lymphatics should likewise improve local control and survival. Fisher's theory considers breast cancer as a systemic disease; therefore, local treatment cannot be expected to improve survival, and only systemic therapy could improve survival. As shown in Table 6.1, an improvement in 10-year survival by either local and/or systemic adjuvant treatment was observed.

The rationale for adjuvant irradiation is supported by the results reported by the Danish randomized trial and others (OVERGAARD et al. 1997; RAGAZ et al. 1997) where a survival benefit was shown following comprehensive chest wall and nodal RT. Tumor cells remaining in the locoregional lymphatics and/or breast or chest wall after mastectomy, chemotherapy and suboptimal RT can be the source of subsequent distant metastases (KOSCIELNY and TUBIANA 1999). Data exist in support of the role of subclinical disease as a source of subsequent metastases in breast cancer patients after mastectomy or breast conserving surgery (FOTTIN et al. 1999; KOSCIELNY and TUBIANA 1999; VERONESI et al. 1995).

Table 6.1. Effect of adjuvant treatment and improvement in 10-year survival in breast cancer patients

Breast cancer patients	Chemotherapy[a]	Radiotherapy[b]
N0 patients	7%	–
Node-positive patients	11%	6% (premenopausal) 9% (postmenopausal)

[a] EARLY BREAST CANCER TRIALISTS' COLLABORATIVE GROUP (1995, 1998)
[b] Danish Breast Cancer Group (OVERGAARD et al. 1997)

The survival benefit provided by adjuvant RT may be attributed to the elimination of occult residual disease in the breast after tylectomy or in the chest wall after mastectomy, and the eradication of occult residual disease in the regional lymphatics. For RT to produce a survival benefit, the following conditions are necessary: occult residual disease is located within the CTV; and distant disease is absent or sufficiently minimal to be efficiently controlled with systemic therapy (Fowble 1999).

6.3 Anatomy and Lymphatics of the Breast

Breast tissue appears to extend from the second or third rib superiorly to the sixth or seventh costal cartilage inferiorly. Medially it extends to the edge of the sternum and laterally to the anterior axillary line. However, breast tissue is found extending beyond these areas, as high as the clavicle and from the midline laterally to the edge of the latissimus dorsi muscle. In the low axilla there is an interpenetration of the breast parenchyma with lymphatic and connective tissue. The axillary tail of Spence is a prolongation of breast tissue upward into the axilla. The amount of breast tissue and its distribution may vary considerably with the age of the patient and the size of the breast. Except for the axillary prolongation, the breast is covered by the superficial fascia. Occasionally, glandular tissue is found in the pectoralis fascia. In the study carried out by Hicken, the incidence of breast carcinoma following prophylactic mastectomy was observed in 94% of cases in the subareolar or skin margin zone. Eighty-eight percent of the patients had incomplete removal of the axillary tail, and in 23% and 11% of cases respectively, the sternal extent and the epigastric ramifications were incompletely removed. Adenocarcinoma occurring in the axillary remnant was also described (Hicken 1940).

The lymphatics of the breast are classified as the external mammary nodes, known as the axillary nodes, and the internal mammary lymph nodes. These are shown in Fig. 6.1.

The anatomical classification of the axillary lymph nodes has been traditionally divided into five groups: the noduli laterales group along the vena axillaris (4–6 nodes), centrales (3–4 nodes), apicales and infraclaviculares (6–12 nodes), and subscapulares (6–7 nodes). In 1955, Berg introduced the three-level classification based on the relative position of

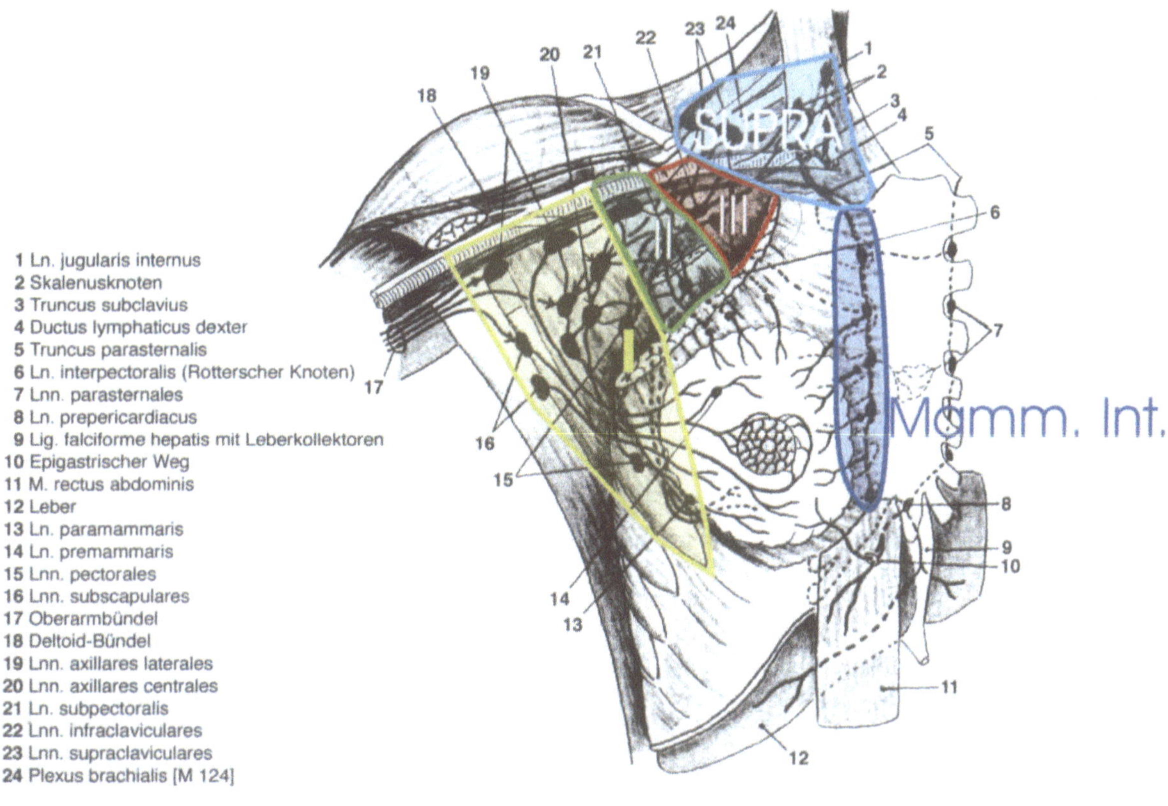

Fig. 6.1. The lymphatics of the breast with the levels according to Berg (from Kubik 1999)

the nodes to the pectoralis minor muscle (Fig. 6.1). Level I contains the lymph nodes situated laterally to the lateral border of the pectoralis minor muscle, and usually contains 10–14 nodes. Level II includes 4–6 nodes located in front of and behind the pectoralis minor muscle, including the Rotter lymph node situated between the pectoralis minor and pectoralis major muscle. Level III includes the nodes medially located from the pectoralis minor muscle, and contains 2–4 nodes.

Veronesi et al. (1990) extensively studied the size and number of the axillary lymph nodes and found an average total number of 20.3 nodes. On 1,446 completed axillary dissections, the average number of lymph nodes was 13.5 in level I, 4.5 in level II, and 2.3 nodes in level III respectively.

The IMC lies parallel to the internal artery and internal vein. Normal internal mammary lymph nodes (IMLN) range from 1–5 mm in diameter, and are not visible by CT or magnetic resonance imaging (MRI). The IMLN are found within each of the first through the fifth or sixth anterior intercostal spaces (ICS), as follows: 91% in the first ICS, 96% in the second ICS, 78% in the third ICS and between 9 and 62% in the fourth to the sixth ICS (Stibbe 1918).

The IMLN are an important site of occult metastases in clinically operable and recurrent breast cancer (Haagensen 1971; Noguchi et al. 1992). Metastases in the IMC can arise from primary lesions in all breast quadrants. The probability of involvement varies and frequently occurs at multiple levels, most often in the second and third intercostal space.

6.3.1 Drainage Patterns

The drainage of different sites of the breast has been extensively studied using node biopsy and nuclear medicine methods such as lymphoscintigraphy.

Over the years, almost every lymphatic basin and region has been explored and documented by lymphoscintigraphy, employing a variety of injection techniques and tracers. In breast cancer patients, Ege (1996) demonstrated via lymphoscintigraphy the drainage to different lymphatic regions and reported her findings as follows: (a) from the mammary and periareolar site to the axillary, supraclavicular, and upper parasternal lymph nodes; (b) from the chest wall, subcutaneous, subperiosteal site to the axillary, supraclavicular, and upper parasternal lymph nodes; (c) from the subcostal posterior rectus sheath to the diaphragmatic, parasternal, internal mammary and mediastinal lymph nodes; and (d) from the peritumoral and intracutaneous site to the superficial lymphatics at risk.

Borgstein (Borgstein 1999; Borgstein et al. 1998) used lymphoscintigraphy to visualize the individual lymph flow to the internal mammary lymph nodes for the different quadrants of the breast. The outer quadrants drain their lymph to the parasternal nodes at a lower level of probability (8–19%) than the inner quadrants and central area (21–31%). In 155 investigated breast cancer patients, lymphoscintigraphy showed in 15% of cases (23/155 patients) drainage to the parasternal nodes. Similar data were reported by Melis et al. (1999), who in 59 patients found drainage to the parasternal nodes in 17% of cases, while Mudum et al. (1999) reported primary parasternal drainage in 30% of cases.

Handley and Thakeray (1954) and Haagensen (1972) extensively studied the lymphatic drainage of each quadrant and the central area in breast cancer patients by performing systematic lymph node dissections of the internal mammary lymph nodes in respectively 800 and 1,001 breast cancer patients. Handley and Thakeray (1954) investigated 800 patients and compared data obtained by lymphadenectomy with that on the patterns of lymphatic drainage from different tumor locations found in 122 examined breast cancer patients obtained through lymphoscintigraphy (parasternal foci) and gamma probe procedure (for axillary SN) as reported by Borgstein et al. (1998). These findings are shown in Fig. 6.2. As demonstrated by the above-mentioned data, the principal drainage is through the axillary nodes, followed by drainage through the parasternal lymphatics.

6.4 The Sentinel Node Concept and the Sentinel Node Procedure

The SNC is fundamentally based on the orderly progression of tumor cells within the lymphatic system. It is the most important new concept in surgical and radiation oncology. A high success rate in the identification of the SN for breast cancer has been reported. The presence or absence of metastases in this node is a very accurate predictor of overall nodal status.

The SNP is at present the most sensitive method of determining the very individual principal drainage of the primary tumor. The SNC is based on a specific lymph node center, called the SN, which appears to be

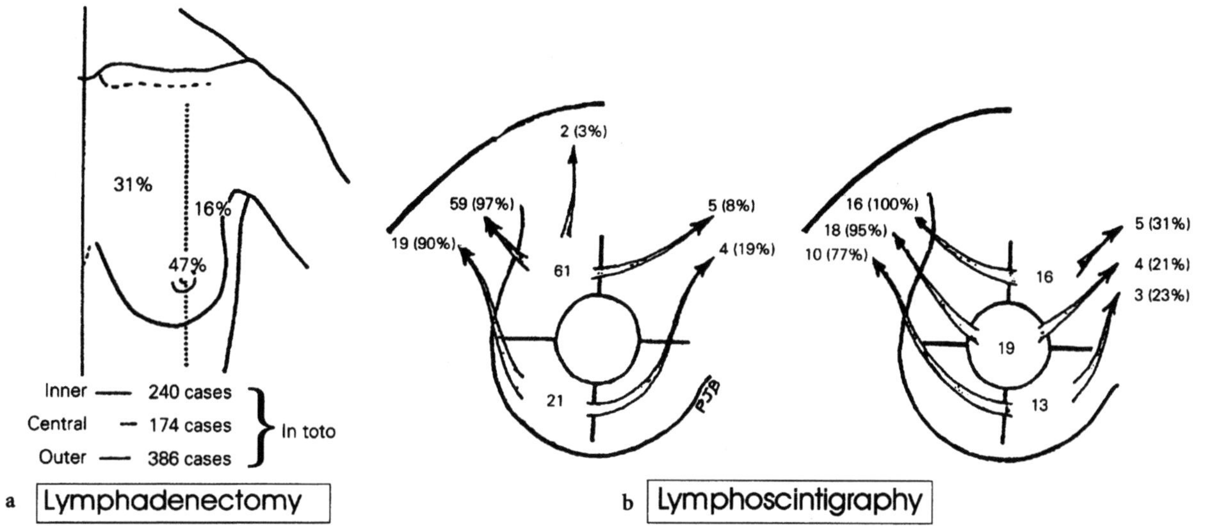

Fig. 6.2. Lymphatic drainage of the different quadrants of the breast studied by a nodal dissection (HANDLEY and THAKERAY 1954) and b lymphoscintigraphy (BORGSTEIN 1999; BORGSTEIN et al. 1998)

the primary site of metastases. The SNP may lead to a more substantiated, systematic approach to adjuvant therapy strategies with low complication rates.

The necessity of examining the SN with the greatest possible degree of accuracy highlights one of the major problems related to SN biopsy. The success of the SNP depends primarily on the adequate functional capacity for sufficient isotope uptake to ensure accurate identification. In SN-negative patients, complete axillary lymph node dissection is avoidable. In SN-positive but clinically negative patients, postoperative RT could permit adequate tumor control. The last two procedures result in a lower morbidity rate.

The definition of a "pN0" patient based on SN biopsy has recently been introduced in the current TNM classification (SOBIN 1999). On this basis, new target volumes can defined for adjuvant RT and the lymphatic basins potentially spared, thereby avoiding unnecessary irradiation.

Randomized trials were set up to validate the SNP and to verify the SNC in breast cancer patients. Important consequences for minimal invasive surgery and adjuvant therapy have resulted. SN biopsy is a highly accurate, minimally invasive method of staging patients and can substantially reduce the morbidity and cost of treatment by avoiding unnecessary complete axillary lymph node dissection or irradiation of the lymphatics.

Identification of the individual lymphatic flow pattern could permit the definition of the CTV and provide indications for irradiation of the individual locoregional lymphatic basin.

6.4.1 Location and Number of Sentinel Nodes in Breast Cancer Patients

The SNP permits the identification of the first echelon lymph node. This node is not infrequently localized in two lymphatic basins or in non-locoregional, anatomically unpredictable lymph node basins as defined by the TNM classification. Examples of the unpredictable lymph node basins are the contralateral parasternal or contralateral axillary nodes in breast cancer patients. Thus, the SNP should reliably indicate which lymphatic basin really is the locoregional one.

In breast cancer patients the SN is found in nodal level I, predominantly in the central group of the axillary lymph nodes. LINEHAN et al. (1999) reported data on 800 SNP in patients with T1–2/N0 invasive breast cancer. In this study, they found the SN in level I in 99% of cases. KRAG et al. (1998) reported that in the 383 patients with a single spot, 365 (95.3%) were in level I, 13 (3.3%) in level II and none in level III. DE CICCO et al. (1998) found that in 108 node-positive patients level I was the only site of metastases in 98 cases (90.7%). A positive SN was found in level II in nine cases (8%) and in level III in one case (0.9%). The location of the primary tumor within specific breast quadrants did not influence the site of the SN, and obvious "skipping" to higher levels was not observed in the study of BORGSTEIN et al. (1998) on 122 patients. In this study, the SN was always found in level I. An average of 1.2 SN were biopsied per patient (range: 1–3): 99 patients (81%) had a single SN, 22 (18%) had two equally radioactive SN, and one patient had three SN.

In 160 examined cases, VERONESI et al. (1997) using the SN probe detected one SN in 104 cases (65%), two SN in 41 cases (25.6%), and three SN in 15 cases (9.4%). RODIER et al. (1999) reported on 74 patients with clinically nodal negative axillary status. The SN was positive in 22.7% of the patients, in 53.5% there was only one node involved, and in 12% the SN was false negative.

Recently, VERONESI et al. (1999) have reported a rate of 5.9% positive in other axillary lymph nodes among patients with a negative SN. The overall agreement between SN and axillary lymph node status was 96.8% (359 out of 371), while the rate of false negative among patients with at least one positive lymph node was 6.7% (12 out of 180). The authors also showed that SN invaded by microfoci of cancer cells are, however, associated with a considerable rate of metastatic involvement (53%) in the rest of the axillary lymph nodes (27 out of 51). They concluded that the presence of microfoci in the SN is an indication for performing a complete axillary dissection. A mathematical model could confirm this conclusion (KIRICUTA 1999).

HAIGH et al. (2000) have reported on the frequency of primary or secondary drainage in the axillary (AX), internal mammary (IM) and infraclavicular (CL) SN found in preoperative lymphoscintigraphy data for 76 cases of breast cancer. Primary drainage to AX only was found in 58 cases, to AX and IM in one case, to AX and IM and CL in one case, and to IM in one case. An additional secondary drainage to a primary drainage was found in eight cases with a primary drainage to AX and a secondary drainage to IM, in two cases with a primary drainage to AX and a secondary drainage to CL, in four cases with a primary drainage to IM and a secondary drainage to AX, and in one case with a primary drainage to CL and a secondary drainage to AX. The frequency of drainage to AX, CL and IM was as follows: 99% to AX, 20% to IM, and 5% to CL.

The data reported on the SNP in regard to the staging and appropriate indications for adjuvant local or systemic treatment has been reconsidered in the TNM classification. Recently the TNM Committee (SOBIN 1999) has proposed that trials should use the following description to record sentinel lymph node status:

- pNX (SN):
  Sentinel lymph node could not be assessed
- pN0 (SN):
  No sentinel lymph node metastasis
- pN1 (SN):
  Sentinel lymph node metastasis

For useful application of the TNM description, standardization of the procedure is mandatory. The clinical consequences of the SNP for target volume selection are as follows:

- It indicates the locoregional lymphatic basin
- It permits the identification of a non-predictable lymphatic basin
- It indicates where to look for and find the SN intraoperatively

The pathological examination of the SN permits the determination of whether the lymphatic basin is involved by tumor cells or not. Thus an appropriate staging is possible.

In selected cases, the degree of involvement of the SN gives information about the degree of involvement of the rest of the lymphatic basin.

It permits tissue sparing in 60% of patients, i.e. complete lymph node dissection could be prevented and the morbidity associated with lymphedema, seroma, and neurological symptoms could be avoided.

If a SN is involved, adequate indications for adjuvant local and systemic treatment exist; furthermore, the SN indicates to the radiation oncologist how to select adequate target volumes for appropriate irradiation.

6.5 Target Volume Selection: the Surgeon's Viewpoint

The radiation oncologist is routinely confronted with the clinical situation of breast cancer patients after ablative or conservative surgery. Several types of breast surgery for the primary tumor with the preservation or removal of different structures are routinely used, as shown in Table 6.2.

6.5.1 Multifocality and Multicentricity of Breast Cancer

Multifocality refers to the presence of cancer in the vicinity of and in continuity with the primary tumor, whereas multicentricity refers to independent cancer foci of cancer unrelated to the primary tumor. The work of HOLLAND et al. (1985) has clarified this issue by studying mastectomy specimens with primary tumors of 2 cm or less in size. In all cases, the tumor was considered unicentric

Table 6.2. Types of breast ablative and breast preserving surgery and structures removed in primary breast cancer

Type of surgery	Structures involved
Ablative surgery	
Standard radical mastectomy	Complete removal of the breast, pectoralis minor, pectoralis major and some axillary nodes
Extended radical mastectomy	Like standard radical mastectomy plus resection of the internal mammary nodes
Modified radical mastectomy	Complete removal of the breast, pectoralis fascia and complete axillary dissection. Resection of the pectoralis minor muscle and preservation of the pectoralis major muscle
Total mastectomy (simple mastectomy)	Removal of the entire breast, including the nipple–areolar complex, but without axillary dissection or removal of the pectoralis muscles
Subcutaneous mastectomy	Removal of the major part of the breast but sparing the nipple–areolar complex
Conservative surgery	
Segmental mastectomy (partial mastectomy)	Removal of a breast segment with the tumor, the overlying skin and with axillary dissection
Quadrantectomy	En bloc excision of the tumor within a quadrant of the breast tissue along with the pectoralis major fascia and overlying skin
Excision (lumpectomy, tumorectomy, tylectomy)	Gross removal of the tumor without attention to margins
Wide excision (limited resection, partial mastectomy)	Excision of the tumor with grossly normal clean margins

based on clinical and radiographic assessment. A precise mapping of the extent and distribution of the residual tumor in relation to the primary was performed. In 41% of cases, no tumor foci were found outside the reference tumor. Tumor foci within 2 cm of the reference tumor were found in 17% of cases. Non-invasive tumor foci extending further than 2 cm from the reference tumor were found in 28% of cases. In 14% of cases, invasive tumor foci extending further than 2 cm from the reference tumor were found (Fig. 6.3). This study demonstrated that breast cancer is very frequently multifocal, but rarely multicentric.

The consequences for target volume designation for postoperative radiotherapy after breast conserving surgery are evident. These findings provide a strong rationale for irradiation of the entire breast and the addition of a boost dose at the primary site after wide local excision. The rate of local recurrence in patients treated by local excision without RT is similar to that of cases with residual cancer more than 2 cm from the reference tumor. Local recurrence in the breast occurs at or near the site of the primary tumor.

6.6 Axillary Dissection

The status of the regional lymph nodes is the most important prognostic factor and a critical component

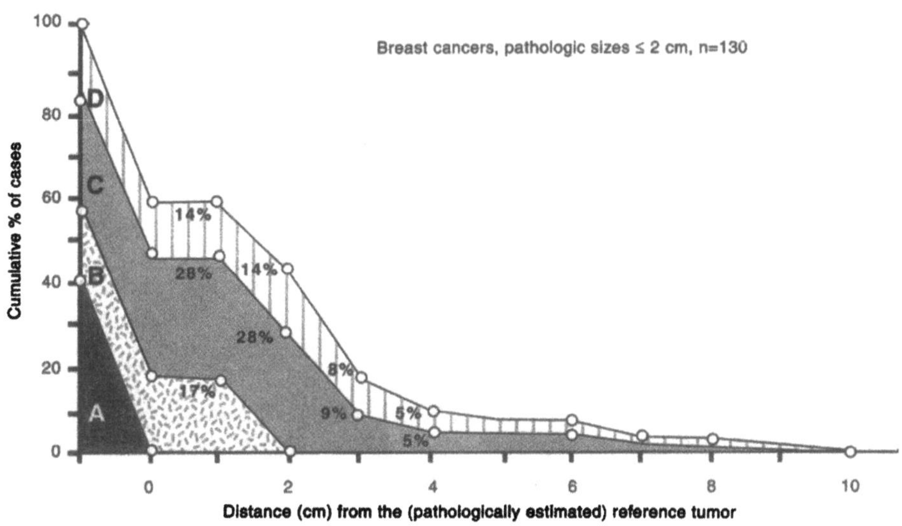

Fig. 6.3. Distribution of tumor foci at different distances from the border of the gross tumor volume in breast cancer with pathological sizes of 2 cm or less than 2 cm (Holland et al. 1985)

for the staging of cancer patients and for indications of adjuvant treatment. The aim of axillary dissection is diagnostic and therapeutic. The management of the regional lymph nodes in breast cancer is a subject of controversy. Recently, increased local control with definitive RT achieved by increasing total doses has been reported to improve survival (Overgaard et al. 1997; Ragaz et al. 1997).

Evaluation of the axillary lymph nodes is carried out by clinical and/or surgical examination. In patients with clinically negative nodes, approximately 35–40% have pathological evidence of lymph node metastases. Even in patients with early stage I and II and clinically negative axillary nodes, failure to perform axillary dissection resulted in about 20% incidence of axillary recurrence. In early breast cancer, for lesions between 1–5 mm in diameter, a 3–28% incidence of axillary node involvement has been described (Carter et al. 1989; Nemoto et al. 1980; Silverstein et al. 1994).

The types of lymphadenectomy in operable breast cancer include: sampling (removal of axillary nodes from the lower axilla without definition of precise anatomical boundaries); low axillary dissection (en bloc excision of level I with clearing of the axillary vein superiorly); levels I and II (en bloc resection of the low and mid portions of the axilla); and complete axillary dissection (en bloc resection of levels I, II and III). A level I and II axillary dissection with at least 10 nodes sampled is considered a standard lymphadenectomy (Urban and Marjani 1971).

6.6.1 How Many Nodes Must Be Examined and Found Uninvolved for a Patient to Be Classified pN0?

According to the TNM Supplement (1993), at least 10 level I and II axillary nodes must be sampled and found uninvolved to describe a patient as pN0. Based on 1,446 complete axillary dissections performed by Veronesi et al. (1990), Kiricuta and Tausch (1992) developed a mathematical model to describe the number of nodes from level I to be examined and found uninvolved in order to describe an axilla as pN0. The model suggests that the number of nodes to be examined from level I and found uninvolved is 11 for T1 and 10 for T2 primaries.

An uninvolved SN or nodes also permit the classification of the axilla as pN0 (Sobin 1999). The investigation of the ipsilateral internal mammary nodes is not considered as standard.

6.6.2 Residual Tumor After Incomplete Axillary Dissection, Extent of Axillary Dissection

The importance of resecting an adequate number of axillary lymph nodes for examination in order to determine true pN0 axillary status was described by Kiricuta et al. (1992) who found poor survival for pN0 patients if fewer axillary lymph nodes were examined. The 10-year survival of pN0 patients in whom less than 5 nodes were examined was around 50%. In pN0 patients in whom more than 9 nodes were examined, a 10-year survival rate of around 90% was noted. These data were similar to the findings of Wilking et al. (1992) who reported an improvement in survival of patients with 1–3 positive nodes when the number of axillary nodes examined increased. With 1–3 positive nodes, the 7-year survival was 45%, 65%, and 80% for patients who had fewer than 5 nodes examined, 5–9 nodes examined, and 10 or more nodes examined respectively. These data reflect a more accurate assessment of the extent of nodal positivity as the number of nodes examined increases. Similar findings were reported by Fisher and Slack (1970). The 5-year survival for patients with 1–3 positive nodes was 44% for 1–5 nodes examined, 58% for 6–10 nodes examined, and 68% for 11–15 nodes examined. These data support the argument that underestimating the number of positive axillary nodes with an axillary sampling results in both an increase in locoregional recurrence and a decrease in survival.

To determine the residual involved axillary nodes after axillary sampling, our mathematical model based on 1,446 complete axillary dissections performed by Veronesi et al. (1990) showed that more than 10 level I nodes have to be examined to assure a 90% probability of true pN0 status (Kiricuta and Tausch 1992).

Based on the same mathematical model using the data on 1,396 complete axillary dissections for T1 and T2 breast tumors performed by Veronesi et al. (1990), it was possible to calculate the maximum number of nodes involved in all levels if 1, 2 or 3 or more level I nodes (*m* is the number of nodes found involved) were found to be involved and an incomplete axillary dissection was performed (*n* nodes is the sample size from only level I). The results are given in Table 6.3.

The numbers are listed depending on the sample size n from level I and the number *m* of involved nodes detected by the pathologist. Firstly, Table 6.3 shows the numbers of nodes that have to be removed

Table 6.3. The maximum number of involved axillary lymph nodes in all levels if for a T1 primary *n* level I nodes were sampled and *m* nodes were found to be involved. The values in parentheses indicate the maximum number of involved axillary lymph nodes in all levels for T2 primaries

n/m	0	1	2	3	4	5	6	7	8	9	10	11	12	13
1	4 (8)	19 (19)												
2	3 (5)	12 (14)	21 (19)											
3	2 (3)	8 (11)	14 (16)	21 (20)										
4	2 (2)	6 (9)	12 (14)	16 (17)	21 (20)									
5	1 (2)	5 (7)	9 (12)	14 (15)	18 (18)	21 (20)								
6	1 (2)	4 (5)	8 (10)	12 (13)	15 (16)	18 (18)	21 (20)							
7	1 (2)	4 (4)	7 (8)	11 (12)	13 (15)	16 (16)	19 (18)	21 (20)						
8	1 (1)	3 (3)	6 (7)	9 (10)	12 (13)	14 (15)	16 (17)	20 (19)	21 (20)					
9	1 (1)	3 (3)	6 (6)	7 (9)	11 (12)	13 (14)	15 (16)	17 (18)	20 (19)	21 (20)				
10	0 (1)	2 (3)	5 (5)	7 (8)	11 (11)	12 (13)	13 (15)	16 (16)	18 (18)	20 (19)	21 (20)			
11	0 (0)	2 (2)	4 (5)	6 (7)	9 (10)	12 (11)	12 (13)	14 (16)	16 (17)	18 (18)	20 (19)	21 (20)		
12	0 (0)	2 (2)	4 (3)	6 (6)	7 (8)	11 (11)	12 (13)	13 (15)	14 (16)	16 (18)	18 (18)	20 (19)	21 (20)	
13	0 (0)	2 (2)	3 (3)	6 (6)	7 (8)	11 (10)	12 (13)	12 (12)	13 (16)	16 (16)	16 (18)	18 (18)	20 (19)	21 (20)

and found to be uninvolved in order to predict a real N0 axillary status. We have to look for the first occurrence of 0 in the first column (m=0). Ten (n=10) axillary lymph nodes from level I have to be removed and found negative for a T1 tumor, and 11 (n=11) nodes for a T2 tumor. Secondly, this table shows the possible number of residual involved nodes after an axillary dissection. Knowing the number of removed lymph nodes, we are now able to predict the amount of positive lymph nodes left in the axilla. As an example, assuming that for a T1 primary the surgeon sampled only 7 nodes from level I (n=7) and the pathologist found 3 of them to be involved (m=3) then from Table 6.3 one can find the possible maximum number of involved nodes =11 written at the intersection of the column at m=3 and the line n=7. In this case of axillary dissection from level I, 8 involved nodes are left in the axilla.

As shown in Table 6.3 for T1 tumors and 1, 2, or 3 positive nodes, the minimum number of nodes to be examined needed for a 90% probability of accuracy is respectively 19, 21 and 21. For T2 tumors and 1, 2, or 3 positive nodes, a minimum number of 19 or 20 nodes is required. The probability of finding 4 or more positive nodes increases as tumor size and the number of reported positive nodes increase, and as the number of examined nodes increases. The accuracy of the extent of axillary nodal positivity is influenced by the number of observed positive nodes, tumor size, and the number of nodes examined. Underestimation of the number of positive nodes will result in errors in the assessment of an individual's risk for locoregional recurrence, distant disease, and breast cancer death, and will adversely impact on treatment recommendations. This model provides the radiation oncologist with a mean for assessing the accuracy of the number of positive nodes if an incomplete axillary dissection is performed. The actual recommendation to examine 10 level I and II axillary nodes suffices only to determine nodal positivity or negativity. Thus, the real number of possible involved nodes is underestimated.

Based on the above-mentioned mathematical model for a T1 primary, if 1–3 positive nodes are found from 10 examined nodes, it can be assumed that 1–4 additional possible involved nodes have not been diagnosed. For a T2 primary, if 1–3 positive nodes are found in 10 examined nodes, then 2–5 additional involved nodes have not been diagnosed. For 4 or more involved nodes found from 10 examined nodes, a maximum of 7 additional involved nodes have not been diagnosed. The predictions of our model have recently been confirmed by Iyer et al. (2000). An inaccurate determination of the number of involved nodes will affect the estimated risk of locoregional recurrence, distant disease and breast cancer death. The therapeutic implications are related to the fact that it is generally accepted that patients with 4 or more involved axillary nodes are candidates for PMRT, whereas in patients with 1–3 involved nodes this recommendation is controversial. To resolve these uncertainties, randomized trials to determine the effect of postoperative RT on these special groups of patients with 1–3 positive nodes are urgently needed.

A strong influence of the number of examined nodes on survival rate as well as on the locoregional recurrence rate in patients with an axillary involvement exists, and is shown in Table 6.4.

Table 6.4. The influence of the number of nodes examined on the survival rate, recurrence-free rate and disease-free survival as well as the locoregional recurrence rate for patients with 1–3 positive nodes or node-positive patients

	Type of axillary involvement	No. of nodes examined 1–5	No. of nodes examined 6–10	No. of nodes examined 11–15	Author
5-year survival rate	1–3	44%	58%	68%	FISHER and SLACK (1970)
5-year recurrence-free survival	1–3	55%	70%	82%	WILKING et al. (1992)
10-year disease-free survival	N+	6.5%	31%	32%	KORZENIOWSKI et al. (1994)
Locoregional recurrence rate	N+	40%	32%	27%	OVERGAARD et al. (1997); chemotherapy only

6.7 Involvement of the Axillary and Internal Mammary Lymph Nodes

Valuable data about the involvement and pattern of metastatic spread to the locoregional lymphatics – axillary and internal mammary nodes – in breast cancer patients are found in the excellent papers by HAAGENSEN (1971), HANDLEY (1975), NOGUCHI et al. (1991), and VERONESI et al. (1990), which are briefly discussed herein.

6.7.1 Axillary Nodes

VERONESI et al. (1990) reported on 1,446 complete axillary dissections, the most detailed report on a large number of complete axillary dissections in breast cancer patients. Metastases confined to level I only were found in 54.2%, the involvement of levels I and II in 22.3%, and of all three levels in 22.3% of cases. The rate of skip metastases (i.e. isolated involvement of higher levels without involvement of lower levels) amounted to 1.2% for level II and 0.1% for level III.

The incidence of involvement of the axillary nodes by level for differing tumor size was extensively examined, and has been presented in Table 6.5.

The involvement of level III in patients with involvement of levels I and II is dependent on the primary tumor size and has been shown in Table 6.6. For primaries larger than 2.0 cm, the involvement of level III nodes is higher than 35% if levels I and II are involved. Level III was found to be involved in 22% of all positive cases. If only one level I node is metastasized, the possibility of second level involvement is low, i.e. around 12.1%, whereas if more than 4 nodes are involved at the first level the other levels are more likely to be involved (83.9%). From these data, the following conclusion can be drawn for target volume selection and delineation: for axillary positive patients with a less than complete axillary dissection, the inclusion in the CTV of the whole axilla or at least the non-dissected levels is indicated.

Table 6.5. The incidence of involvement of the axillary nodes by level for different tumor size (data from VERONESI et al. 1990)

Level	T1	T2	T3
I	263 (64.8%)	182 (46.2%)	10 (25.6%)
I+II	68 (16.7%)	107 (27.1%)	12 (30.8%)
I+II+III	67 (16.5%)	102 (25.9%)	17 (43.6%)
Skip level	8 (2.0%)	3 (0.8%)	0
Total	406 (100%)	394 (100%)	39 (100%)

Table 6.6. Risk of metastases at the third level in cases of metastatic involvement of the first and second levels, according to size of the primary carcinoma (data from VERONESI et al. 1990)

Size of primary carcinoma	Risk of metastases at the third level (%)
<2 cm	35.2
3.1– 5.0 cm	53.8
>5.0 cm	74.7
Total	45.7

VERONESI et al. (1990) examined in 1,446 complete axillary dissections the relation between involvement of the axillary lymph nodes and tumor size. The number of involved axillary nodes is dependent on the size of the primary cancer, as shown in Table 6.7. One to 3 involved axillary nodes were found in 30.3% of T1 primaries, 29.9% of T2 primaries and 18% of T3 primaries. The involvement of 4 or more axillary lymph nodes was as follows: 18.5% of T1, 39.8% of T2 and 60% of T3 primaries.

6.7.2 Internal Mammary Lymph Nodes

The IMLN are largest and most numerous in the upper three intercostal spaces. In one study, all of the

Table 6.7. Number of positive axillary lymph nodes depending on tumor size in operable breast cancer patients (data from VERONESI et al. 1990)

No. of positive nodes	T1 (<2 cm)	T2 (>2<5 cm)	T3 (<5 cm)	Total
0	425 (51.1%)	171 (30.3%)	11 (22.0%)	607 (42.0%)
1	138 (16.6%)	72 (12.7%)	5 (10.0%)	215 (14.9%)
2–3	114 (13.7%)	97 (17.2%)	4 (8.0%)	215 (14.9%)
4–10	95 (11.4%)	114 (20.2%)	11 (22.0%)	220 (15.2%)
>10	59 (7.1%)	11 (19.6%)	19 (38.0%)	189 (13.0%)
Total	831	565	50	1446

nodes identified in the lower three spaces were solitary, while multiple nodes were often present in the upper spaces. NOGUCHI et al. (1991, 1992) reported that of the 521 nodes identified, approximately 80% were recovered from the upper three spaces versus approximately 20% from the lower three spaces. The same authors reported similar results for patients undergoing extended radical mastectomy. Sixty-five percent of the nodes recovered from the upper three spaces contained cancer cells versus only 5% of the nodes removed from the fourth space.

The location and incidence of metastatic IMLN has been described by NOGUCHI et al. (1991, 1992). The authors found the involvement of the first intercostal space (ICS) in 90% (in 19 patients out of 21) of cases, of the second ICS in 81% (17/21), of the third ICS in 48% (10/21), and of the fourth ICS in only 10% (2/21) of patients.

Based on these data, the CTV should include the IMC nodes of only the first four ICS. In early studies, the late side-effects of non-optimized irradiation techniques for IMLN irradiation were responsible for reduced survival (CUZICK et al. 1997). The anatomical relationship between the CTV for IMLN so defined and the myocardium in two entirely different gantry positions has been shown in Fig. 6.4. If only the first four ICS are included in the target volume, no irradiation of the myocardium is necessary or possible (SMITT and GOFFINET 1999).

A close correlation between axillary and internal mammary lymph node metastases has been shown. Even in patients with a negative axilla, 5–10% have been shown to have positive ILMN (MORROW and FOSTER 1981; VERONESI et al. 1985).

The incidence of nodal metastases of the IMLN chain is dependent on the location of the primary tumor in the outer or inner quadrants and on the axillary status, as shown in Table 6.8. The probability of involvement of the parasternal nodes is higher if the axillary nodes are involved.

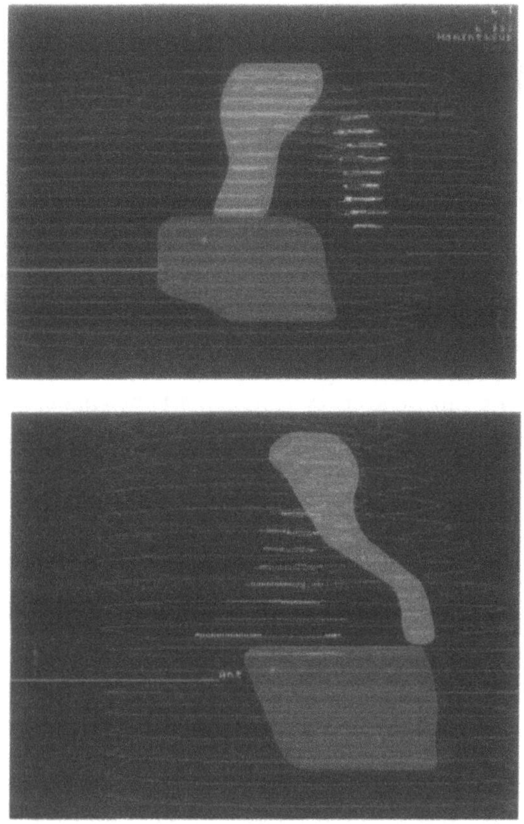

a

b

Fig. 6.4. Beam's eye view of the clinical target volume of the IMLN chain (ICS 1–4) and supraclavicular nodes (*blue*) and the heart (*dark blue*) at gantry positions **a** 0 degree and **b** 270 degrees. The other contours are: body outline (*gray*), and axillary level I (*white*), level II (*red*), level III (*green*). No superposition of the IMLN chain target volume and the heart exists

Table 6.8. The involvement of the internal mammary lymph nodes depending on axillary status, tumor size and tumor location. (Data from 3,495 internal mammary lymphadenectomies reviewed by WILLNER and FLENTJE 1998)

Axillary status		Tumor in outer quadrants		Tumor in inner quadrants	
		T1–2	T3	T1–2	T3
N0	(a)	7% (45/643)		13% (126/998)	
	(b)	5% (17/328)	19% (16/82)	10% (28/271)	9% (8/85)
N+	(a)	23% (197/861)		45% (446/993)	
	(b)	18% (70/390)	33% (57/171)	33% (83/255)	42% (4/151)

Data from:
(a) VERONESI and VALAGUSSA (1981); LACOUR et al. (1976); HANDLEY and THAKERAY (1954); URBAN and MARJANI (1971)
(b) VERONESI and VALAGUSSA (1981); LACOUR et al. (1976)

6.8 Historical View of Field Selection in Postmastectomy Radiotherapy

Target volume selection for breast cancer after mastectomy remains a subject of controversy. A review of the fields used to irradiate different anatomical regions (chest wall, axillary nodes, internal mammary nodes, supraclavicular nodes) in the most important trials involving postoperative RT and their effects on local recurrence, disease-free survival and survival overall is given in Table 6.9.

As can be seen in Table 6.9, a beneficial effect of postoperative RT on survival rate in node-positive patients was obtained only in the Danish (Overgaard et al. 1997) and the British Columbia (Ragaz et al. 1997) trials. Each of these postmastectomy irradiation trials included the chest wall and all lymphatic areas within their target volumes.

6.8.1 Patterns of Recurrence

In general, the term "isolated locoregional recurrence" refers to the first site of failure in the chest wall or axillary, internal mammary or supraclavicular nodes, without the simultaneous presence of distant metastases. The term "locoregional recurrence" includes cancers in patients who present with simultaneous distant metastases. Differences in reporting local failure have varied, however, because of the definition of locoregional recurrence that has been used. Some authors included only the chest wall and the axillary failures, whereas most of the other authors included the supraclavicular recurrences. In some reports, local recurrence was classified as such only in the case of the first site of failure, whereas in others any local recurrences were enumerated.

Reported local recurrence rates after radical mastectomy and modified radical mastectomy alone varied from 4%–26%, although the incidence of nodal positivity was similar in that series, ranging from 38%–53% (Morrow 1999).

The presence of axillary nodal metastases and the number of involved axillary nodes appear to be the most reliable predictors of the risk of locoregional recurrence, as shown in Table 6.10.

Urban and Castro (1971) described an increased risk of internal mammary nodal metastases with the extent of axillary nodal involvement. A 25% risk of internal mammary nodal metastases existed if only level I of the axilla was involved, whereas an increase to 67% was observed if level III was involved.

Table 6.10. The risk of locoregional recurrence depending on the type of axillary nodal involvement

Authors	Type of axillary involvement	Locoregional recurrence (%)
Urban and Castro (1971)	0	2
	Axilla involved	8
	Level I	8
	Level II	19
	Level III	27
Haagensen and Bodian (1984)		Chest wall
	0	2.7
	1–3 nodes involved	4.5
	4–7 nodes involved	10.4
	8 or more nodes involved	33.8

Table 6.9. The fields used in the most important trials examining the role of postoperative RT

Trials	Fields used	Results
Manchester Q (Patterson and Russel 1959; Easson 1968)	CW+Ax. Apex	LC improved
Manchester P	Ax.+Supra+MI	LC improved
CRC (Brinkley et al. 1984)	CW+Ax.+Supra+MI	LC improved
NSABP 04 (Fisher et al. 1985)	CW+Ax.+Supra+MI	Disadvantage of RT
OSLO I (Host and Brennhovd 1975)	CW+Ax.+Supra+MI	MFS and OS improved
OSLO II (Host et al. 1986)	Ax.+Supra+MI	LC improved
Stockholm (Wallgren et al. 1986)	CW+Ax.+Supra+MI	MFS and OS improved
Danish Trial (N+/1–3 nodes involved) (Overgaard et al. 1997)	CW+Ax.+Supra+MI	LC improved, OS improved
British Columbia Trial (Ragaz et al. 1997)	CW+Ax.+Supra+MI	OS benefit
EORTC (1996)	Supra (medial)+MI	Trial not finished

CW, chest wall; Ax., axilla; MI, internal mammary; Supra, supraclavicular nodes; LC, local control; RT, radiotherapy; MFS, metastasis-free survival; OS, overall survival

The risk of supraclavicular node involvement and its dependence on axillary nodal involvement was described by DAHL IVERSEN (cited by HAAGENSEN 1972) as 0% if the axilla was found to be uninvolved and 18% if the axilla was found to be involved. HAAGENSEN (1971) reported 18% supraclavicular involvement if the internal mammary nodes were involved.

The frequency and location of locoregional recurrence (first site of failure) as a function of RT reported in the Danish trial (OVERGAARD et al. 1997) is summarized in Table 6.11.

Based on the data from the Danish trial (OVERGAARD et al. 1997), the extent of axillary surgery is the most important factor for the prevention of locoregional failure. The dependence of locoregional failure on the extent of axillary surgery is shown in Table 6.12.

The effect of systemic therapy on patterns of local recurrence following radical or modified radical mastectomy is limited. The data of FOWBLE et al. (1988) and those of the Milan trial (BONADONNA et al. 1985) confirmed the limited effect of systemic treatment on the incidence of local recurrence, as shown in Table 6.13.

Table 6.11. The frequency and location of locoregional recurrence (first site of failure) as a function of RT (in parentheses, the percentage of patients with concomitant metastases; data from OVERGAARD et al. 1997)

Treatment	No local recurrence (%)	Chest wall (%)	Axilla (%)	Supra/infra. clavicular (%)	All recurrences (%)
RT	92	5 (2)	2 (1)	2 (1)	8 (3)
No RT	67	16 (3)	13 (2)	5 (2)	33 (6)

Table 6.12. Locoregional failure depending on the extent of axillary surgery (OVERGAARD et al. 1997)

Primary treatment	No. of nodes removed	Locoregional recurrence (%)
Axillary dissection and only CMF	1–3 nodes	40
	>9 nodes	27
Complete axillary dissection		Rare

Table 6.13. The effect of systemic therapy on patterns of local recurrence following radical or modified radical mastectomy in breast cancer patients

Author	Type of systemic treatment	Locoregional recurrence		
		Isolated (%)	Plus distant disease(%)	Only distant disease (%)
VALAGUSSA et al. (1978)	No	14.5	6.8	27.2
FOWBLE et al. (1988)	CMF	10	4	18
Milan Trial (BONADONNA et al. 1985)	Control group	14.5		
	CMF	11.6		

6.9 CT Anatomy of the Glandular Breast and Locoregional Lymph Nodes

There is a large variability in the glandular breast tissue (GBT) and in the location of the IMLN chain visualized by CT scan. The use of CT as an aid to treatment planning in patients with breast cancer is limited by the ability to radiographically identify GBT. This is a problem, especially in older women. Tissues of increased density are commonly seen on CT images, and likely correspond to GBT. The radiographically visible tissue like GBT does not represent the full extent of GBT, but does provide, as described in the paper by BENTEL et al. (1999), anatomical information that may be useful in designating target volumes. Large variations have been found in the location of GBT. The midline border was appropriate in only 10%, "inadequate" in nearly half (44.5%), and the applied fields included "excessive," non-target tissues in 45.5% of the patients.

CT scans are also useful as regards placement of the boost volume, localization of the excision cavity, determination of the electron energy, and localization of the clips (MESSER et al. 1997).

BENTEL et al. (1999) determined the variability of GBT and the location of the internal mammary vessels (IMV) in patients undergoing breast-conserving and CT-based RT. They found that the position of IMV and GBT varied widely in breast cancer patients, as shown in Table 6.14.

It is essential to have a knowledge of the anatomical distribution of the axillary, internal mammary and supraclavicular lymph nodes in CT axial slices at different anatomical levels for CTV delineation. The axillary levels are based on the relative position of the lymph nodes to the pectoralis minor muscle. The nodes within the area for standard axillary dissection as well as the internal mammary chain and the supraclavicular nodes are shown in Fig. 6.5. Clinical examples of the involvement and localization of lymph node metastases in breast cancer patients are shown in Fig. 6.6a–f.

An orientation plain view of the locoregional lymphatics and the breast or chest wall which

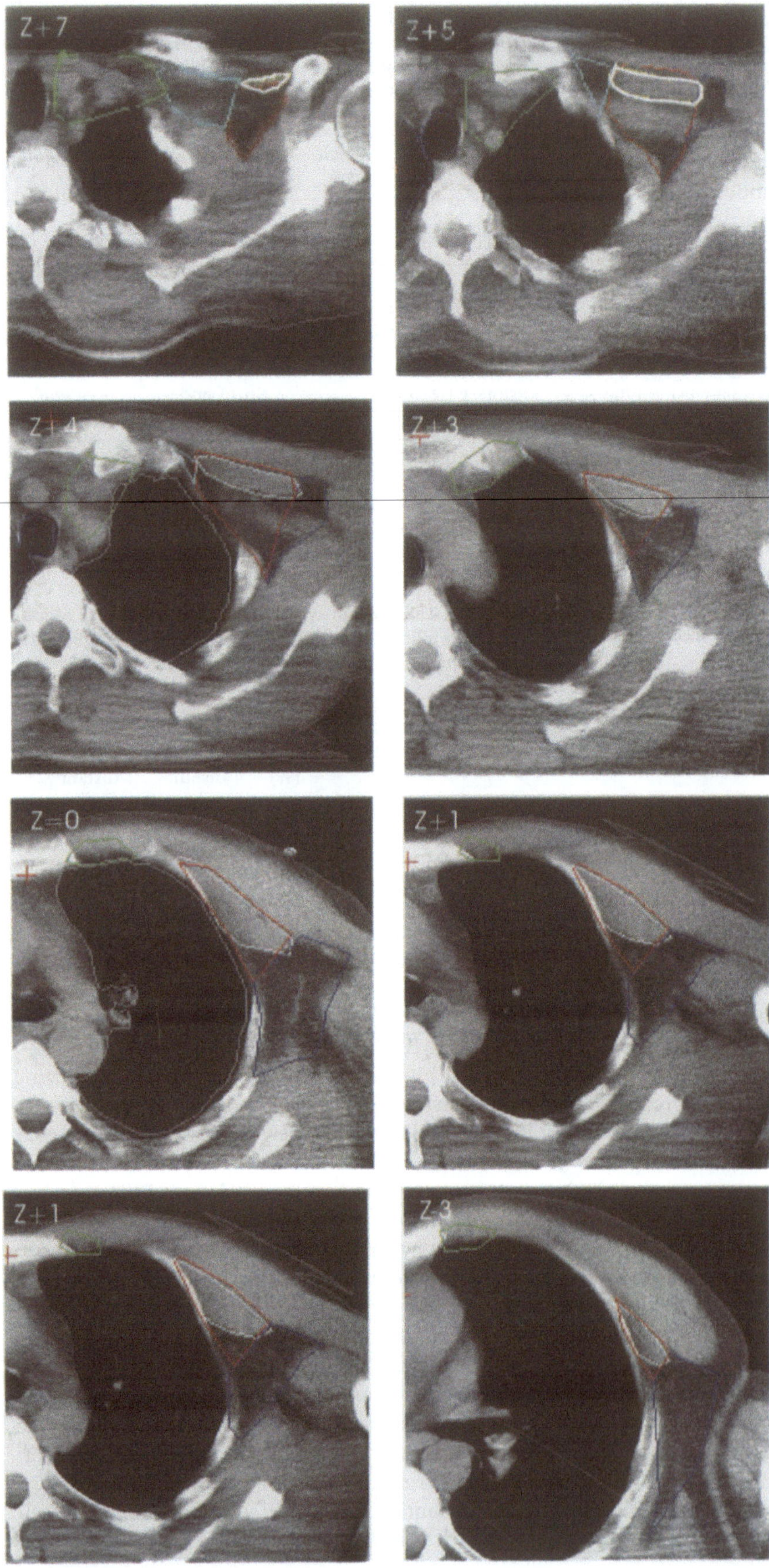

Fig. 6.5. CT based nodal classification of the locoregional lymph nodes: axillary, internal mammary (*green*) and supraclavicular nodes (*green*). The nodes belonging to the area considered for standard complete lymphadenectomy are: level I (*dark blue*), level II (*red*) and level III (*blue*). The pectoralis minor is contoured in *white*

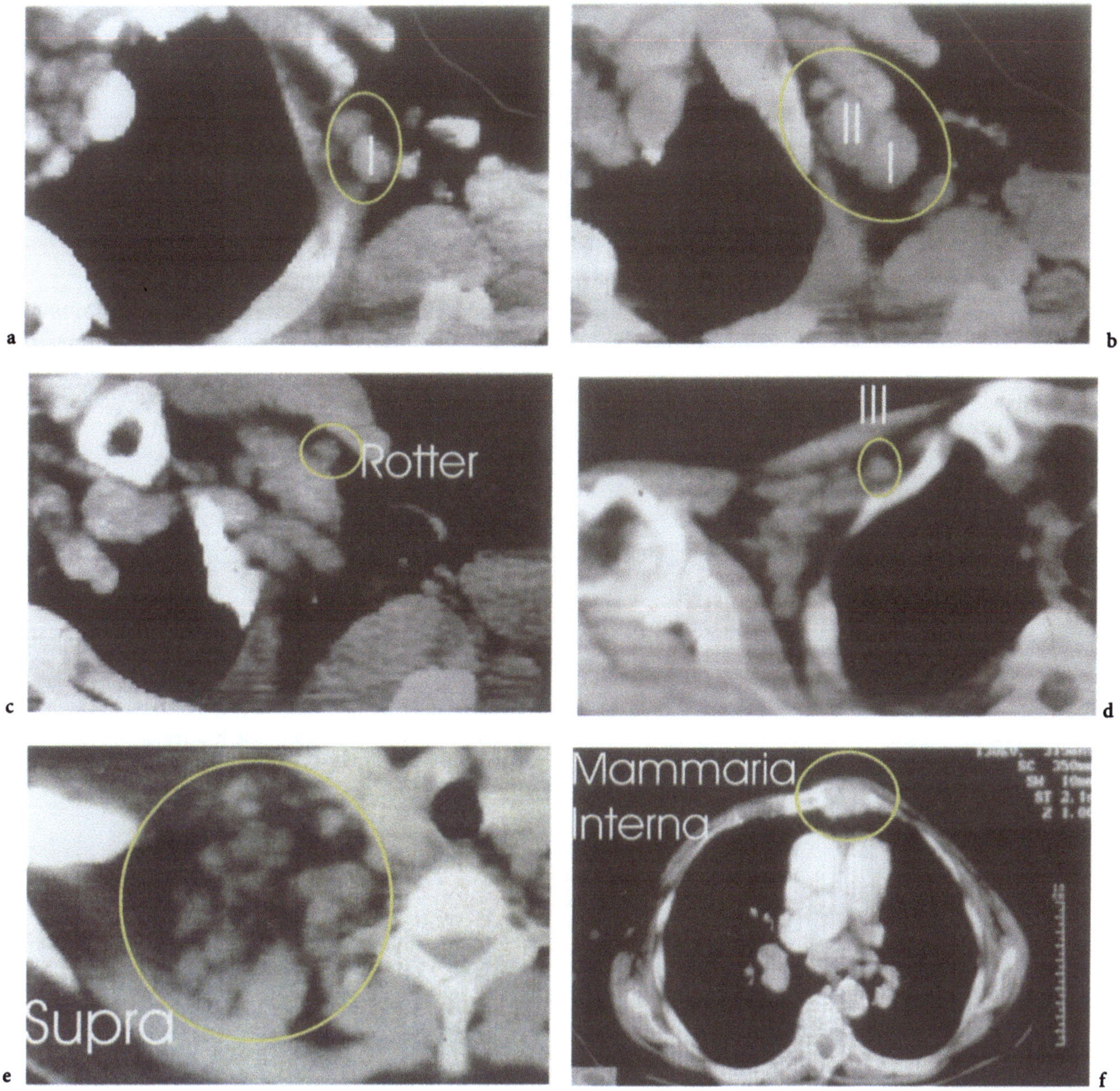

Fig. 6.6. Type of involvement of: **a** level I; **b** level I and level II; **c** level II with the Rotter lymph node; **d** level III; **e** supraclavicular nodes; and **f** internal mammary nodes

Table 6.14. Frequency and magnitude of the difference between surface-based and CT-based tangential field borders (from Bentel et al. 1999)

	All patients[a] (n=254)			GTB only[a] (n=168)	GBT+IMN[a] (n=63)
	Frequency (%)	Median shift (mm)	Range of shift (mm)	Frequency (%)	Frequency (%)
Patients with shifts of one of two borders	65	10	5–60	60	75
Medial border shifted	30				
Ipsilaterally	12	10	5–30	12	11
Contralaterally	18	10	5–60	12	38
Lateral border shifted	56				
Anteriorly	18	10	5–20	20	17
Posteriorly	38	15	5–40	36	38

[a] There were 254 patients in the whole group, and when they were segregated depending on IMN treatment, 23 subjects with a separate IMN field were excluded

are included in the CTV is presented in Fig. 6.7a (KIRICUTA et al. 2000).

The CTV in each CT slice is underlined by a red contour throughout the entire target volume, starting from the supraclavicular region and ending 1 cm under the breast (Fig. 6.7b). The upper part includes the lymphatics of the supraclavicular groove and the apex axilla (level III); in the middle and lower part, the lymphatics of levels I and II are included, as well as the internal mammary nodes and/or the breast after conserving surgery or the chest wall following mastectomy.

6.10 ICRU 62 Recommendations

The recommendations of the ICRU REPORT 62 (1999) include definitions for target volumes, volumes of

a

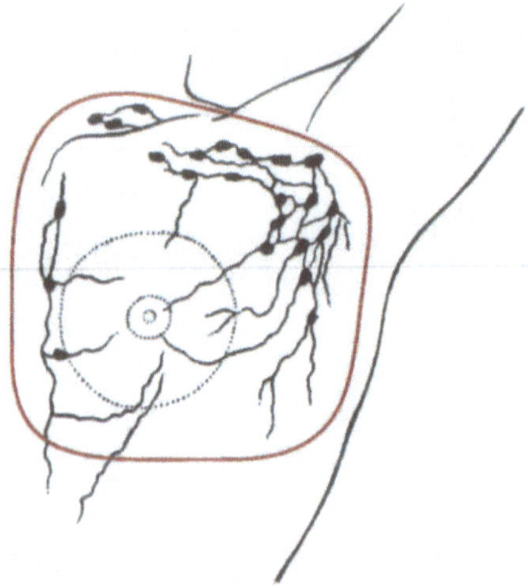

Fig. 6.7a, b. Orientation view and CTV for postoperative RT. **a** Plain view of the planning target volume including the breast and/or chest wall and the locoregional lymphatics (internal mammary, axillary and supraclavicular lymphatics); and **b** the CTV in nine representative CT axial sections through the planning volume. The locoregional lymphatics are marked as *dark spots*. (The CT slices are from RICHTER and FEYERABEND 1991)

b

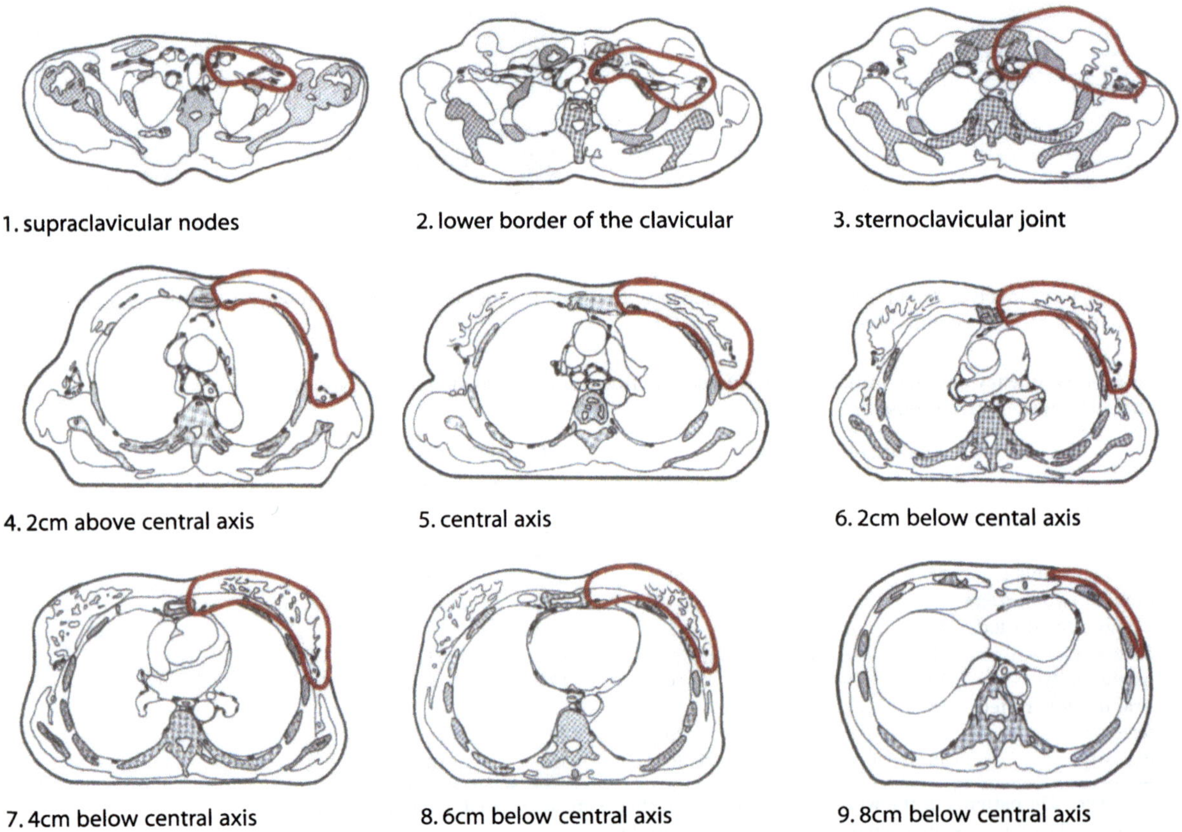

interest, organs at risk, and other definitions such as setup margins (SU) and internal margins (IM). The gross tumor volume (GTV) or macroscopic disease and CTV which include possible microscopic disease are presented as a clinical-oncological concept. Other descriptions such as the planning target volume (PTV), IM, and SM are viewed as a geometrical concept, aiding in the selection of appropriate beam size and beam arrangements to ensure that the prescribed dose is actually delivered to the CTV. In this paper, the defined target volume is the GTV and/or the CTV only, without considering the PTV and the other defined volumes. The risk of overlooking part of the microscopic disease must be counterbalanced against a reduction of the risk of acute or late severe normal tissue reactions (lung and cardiac complications). The selection of a composite margin and the delineation of the border of the PTV are based on a compromise involving the experience and judgment of the radiation-oncology team (Landberg 2001).

6.11 Consensus Statements for Postoperative Radiotherapy

In this presentation, the selection of CTV for postoperative RT after ablative or breast conserving surgery is based on currently well accepted consensus statements. In the consensus statements of the 1998 International St. Gallen Consensus Panel (Goldhirsch et al. 1998), the American Society for Therapeutic Radiology and Oncology (Harris et al. 1999; Recht et al. 1998) and the German Society of Senology (Sauer et al. 2001), the importance of PMRT is to reduce the recurrence rate and to improve overall survival.

6.11.1 Postmastectomy Radiotherapy

Based on the above-mentioned consensus statements, the indications for PMRT are as follows:

- An optimally performed mastectomy is a major prerequisite for curative surgery.
- Radical (R0) resection of the tumor as well as dissection of at least 10 level I and II axillary lymph nodes should be carried out.
- Patients with 4 or more positive lymph nodes should be given RT.

All patients with pT2 (>3 cm) or pT3–4, and/or multicentric tumor growth, lymphangiosis carcinomatosa or vessel involvement, involvement of the pectoralis fascia, a safety margin of <5 mm, R1 or R2 resection, extensive intraductal component, negative hormone receptor status, G-3 differentiation grade, diffuse microcalcifications, non-complete biopsies or age <35 years should be treated by RT.

The EORTC inclusion criteria of the EORTC Protocol (1996) for irradiation of the internal mammary lymph node chain and the medial supraclavicular lymph nodes are as follows: non-metastatic breast cancer, women aged 75 years or under with operable breast cancer (TX, T0–T3, N0–N2), central or medial location in the breast, regardless of axillary lymph node status, central tumors underlying the areola, medial tumors occupying at least part of the upper or lower medial quadrants of the breast. The results of this study are forthcoming.

Patients with 1–3 positive nodes should receive RT as part of the treatment strategy in randomized trials.

Suggested guidelines for CTV selection for possible PMRT based on the above-mentioned consensus statements are presented in Table 6.15.

6.11.1.1 Selection and Delineation of Clinical Target Volumes for Postmastectomy Irradiation

Based on the above-described clinical and pathological data as well as the CT-based nodal classification, the selection and delineation of CTV for different postmastectomy situations is possible. Well defined target volumes (CTV only) for different clinical situations are shown in Fig. 6.8a–d.

The supraclavicular lymph nodes should not be included in the CTV for adjuvant treatment. The involvement of this area is similar to that of distant metastasized disease (Kiricuta 1993; Kiricuta et al. 1994). The irradiation of this lymphatic area should improve local control. The improvement of survival remains questionable.

6.11.2 Radiotherapy After Breast Conserving Surgery

Breast conserving surgery associated with planned RT for the conserved breast is the treatment of choice for unifocal invasive breast cancer that can be excised with clear margins. For a reduced local recurrence rate, the importance of clear margins (defined as normal tissue of about 1 cm surrounding the tumor)

Table 6.15. Suggested guidelines for CTV selection for PMRT based on most recent consensus statements

Axillary status	TVD Primary in the inner quadrant		TVD Primary in the outer quadrant		TVD Primary in the central area		TVD Multicentric primary
	T1–T2	T3–4	T1–T2	T3–T4	T1–T2	T3–4	
N0 (>10 Level I nodes examined)	Chest wall	Chest wall+MI	Chest wall	Chest wall+MI	Chest wall	Chest wall+MI	Chest wall+MI[a]
	T2>3 cm		T2>3 cm		T2>3 cm		
N0 (<10 Level I nodes examined)	Chest wall	Chest wall	Chest wall	Chest wall	Chest wall	Chest wall	Chest wall
	T2>3 cm		T2>3 cm		T2>3 cm		
	Ax.+MI[a]	Ax.+MI	Ax.	Ax.+MI	Ax.+MI*	Ax.+MI	Ax.+MI[a]
N+ (1–3 nodes involved, CAD)[a]	Chest wall	Chest wall	Chest wall	Chest wall	Chest wall	Chest wall	Chest wall
	T2>3 cm		T2>3 cm		T2>3 cm		
	MI[a]	MI		MI	MI[a]	MI	MI
N+ (>4 nodes involved, CAD, no CD, no LCM)	Chest wall	Chest wall	Chest wall	Chest wall	Chest wall	Chest wall	Chest wall
	MI	MI	MI	MI	MI	MI	MI
N+ (>4 nodes involved, CAD, CD and/or LCM)	Chest wall	Chest wall	Chest wall	Chest wall	Chest wall	Chest wall	Chest wall
	Ax.	Ax.	Ax.	Ax.	Ax.	Ax.	Ax.
	MI	MI	MI	MI	MI	MI	MI

CAD, complete axillary dissection; CD, lymph node capsule disruption; LCM, lymphangiosis carcinomatosa in the axilla
[a] Irradiation should be performed as part of randomized trials

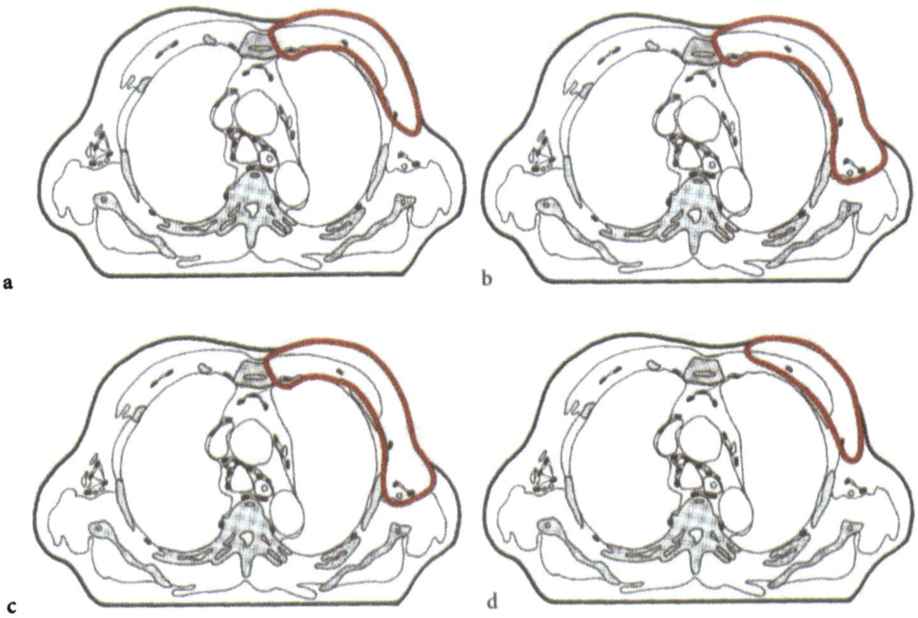

Fig. 6.8a–d. Target volume definition in only one representative CT axial slice for different clinical situations of a left localized breast cancer. **a** pT3 (inner quadrant) pN0 (11 level I examined nodes) node negative breast cancer; **b** pT2 (4.5 cm diameter) pN0 (only 5 nodes examined) multicentric cancer; **c** pT3 in the external quadrant and pN+ (4 involved nodes from 12 examined nodes) localized cancer; **d** pT1 R1 (pectoralis major infiltration) pN0 (20 examined nodes) resected cancer

has been demonstrated, although clear margins do not guarantee freedom from local recurrence. The remaining GBT should always be included in the CTV as well as the anterior face of the pectoralis fascia. At least 0.5 cm of the pectoralis muscle should also be included in the CTV.

6.11.2.1
Selection and Delineation of Clinical Target Volumes After Breast Conserving Surgery

Given the concepts of multifocality and multicentricity, the number of breast preservation procedures described (Table 6.2), the consensus statements and the ICRU 62 recommendations, the selection and delineation of GTV and/or CTV are not simple. The use of CT planning for patients after conservative surgery is limited by two factors: (1) the ability to radiographically identify GBT which is age-dependent; and (2) positioning of the patient for the scanning for CT planning, and during irradiation. The first factor constitutes a problem, especially in older women. In younger patients, tissues of increased density are commonly seen on CT images and likely correspond to GBT. The radiographically visible tissue most likely does not represent the full extent of GBT, but provides anatomical information that may be useful in designating CTV. As mentioned before, there were large variations in the location of GBT (Bentel et al. 1999). GBT seen on CT slices for three clinical situations is shown in Fig. 6.9: (a) well represented GBT in a 35-year-old woman; (b) GBT in a patient with partial glandular atrophy; and (c) no GBT visible in an "empty breast". The second problem is related to positioning of the ipsilateral arm during immobilization, determined by the diameter of the CT scanner, by the irradiation technique, or by the mobility of the shoulder itself. In patients with the arm abducted more than 90 degrees and with their hand placed above or on their head, recognition of the anatomical structures in the axilla or the supraclavicular groove is quite difficult. The axillary apex and the supraclavicular lymph nodes are shifted cranially so that the content of the axilla is at least at the level of the supraclavicular nodes and is not easy to identify. In this position, irradiation of the axillary and the supraclavicular lymph nodes is quite impossible.

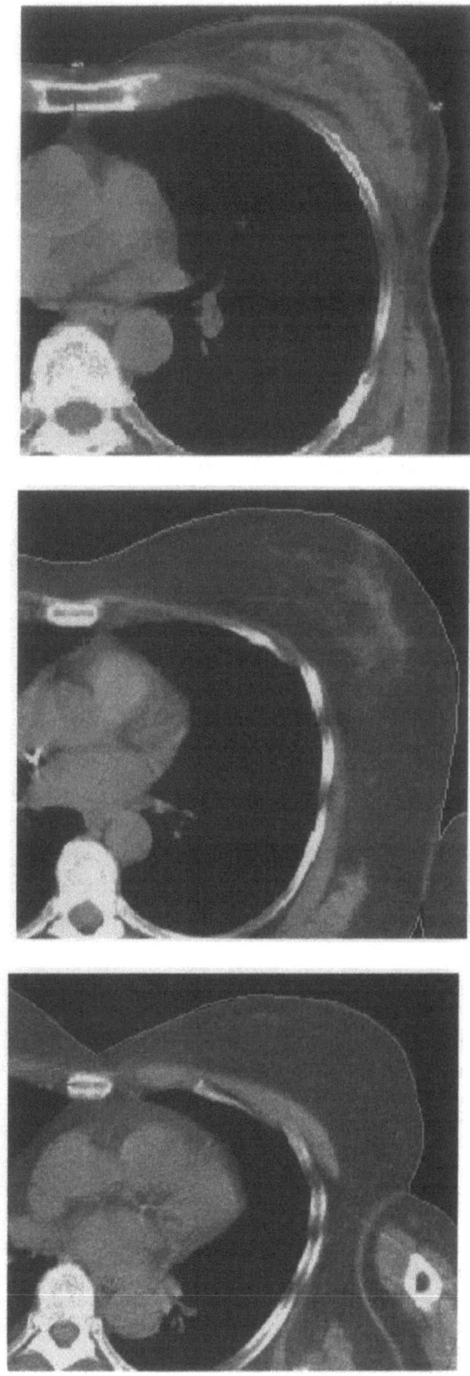
a b c

Fig. 6.9a–c. GBT seen on CT slices for three clinical situations. **a** Well-represented GBT in a 35-year-old woman; **b** GBT in a patient with partial glandular atrophy; and (**c**) no GBT visible in an "empty breast"

6.11.3
Selection and Delineation of Clinical Target Volume After Sentinel Node Procedure

Based on the new data obtained with the SNP, a new selection of lymphatics for the CTV for adjuvant RT is possible, as shown in Table 6.16. For instance, for a primary breast tumor, regardless of the location in one of the quadrants of the breast or centrally, and independent of the status of the axillary lymph nodes where no drainage to the parasternal nodes is visible by gamma probe, avoidance of irradiation of these regions is indicated. If only drainage to the ipsilateral parasternal nodes is evident by SNP, avoidance of an axillary dissection is indicated. Irradiation of only the ipsilateral parasternal lymph nodes should be carried out. If simultaneous drainage to the parasternal and axillary nodes is evident and no nodes are clinically palpable in the axilla or enlarged parasternal nodes visible by imaging, only adjuvant irradiation of these areas is indicated. If only drainage to the contralateral parasternal lymph nodes is present, that site should be included in the CTV. The CTV delineation for different clinical situations in which SNP was performed is shown in Fig. 6.10.

Galper et al. (2000) estimated the possible efficacy of axillary RT following a positive SN biopsy by evaluating the risk of regional failure for patients with clinical stage I or II, clinically node-negative invasive breast cancer treated either by no dissection or by limited dissection, defined as removal of 5 nodes or less, followed by axillary RT. A regional nodal failure of 1% was noted in the no axillary dissection group. The regional nodal failure was 7% in the pathologically-involved node group and 0% in the node-negative group. These results imply that axillary RT may be an effective and safe alternative to complete dissection for treatment of the axilla following a positive SN biopsy.

6.12
Conclusions

The selection and delineation of CTV in axial CT slices can be made according to the stage of the primary breast cancer and the surgery performed. The anatomy and the CT based nodal classification of the lymphatics of the breast have been reviewed, and recommendations for delineation of the CTV have been adapted to take into account specific radiological landmarks that are more easily identifiable on CT slices. Guidelines considering consensus statements and the results of the SNP for the selection of CTV to include or exclude the chest wall, the conserved breast and regional lymphatics such as the axillary, internal mammary and supraclavicular nodes for irradiation have been proposed.

Table 6.16. Suggested guidelines for CTV selection of lymphatic areas for postoperative RT based on the SNP (followed by breast conserving surgery or mastectomy)[a]. The rules for the inclusion of the chest wall or breast are similar to those presented in Table 6.15

Axillary status	TVD Primary in the inner quadrant		TVD Primary in the outer quadrant		TVD Primary in the central area		TVD Multicentric primary
	T1–T2	T3–4	T1–T2	T3–T4	T1–T2	T3–4	
SNP (axilla) Negative, only axillary drainage							
Axillary and internal mammary drainage	MI	MI	MI	MI	MI	MI	MI
SNP (axilla) positive							
Only axillary drainage (no CAD)	Ax.	Ax.	Ax.	Ax.	Ax.	Ax.	Ax.
Axillary and internal mammary drainage	Ax.	Ax.	Ax.	Ax.	Ax.	Ax.	Ax.
No axillary drainage							
Only internal mammary drainage (no dissection of IM nodes)[b]	MI	MI	MI	MI	MI	MI	MI

CAD, complete axillary dissection.
[a] CTV after breast conserving surgery should always include the breast.
[b] Irradiation should be performed in randomized trials

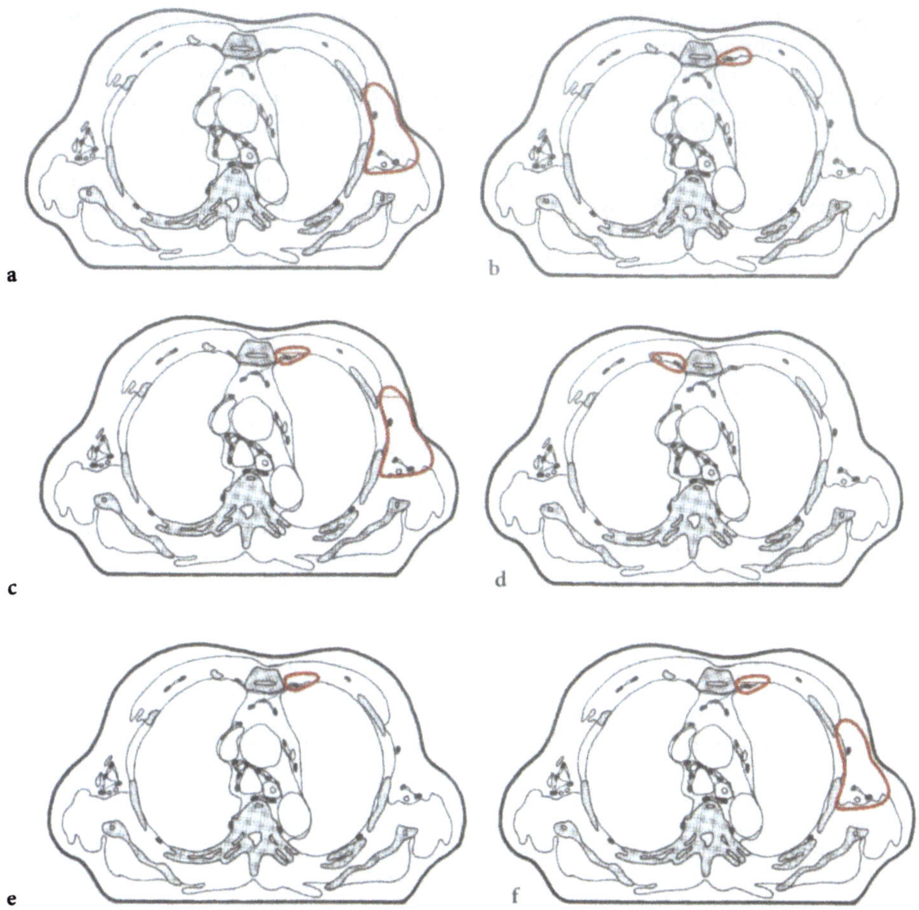

Fig. 6.10a–f. CTV selection and delineation for lymphatic areas only for different clinical situations of a left located breast cancer when SNP was performed. **a** For a primary in the breast independent of the location in one of the quadrants of the breast or centrally and with a positive SNP in the axilla and no axillary dissection, and no visible gamma probe drainage to the parasternal nodes; **b** if only drainage to the ipsilateral parasternal nodes is evident by SNP; **c** if simultaneous drainage to the parasternal and axillary nodes is evident and no nodes are clinically palpable in the axilla or enlarged parasternal nodes visible by an imaging method; **d** if only drainage to the contralateral parasternal lymph nodes exists; **e** if there is a primary pT3 in the outer quadrant with negative axilla (pN0–12 nodes were examined) and evident SNP for ipsilateral mammary internal nodes; **f** if there is a primary in the upper external quadrant and SNP positive in the infraclavicular area the CTV should include levels I, II and III

References

Bentel G, Marks LB, Hardenberg P et al (1999) Variability of the location of internal mammary vessels and glandular breast tissue (GBT) in breast cancer patients undergoing routine CT-based treatment planning. Int J Radiat Oncol Biol Phys 44:1017–1025

Berg JW (1955) The significance of axillary node levels in the study of breast cancer. Cancer 63:776–778

Bonadonna G, Valagussa P, Rossi A et al (1985) Ten-year experience with CMF-based adjuvant chemotherapy in resectable breast cancer. Breast Cancer Res Treat 5:95–115

Borgstein PJ (1999) The sentinel node concept. Consequences of lymphatic tumor spread in melanoma and breast cancer. Thesis, Vrije Universiteit, Amsterdam

Borgstein PJ, Pijpers R, Comans EF et al (1998) Sentinel lymph node biopsy in breast cancer: guidelines and pitfalls of lymphoscintigraphy and gamma probe detection. J Am Coll Surg 186:275–283

Brinkley D, Aybitte JL, Houghton J (1984) The cancer research campaign (King's/Cambridge) trial for early breast cancer: an analysis of the radiotherapy data. Br J Radiol 57:309–316

Carter CL, Allen C, Henson D (1989) Relation of tumor size, lymph node status and survival in 24,740 breast cancer cases. Cancer 63:181–187

Cuzick J, Stewart H., Rutquist L et al (1997) Cause specific mortality in long-term survivors of breast cancer who participated in trials of radiotherapy. J Clin Oncol 12:447–453

De Cicco C, Cremonesi M, Luini A et al (1998) Lymphoscintigraphy and radioguided biopsy of the sentinel axillary lymph node in breast cancer. Eur J Nucl Med 39:2080–2084

Early Breast Cancer Trialist's Collaborative Group (1995) Effects of radiotherapy and surgery in early breast cancer. An overview of the randomized trials. N Engl J Med 333: 1444–1445

Early Breast Cancer Trialists' Collaborative Group (1998) Polychemotherapy for early breast cancer: an overview of the randomized trials. Lancet 352:930–942

Easson EC (1968) Postoperative radiotherapy in breast cancer. In: Forrest APM, Kunkler PB (eds) Prognostic factors in breast cancer. Livingstone, Edinburgh, pp 118–127

Ege GN (1996) Lymphoscintigraphy in oncology. In: Henkin RE, Boles EM (eds) Nuclear medicine: principles and practice, vol II. Mosby, St Louis, pp 1505–1523

EORTC (1996) EORTC cooperative group for breast cancer. Internal mammary and medial supraclavicular lymph node chain irradiation in stage I–III breast cancer. Protocol 22922/10925, May 1996

Fisher B (1998) The effect of recent findings from NSABP clinical trials on paradigms governing the therapy of primary invasive breast cancer. In: Untch M, Konecny G, Sittek H, Kessler M, Reiser M, Hepp H (eds) Diagnostik und Therapie des Mammakarzinoms. State of the art. Zuckschwerdt, Munich, pp 193–220

Fisher B, Slack NH (1970) Number of lymph nodes examined and the prognosis of breast carcinoma. Surg Gynecol Obstet 131:79–88

Fisher B, Redmond C, Fisher ER et al (1985) Ten-year results of a randomized clinical trial comparing radical mastectomy and total mastectomy with or without radiation. N Engl J Med 312:674–681

Fottin A, Larochelle M, Lavertu S et al (1999) Local failure is responsible for the decrease in survival for patients with breast cancer treated with conservative surgery and postoperative radiotherapy. J Clin Oncol 17:101–109

Fowble B (1999) Postmastectomy radiation in patients with one to three positive axillary nodes receiving adjuvant chemotherapy: an unresolved issue. Semin Radiat Oncol 9:230–240

Fowble B, Gray R, Gilchrist K et al (1988) Identification of a subgroup of patients with breast cancer and histologically positive axillary nodes receiving adjuvant chemotherapy who may benefit from postoperative radiotherapy. J Clin Oncol 6:1107–1117

Galper S, Recht A, Silver B et al (2000) Is radiation alone adequate to the axilla for patients with limited axillary surgery? Implications for treatment after a positive sentinel node biopsy. Int J Radiat Oncol Biol Phys 48:125–132

Goldhirsch A, Glick JH, Gelber RD et al (1998) Meeting highlights: International Consensus Panel on the treatment of primary breast cancer. J Natl Cancer Inst 90:1601–1608

Haagensen CD (1971) The natural history of breast cancer. In: Diseases of the breast, 2nd edn. WB Saunders, Philadelphia, pp 411–413

Haagensen CD (1972) General anatomy of the lymphatic system. The lymphatics of the trunk. In: Haagensen CD, Feind CR, Herter FP et al (eds) The lymphatics in cancer. Saunders, Philadelphia, pp 300–398

Haagensen CD, Bodian C (1984) A personal experience with Halstead's radical mastectomy. Ann Surg 199:143–150

Haigh PI, Hansen NM, Giuliano AE et al (2000) Factors affecting sentinel node localization during preoperative breast lymphoscintigraphy. J Nucl Med 41:1682–1688

Halsted WS (1907) The results of radical operations for the cure of cancer of the breast. Ann Surg 46:1–5

Handley RSA (1975) Carcinoma of the breast. Ann R Coll Surg (Engl) 57:59–66

Handley RSA, Thakeray AC (1954) Invasion of the internal mammary lymph gland in carcinoma of the breast. Br Med J 1:61–68

Harris J, Halpin-Murray P, McNeese M et al (1999) Consensus statement on postmastectomy radiation therapy. Int J Radiat Oncol Biol Phys 44:989–990

Hicken FN (1940) Mastectomy: a clinical pathologic study demonstrating why most mastectomies result in incomplete removal of the mammary gland. Arch Surg 40:6–7

Holland R, Veling SHJ, Matrunac M et al (1985) Histologic multifocality of Tis, T1–2 breast carcinoma. Cancer 56: 979–990

Host H, Brennhovd IO (1975) Combined surgery and radiation therapy versus surgery alone in primary mammary carcinoma. I. The effect of orthovoltage radiation. Acta Radiol Ther Phys Biol 14:25–32

Host H, Brenhovd IO, Loeb M (1986) Post-operative radiotherapy in breast cancer: long-term results from the Oslo study. Int J Radiat Biol Phys 12:727–732

ICRU Report 62 (1999) Prescribing, recording and reporting photon beam therapy [supplement to ICRU 50]

Iyer RV, Hanlon A, Fowble B et al (2000) Accuracy of the extent of axillary nodal positivity related to primary tumor size, number of involved nodes, and number of nodes examined. Int J Radiat Oncol Biol Phys 47:1177–1183

Kiricuta IC (1993) TNM-system [letter to editor]. Eur J Surg Oncol 19:393–395

Kiricuta IC (1999) If one obtains a positive report from the sentinel node biopsy, should one go ahead and perform a complete dissection? Eur J Nucl Med 26 [Suppl]: P08.09

Kiricuta IC, Tausch J (1992) A mathematical model of axillary lymph node involvement based on 1446 complete axillary dissections in patients with breast cancer. Cancer 69:2496–2501

Kiricuta IC, Willner J, Kölbl O, Bohndorf W (1992) Die Bedeutung der Axilladiagnostik beim Mammakarzinom aus der Sicht des Strahlentherapeuten. Strahlenther Onkol 169: 390–396

Kiricuta IC, Willner J, Koelbl O et al (1994) The diagnostic significance of the supraclavicular lymph node metastases in breast cancer patients. Int J Radiat Oncol Biol Phys 28: 387–393

Kiricuta IC, Götz U, Schwab F et al (2000) Target volume definition and target conformal irradiation technique for breast cancer patients. Acta Oncol 39:429–436

Krag DN, Weaver D, Ashikaga T et al (1998) The sentinel node in breast cancer. A multicenter validation study. N Engl J Med 339:941–946

Korzeniowski S, Dyba T, Skolyszewski J (1994) Classical prognostic factors for survival and locoregional control in breast cancer patients treated with radical mastectomy alone. Acta Oncol 33:759–765

Koscielny S, Tubiana M (1999) The link between local recurrence and distant metastases. Int J Radiat Oncol Biol Phys 43:11–24

Kubik S (1999) Efferente Lymphgefäße und die regionalen Lymphknoten der Brustdrüse. In: Földi M, Kubik S (eds)

Lehrbuch der Lymphologie, 4th edn. Fischer, Stuttgart Jena Lübeck Ulm Chap 1.7.7, p 135
Kuske R (1998) Adjuvant chest wall and nodal irradiation: maximize cure, minimize late cardiac toxicity. J Clin Oncol 16:2579–2582
Lacour J, Bucalossi P, Caceres E et al (1976) Radical mastectomy versus radical mastectomy plus internal mammary dissection. Five-year results of an international cooperative study. Cancer 37:206–214
Landberg T (2001) New supplement to ICRU 50, ICRU 62. First international symposium on target volume definition in radiation oncology, Limburg, Germany, 24–26 May
Linehan DC, Hill ADK, Tran KN et al (1999) Sentinel lymph node biopsy in breast cancer: the Memorial Hospital experience of 800 cases. Eur J Nucl Med 26 [Suppl]:S11.06
Melis K, Makar A, Van Leuven L et al (1999) Lymphoscintigraphic and gamma probe guided intraoperative localisation of the sentinel node in breast cancer. Eur J Nucl Med 26 [Suppl]:P03.10
Messer PM, Kiricuta IC, Bratengeier K, Flentje M (1997) CT planning of boost irradiation in radiotherapy of breast cancer after conservative surgery. Radiother Oncol 42:239–243
Morrow M (1999) Postmastectomy radiation therapy: a surgical perspective. Semin Radiat Oncol 9:269–274
Morrow M, Foster RS (1981) Staging for breast cancer. Arch Surg 116:748–751
Mudum A, Aygen M, Aslay Y et al (1999) Preoperative lymphatic mapping and sentinel node localisation as a useful guide in patients with breast cancer. Eur J Nucl Med 26 [Suppl]:P13.14
Nemoto T, Vana J, Bedwani RN et al (1980) Management and results of a national survey by the American College of Surgeons. Cancer 45:2917–2924
Noguchi M, Ohta N, Koyasaki N et al (1991) Reappraisal of internal mammary node metastases as a prognostic factor in patients with breast cancer. Cancer 68:1918–1925
Noguchi M, Taniya T, Koyasaki N et al (1992) A multivariate analysis of en bloc extended radical mastectomy versus conventional radical mastectomy in operable breast cancer. Int Surg 77:48–54
Overgaard M, Hansen PS, Overgaard J et al of the Danish Breast Cancer Cooperative Group (1997) Postoperative radiotherapy in high-risk premenopausal women with breast cancer who receive adjuvant chemotherapy. N Engl J Med 337:949–955
Paterson R, Russell MH (1959) Breast cancer: evaluation of postoperative radiotherapy. J Fac Radiol 10:174–180
Perez CA, Garcia DM, Kuske RR et al (1992) Breast: stage Tis, T1, and T2 tumors. In: Perez CA, Brady LW (eds) Principles and practice of radiation oncology. Lippincott, Philadelphia, , chap 42, pp 877–889
Ragaz J, Jackson SM, Le N et al (1997) Adjuvant radiotherapy and chemotherapy in node positive premenopausal women with breast cancer. N Engl J Med 337:956–962
Recht A, Bartelink H, Fourquet A et al (1998) Postmastectomy radiotherapy: questions for the twenty-first century. J Clin Oncol 16:2886–2889
Richter E, Feyerabend T (1991) Normal lymph node topography – CT atlas of lymphatics. Springer, Berlin Heidelberg New York
Rodier JF, Mignotte H, Janser JC et al (1999) Sentinel node biopsy in breast cancer: preliminary analysis of the French cooperative multicenter study. Eur J Nucl Med 26 [Suppl]: P08.05
Sauer R, Schulz K-D, Hellriegel K-P (2001) Radiation therapy after mastectomy – interdisciplinary consensus puts end to a controversy. Strahlenther Onkol 177:1–9
Silverstein MJ, Gierson ED, Waisman JR et al (1994) Lymph node dissection for T1 breast carcinoma – is it indicated? Cancer 73:664–667
Smitt MC, Goffinet DR (1999) Utility of three-dimensional planning for axillary node coverage with breast-conserving radiation therapy: early experience. Radiology 210:221–226
Sobin LH (1999) Frequently asked questions regarding the application of of the TNM classification. Cancer 85: 1405–1146
Stibbe EP (1918) The internal mammary lymphatic glands. J Anat 52:257–261
TNM Atlas (1998) 4th edn. Springer, Berlin Heidelberg New York
TNM Supplement (1993) A commentary on uniform use. Springer, Berlin Heidelberg New York
Urban JA, Castro EB (1971) Selecting variations in extent of surgical procedure for breast cancer. Cancer 28:1615–1623
Urban JA, Marjani MA (1971) Significance of internal mammary lymph node metastases in breast cancer. Am J Roentgenol Radium Ther Nucl Med 111:130–136
Valagussa P, Bonadonna G, Veronesi U (1978) Patterns of relapse and survival following radical mastectomy: analysis of 716 consecutive patients. Cancer 41:1170–1176
Veronesi U, Valagussa P (1981) Inefficacy of internal mammary nodes dissection in breast cancer surgery. Cancer 47:170–175
Veronesi U, Cascinely N, Greco M et al (1985) Prognosis of breast cancer patients after mastectomy and dissection of the internal mammary nodes. Ann Surg 202:702–707
Veronesi U, Luini A, Galimberti V et al (1990) Extent of metastatic axillary involvement in 1,446 cases of breast cancer. Eur J Surg Oncol 16:127–133
Veronesi U, Marubini E, Del Vechio M, Manzari A, Andreola S, Greco M, Luini A, Merson M, Saccozzi R, Rilke F, Salvadori B (1995) Local recurrences and distant metastases after conservative breast cancer treatments: partially independent events. J Natl Cancer Inst 87:19–27
Veronesi U, Paganelli G, Galimberti V et al (1997) Sentinel node biopsy to avoid axillary dissection in breast cancer with clinically negative lymph-nodes. Lancet 349:1864–1867
Veronesi U, Paganelli G, Viale G et al (1999) Sentinel node biopsy and axillary dissection in breast cancer: results in a large series. J Natl Cancer Instit 91:368–373
Wallgren A, Arner O, Bergstrom J et al (1986) Radiation therapy in operable breast cancer: results from the Stockholm trial on adjuvant therapy. Int J Radiat Biol Phys 12: 533–537
Wilking N, Rutqvist LE, Carstensen J et al (1992) Prognostic significance of axillary nodal status in primary breast cancer in relation to the number of resected nodes. Acta Oncol 31:29–35
Willner J, Flentje M (1998) Adjuvante Strahlentherapie beim operablen Mammakarzinom. Onkologe 4:923–935

7 CTV for Lymphatics in Prostate Adenocarcinoma: an Anatomical Description and Clinical Discussion

P. Scalliet, L. Renard, B. Lengelé, B. Tombal

CONTENTS

The presentation of a definite outlook is of more value than the discussion of different principles and practices. It does not mean to imply that it is the only way, or the best, or the most correct method but may leave the reader with something concrete

R. Paterson (1948)

7.1 Introduction

The prognosis for patients diagnosed as having prostate cancer is influenced by several factors: the grade of differentiation (Gleason grade), the tumour size and its extension into the periprostatic tissue, any extension in the proximal lymphatics, and the possible presence of metastases (usually in the bones, but sometimes in the extra-pelvic lymph nodes).

P. Scalliet, MD, PhD; L. Renard, MD
Department of Radiation Oncology, University Hospital Saint Luc, Université Catholique de Louvain, 10 Avenue Hippocrate, 1200 Brussels, Belgium
B. Lengelé, MD, PhD
Department of Anatomy, University Hospital Saint Luc, Université Catholique de Louvain, 10 Avenue Hippocrate, 1200 Brussels, Belgium
B. Tombal, MD, PhD
Department of Urology, University Hospital Saint Luc, Université Catholique de Louvain, 10 Avenue Hippocrate, 1200 Brussels, Belgium

Lymph node invasion can be detected either clinically (computed tomography, CT scan is the standard detection method) or surgically (by laparoscopy or laparotomy). Whether a curative approach to pelvic node metastasis is of any benefit remains a matter of debate; there is no level 1 or 2 evidence yet available to settle this issue.

Interestingly, most urologists share the opinion that prostate cancer spreads first through the pelvic lymph nodes and therefore they usually consider lymph node metastasis as an early marker of systemic dissemination. That is why lymph node dissection is usually performed with immediate pathological verification (frozen sections) before radical prostatectomy is carried out. Whenever the lymph nodes harbour cancer cells, then prostatectomy is counterindicated and the patient is switched to palliative hormonal treatment. Less often, the procedure is completed and the patient is administered adjuvant hormonotherapy. In contrast, extensive nodal dissections, as advocated in the case of cervical or bladder cancer, are not recommended by the urologist since this approach would only increase morbidity without improving survival.

Radiation oncologists hold a different opinion. Prostate cancer may or may not spread through the blood vessels and result in bone metastases, independently of lymphatic invasion. Subsequently, the type of case can be divided into four categories: (1) no lymphatic invasion; (2) invasion of the pelvic nodes; (3) invasion of the blood vessels (with subsequent spread to the bones); and (4) invasion of both the lymph nodes and the blood vessels. Adopting the argument that patients in categories 1 and 2 can theoretically be cured by a loco-regional therapeutic approach, it has been routine procedure for several decades to include the pelvis in the treated volume for "prophylactic" nodal irradiation.

There is thus a marked and enduring misunderstanding between urologists and radiation oncologists regarding the clinical significance of lymph node metastases.

The present chapter will successively address two issues: (1) delineation of the lymphatic clinical target volume (CTV) in prostate cancer; and (2) whether lymphatic irradiation modifies the course of the disease.

7.2 The Normal Prostate and Its Lymphatic Drainage

Not withstanding the uniform aspect of the normal adult prostate, pathological studies have suggested for quite some time the existence of different areas. Mc Neal's model is currently the most widely used (Mc Neal 1968). The axis of reference is the urethra, which divides the prostate into two distinct segments - proximal and distal - of approximately equal length, differentiated by an abrupt anterior angulation. Two major areas can be identified: the non-glandular component (33% of the total organ volume) and the epithelial (glandular) part (66%).

The glandular part is divided into three zones: central, transitional and peripheral. The central zone represents approximately 25% of the glandular component. It is conically shaped with its base at the neck of the bladder and the vertex toward the urethra, surrounding part of the proximal urethra, and it is traversed by the ejaculatory ducts. In the young adult, the transitional zone (TZ) is located around the proximal part of the urethra; it represents 5% to 10% of the glandular component. The peripheral zone is the largest (about 70% of the gland); it is pear-shaped in form, located posteriorly and laterally, surrounding the two other areas and extending down to the apex of the gland. By the age of 45–50, the TZ volume begins to increase as a result of benign prostate hyperplasia (BPH). In elderly men, the TZ/BPH might represent up to 75% of the prostatic volume. In contrast, 86% of the cancers develop in the peripheral zone (Mc Neal et al. 1988).

Lymphatic vessels emerging from the prostate insterstitium collect around the gland and progressively converge in four distinct drainage paths (Poirier et al. 1903; Testut and Latarjet 1931).

- The first drainage path is constituted by the lymphatics from the anterior and lateral part of the prostate; it follows the vas deferens and drains towards the external iliac nodes, a few centimetres below the bifurcation of the common iliac artery.
- The second path drains the postero-lateral part of the gland; it follows the vesico-genital vessels, running posteriorly and laterally, directly into the internal iliac nodes.
- The third path drains the postero-median part of the prostate; it runs posteriorly in the sacro-recto-genito-pubic fascia, along the lateral wall of the rectum, reaching the pre-sacral lymphatics, and extending up to the promontorium.
- The fourth path originates from the infero-anterior part of the gland. It runs along the internal pudendal vessels, within Alcock's canal, merging eventually with the internal iliac chain.

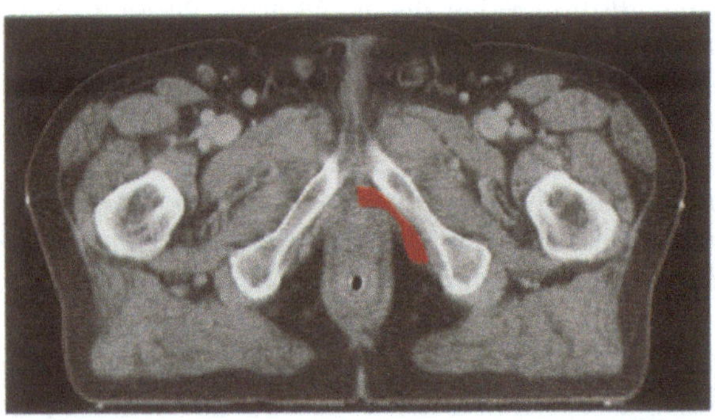
1

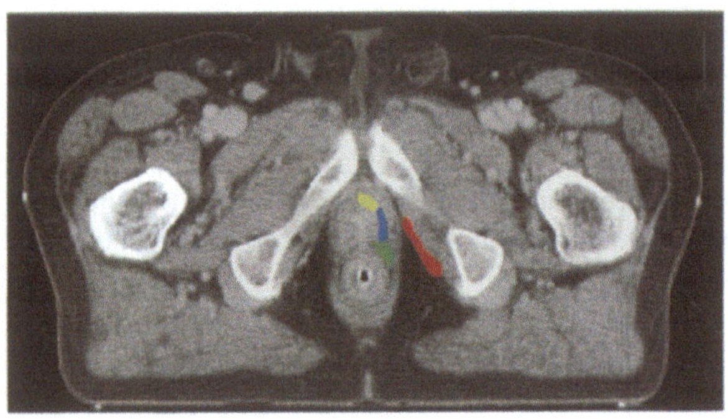
2

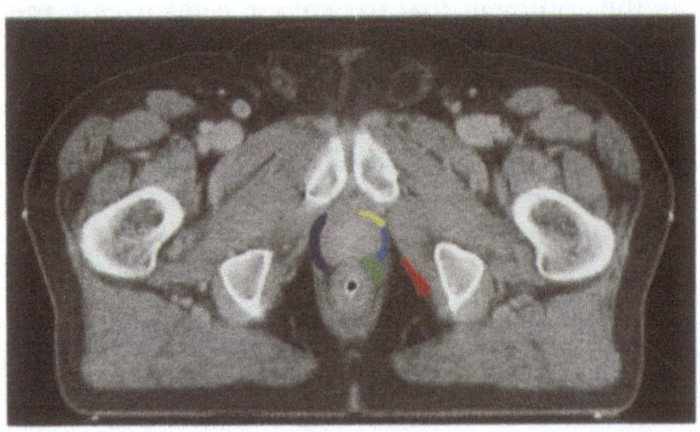
3

Fig. 7.1. CT images of a male pelvis with identification of the four lymphatic pathways, shown on the left side of the patient (*right side of the figure*). CT slices are separated by 1 cm. Each coloured area corresponds to one of the four paths. None of these paths bear a specific name, but are simply described according to their traject. 1. The first path (*in yellow*) follows the deferens. It drains toward the external iliac lymph nodes. 2. The second path (*in light blue*) drains directly toward the internal iliac lymph nodes. 3. The third path (*in green*) runs along the lateral wall of the rectum toward the promontorium. ▷

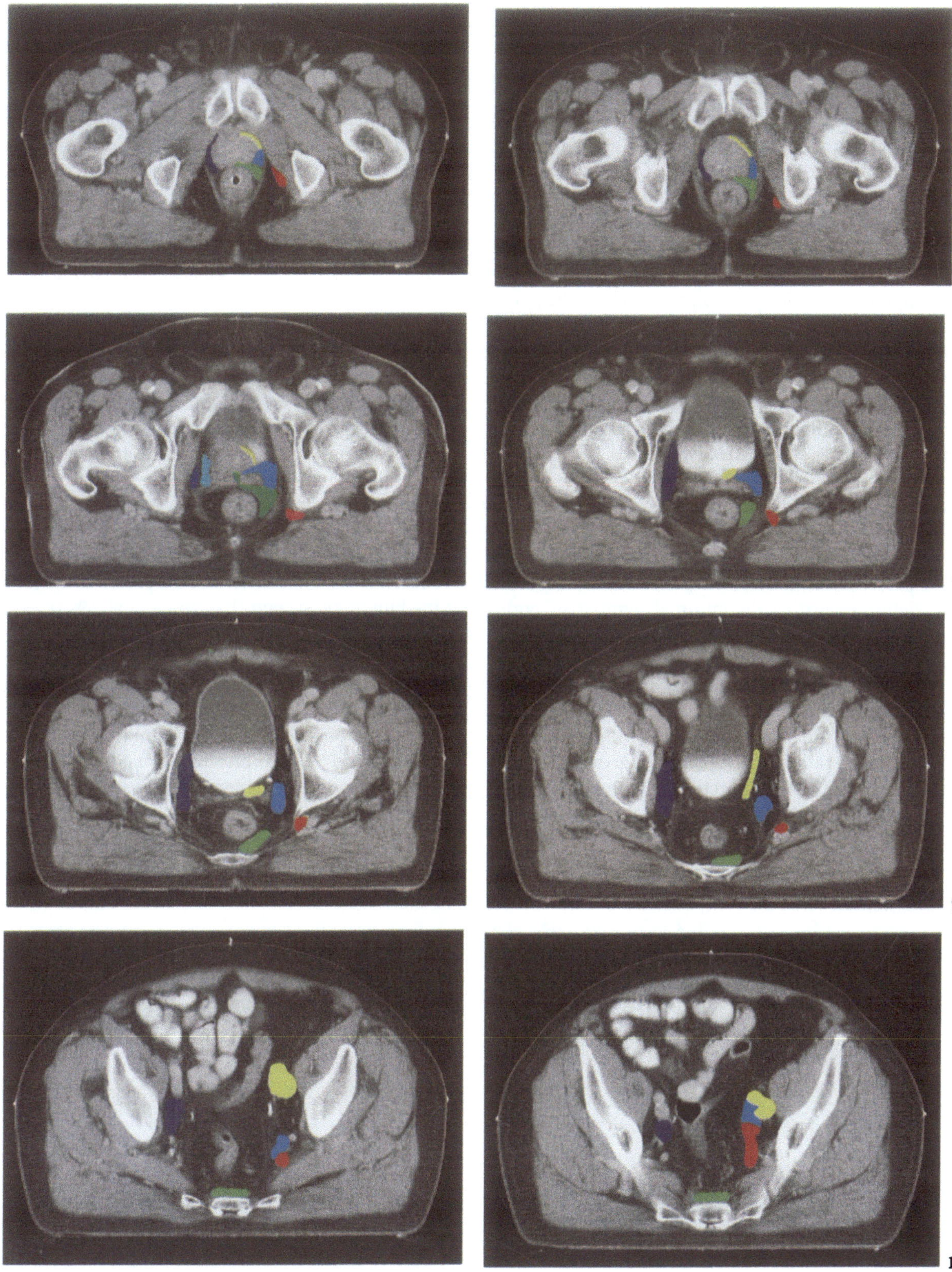

4. The fourth path (*in red*) follows the internal pudendal artery and eventually merges with the internal iliac lymphatics. On the right side of the patient (*left of the figure*), the area concerned by the lymph node dissection during a radical prostatectomy procedure is illustrated in *dark blue*. In a nerve-sparing operation, the dissection would not extend to the prostate, but leave behind the proximal part of the lymphatics (*sky blue*). It is not inconceivable that skip metastases could be left behind in the proximal lymphatics

7.3 The Surgical Perspective

There is no international nomenclature for these lymphatic paths as is the case, for instance, in the head and neck or the thoracic region. When urologists refer to pre-prostatectomy lymph node dissection, they usually only consider the ilio-obturator nodes and disregard the other lymphatic drainage routes.

Dissection starts at the external iliac vein, extending down to Cooper's ligament. At this point, dissection is carried out posteriorly and also laterally to the pelvic side wall. The posterior extent is the obturator nerve and vessels. The entire nodal package is then dissected superiorly to the bifurcation of the common iliac artery. In fact, this ilio-obturator lymphadenectomy removes lymph nodes within the second path, whereas the third path is systematically ignored.

Surgical lymph node staging in prostate cancer, therefore, is an approximation to "real" lymphatic staging. It is thus not inconceivable to think that a patient may be staged pN0, whereas positive nodes are present elsewhere in the pelvis. Also, there is no guideline regarding the minimal number of nodes removed and/or examined by the pathologist as there is, for instance in cases of breast or rectal cancer.

Nerve-sparing prostatectomy is a new approach to the treatment of prostate cancer, designed to preserve sexual function (Walsh and Mostwin 1984). The success rate of this technique greatly depends on the quality of the dissection of the neurovascular bundles. The erectile nerves run along the vesicogenital vessels, together with the lymphatics from the second drainage path. Thus a nerve-sparing procedure can also be viewed as a proximal lymphatic sparing procedure.

The higher risk of local recurrence associated with this technique has commonly been interpreted in terms of positive margins along the prostate capsule, but proximal lymphatic invasion could also explain this occurrence.

7.4 The Radiotherapeutic Perspective

When radiotherapy entered into common use for the treatment of prostate cancer, CT reconstruction of the prostate was not yet available. In addition, most patients were diagnosed as having large bulky prostate cancer invading the seminal vesicles, and quite often the lymphatic nodes of the prostate were also involved. Therefore, the treatment volumes were usually extended to include at least the proximal stations of the lymphatic system (Bagshaw et al. 1993).

The problem of including lymph nodes in the target volume has become much more complex since the introduction and generalized use of PSA testing (Catalona et al. 1993; Polascik et al. 1999) and the introduction of CT-based target definition.

The use of PSA has introduced major changes in the clinical profile of patients diagnosed with prostate cancer:

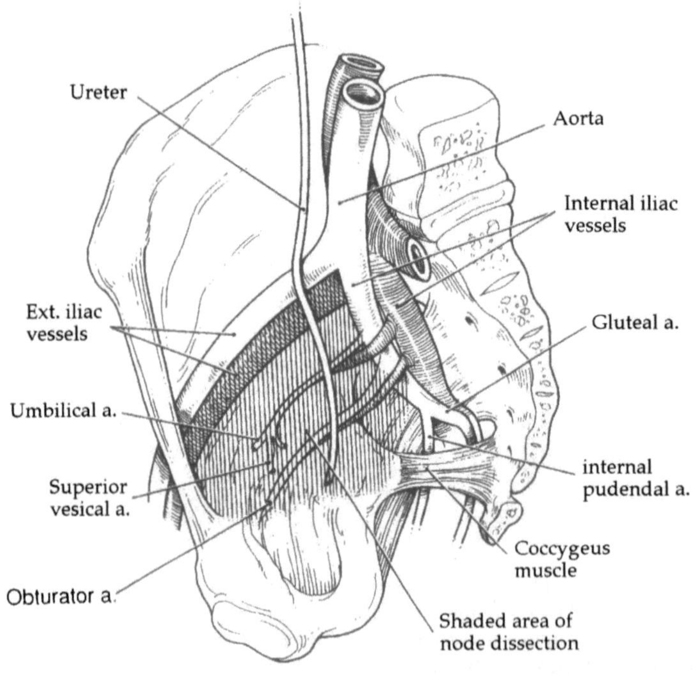

Fig. 7.2. Lateral and oblique view of the pelvic wall showing the region for lymphatic dissection (*shaded area*). It shows that only the second path is entirely removed for pathological staging. The third path is systematically ignored, and the first and the fourth paths are only partially explored.

1. The disease is now diagnosed much earlier on and the proportion of patients with detectable lymph node metastases on preoperative CT scan or magnetic resonance imaging (MRI) has decreased dramatically (Danella et al. 1993; Polascik et al. 1999; Rietbergen et al. 1999; Schröder et al. 1999). In 1997, the number of organ-confined prostate cancers diagnosed in the USA was 8 times greater than the number of those that were locally advanced or with distant spread at the time of diagnosis. This can be compared with a ratio of 5.4:1 in the USA some 10 years ago and the current ratio of around 4:1 in many European countries (Polascik et al. 1999).
2. Most patients are diagnosed as having prostate cancer when they are in their early fifties or sixties, and expect effective treatment with a very low rate of morbidity.
3. The usual definition of advanced prostate cancer has changed radically: that is to say, from high volume M+ or N+ disease to a much lower tumour burden such as T3 cases, a high Gleason score, or high PSA.

Prophylactic nodal irradiation is widely used in the treatment of prostate cancer. There is, however, still no consensus regarding its precise therapeutic value.

Let us examine the underlying assumptions. The first and most important of these is that information on the N stage is needed as irradiation of the pelvis is indicated if the lymph nodes contain metastases. This will be further discussed below. Another assumption is that the probability scores apply to patients with normal CT staging in the absence of pathological staging. Patients with positive nodes on CT scan are obviously not concerned. This is not an unimportant point since it leads to the issue of the degree of lymph node invasion (microscopic vs. bulky) and its relevance to prognosis and treatment. Unfortunately, only limited data are available on this subject. There is therefore a clear interest in identifying those patients at risk of lymph node micrometastases.

7.5 Pathological and Radiological Lymph Node Staging

A patient with prostate cancer may or may not harbor lymph node metastases. Unfortunately, neither pathological nor clinical staging is 100% reliable in detecting the smallest invasion. Actually, both methods can be considered inaccurate.

Surgical pelvic lymphadenectomy combined with pathological examination of lymph node tissue has remained the golden standard for determining whether lymph node metastasis is present. It is a surgical procedure that requires general anaesthesia, hospitalisation and which has its own morbidity. Lymph node metastases may be detected by methods other than open pelvic lymph node dissection. Minimally invasive techniques such as laparoscopic and mini-laparotomy pelvic lymph node dissection have been well described and provide comparable information while improving patient prognosis (Parra et al. 1992; Perrotti et al. 1996; Rukstalis et al. 1994). These techniques, however, offer no advantage with respect to operative time and cost. However, certain groups routinely perform lymphadenectomy to select pathologically node negative patients (Dinges et al. 1998), although this approach is based more on assumption rather than on established evidence.

In a pooled analysis of two RTOG trials (75-06 and 77-06), the staging of lymph nodes by lymphangiography or CT scan was not predictive of loco-regional control or survival, whereas lymphadenectomy was (Hanks et al. 1992). Other authors have not confirmed this observation. For example, Gerber et al. (1996) reported that patients classified as pN0 did not fare better than unselected patients with a similar Gleason grade. However, this observation could be interpreted as the limitations of laparoscopic lymph node staging in accurately diagnosing lymphatic invasion.

In addition, it is worth noting that lymph node dissection can be the source of abnormal CT findings such as necrotic nodes (low attenuation masses). In a series of 73 patients, 42 subjects were found at CT to have such abnormalities. This can be somewhat distressing to the radiation oncologist when planning treatment on pelvic CT (Glajchen et al. 1996).

Over the years, several non-surgical techniques have been used to avoid surgical pelvic lymph node dissection. The American College of Radiology appropriateness criteria for clinical staging are available on the Internet (www.acr.org).

Pedal lymphangiography has only been routinely performed by a few centres. Due to its very low level of detection and its relative invasiveness, it should be now considered of no further use.

Since its introduction in the early eighties, pelvic CT has been used on a widespread basis to detect lymph node metastases. However, several studies have reported its insufficient accuracy, both as regards tumour invasion and nodal staging. CT imaging can detect only abnormalities in lymph node size that may result from extensive tumour involvement (=1 cm). Therefore the diagnostic sensitivity of this procedure with respect to lymph node assessment is poor (about 25%) (Engeler et al. 1992; Flanigan et al. 1996; Huncharek and Muscat 1996; Levran et al. 1995). However, a recent study reported a 93.7% accuracy for CT in detecting positive nodes, which increased to 96.5% if CT-guided fine needle aspiration biopsy was also used (Clements et al. 1992). This degree of accuracy was obtained by considering every node of 6 millimetres or larger as pathological. This is a departure from previous CT assessment criteria for positive nodes. In patients who are allergic to contrast medium, body coil MRI is roughly equivalent to CT imaging.

ProstaScint® is a popular radioimmunoscintigraphic agent targetted against PSMA, a prostate-specific cell surface antigen that is highly expressed in prostate cancer cells, especially in the case of metastases. Theoretically, this approach should be helpful in providing information on the presence of lymph node and bone metastasis with a single test (Lamb and Faulds 1998). It is not yet widely used and whether it provides additional information which cannot be obtained by other methods has not yet been determined.

More recently, there have been some interesting preliminary observations on the use of ultrasmall superparamagnetic iron oxide (Combidex)-enhanced MRI of pelvic lymph nodes which appears to be a very promising technique (Harisinghani et al. 1997).

7.6 Statistical Prediction of Lymph Node Involvement

With the widespread use of radical prostatectomy, many centres have generated large pathological databases. These are extensively used to generate algorithms to predict pathological extension and survival following radical prostatectomy. They have also been successfully used by surgeons to identify patients for whom the increased time, cost and potential morbidity of lymph node dissection could be avoided (Alagiri et al. 1997; Bishoff et al. 1995; Campbell et al. 1995; Danella et al. 1993; Spevack et al. 1996). To some extent at least, these algorithms also apply to patients treated by radiotherapy.

Amongst these, multiple methods exist to accurately predict the probability of nodal invasion. Multiple models and nomograms combining PSA, clinical stage and Gleason score have been developed (Bishoff et al. 1995; Bluestein et al. 1994; Partin et al. 1997). Others have proposed PSA and Gleason grade cut-off points for selecting patients in whom the risk of nodal disease is low, obviating the need for pelvic lymph node dissection. Basically these cut-off points would define an acceptable proportion of patients with potentially detectable metastatic disease who would nevertheless undergo radical prostatectomy or, in case of radiotherapy, not receive prophylactic irradiation of the lymph nodes.

Using a false-positive rate of 3%, Bluestein et al. (1994) estimated that 25% of patients with clinically localised disease could be spared lymph node dissection. Rees et al. (1997) constructed a predictive model to identify patients with less than a 3% likelihood of harbouring lymph node disease. They validated this model in several series. Approximately 50% of their patients met certain criteria, including PSA not greater than 5 ng/ml, Gleason score not higher than 5 or the combination of PSA not greater than 25 ng/ml, Gleason score not higher than 7 and negative digital rectal examination (Rees et al. 1997). Campbell et al. reported similar results: 73% of their patients were in the low risk category and the actual rate of positive lymph nodes only amounted to 2.2% (Campbell et al. 1995).

One of the most commonly used nomograms is that of Partin, proposed by Partin et al. (1997) from Johns Hopkins University School of Medicine. They used clinical stage, Gleason score and PSA levels to predict the pathological stage in patients with localised prostate cancer. All patients were assigned a clinical stage by one urologist. The Gleason score was determined from preoperative needle biopsy, and serum PSA levels were measured on an ambulatory basis. Final pathological stage was determined to be either organ-confined established capsular penetration, seminal vesicle involvement or lymph node involvement. From these analyses probability plots and nomograms were constructed to predict the final pathological stage of prostate cancer. Only 1 out of 64 men (less than 1%) with a Gleason score of 2–4 had positive lymph nodes while 42% of those with a Gleason score of 8–10 had positive pelvic lymph nodes. Positive pelvic lymph nodes were an infrequent finding (<6%) for patients with clinical stage T1a, T1b or T2a disease. All levels of pathological stage were accurately predicted by the various combinations of the 3 variables with P values <0.00001.

Table 7.1. Patients enrolled in various studies involving predictive algorithms

Senior author: institution	No. of patients	Reference
Partin (new): Hopkins, Baylor, Michigan	4,133	PARTIN et al. (2001)
Bluestein: Mayo	1,632	BLUESTEIN et al. (1994)
Lerner: Mayo	904	LERNER et al. (1996)
Narayan: Univ. Florida	813	NARAYAN et al. (1995)
Eastham: Baylor	766	EASTHAM et al. (1999)
Partin (II): Hopkins	542	PARTIN et al. (1997)
Pisansky: Mayo	500	PISANSKY et al. (1997)
D'Amico: Harvard	480	D'AMICO et al. (1996)
Dugan: Mayo	337	DUGAN et al. (1996)
Huncharek: Mass. General	300	HUNCHAREK and MUSCAT (1995)
Bostwick: Mayo, Baylor, Univ. Wash., Laval	186	BOSTWICK et al. (1996)
Oesterling: Mayo	852	OESTERLING et al. (1993)
Powell: Wayne State, Michigan	369	POWELL et al. (1997)
Kleer: Mayo	945	KLEER et al. (1993)
Total	12,759	

All combinations predicted pathological stage better than any single variable alone. Probability plots were constructed for the prediction of final pathological stage by the combination of serum PSA with Gleason score and clinical stage. The slope of the probability curves increased with increasing Gleason score as well as with advancing clinical stage for each pathological stage. Several other authors have evaluated the utility of the original Partin's nomograms on their own dataset, and the predictions were compared with actual outcomes of the author's patients. Interestingly, in all cases these were highly reproducible (KATTAN et al. 1997; PARTIN et al. 2001).

Since then, Partin et al. have combined the clinical data from 3 academic institutions and developed a multi-institutional model combining PSA level, clinical stage, and Gleason score to predict pathological stage for 4,133 men with clinically localised prostate cancer.

The Partin tables are available in various forms, including on the Internet, and allow each physician to make predictions for individual patients. The Internet address is www.prostatecalculator.org. For example, a T1c, Gleason 6 prostate carcinoma with a PSA of 5 ng/ml has less than a 1% probability of nodal involvement. A T2b, Gleason 7 with a PSA of 9 ng/ml has a 17.8% probability.

These models and nomograms show that a small percentage still remains of patients harbouring positive lymph nodes in the low risk group. The problem then arises of how to define an acceptable false-negative rate if pelvic lymphadenectomy or lymph node irradiation is not done.

It seems acceptable that the benefit of omitting pelvic lymph node radiation in 50% to 70% of patients would outweigh the 2% to 5% of patients in whom positive lymph nodes have been overlooked. REES et al. (1997) stated that physicians evaluating patients with newly diagnosed prostate cancer should be willing to accept a false negative rate of 1.8% or less when deciding whether to perform pelvic lymph node dissection for evaluation. Nevertheless, to our knowledge this threshold has not been evaluated objectively as regards its potential impact on survival.

Table 7.2. Example of a Partin table combining Gleason grade with stage. The numbers represent percentage probability of nodal involvement

Gleason	2–4	5	6	7	8–10
T1a	0	3	–	18	–
T1b	2	5	13	24	40
T1c	0	1	3	8	16
T2a	1	–	4	9	17
T2b	1	4	10	17	29
T2c	1	4	10	18	29
T3a	–	7	18	26	37

7.7 Arguments for Lymphatic Irradiation

It is logical that if a patient has a prostate cancer with lymph node metastases, it makes little sense to focus treatment on the gland and to leave cancer cells behind in the nodes.

Nodal invasion is a strong marker for bad prognosis because bone metastases, whether occult or not, are frequently present when lymph nodes are invaded. Nodal irradiation is therefore considered of little use by some authors as survival in node-positive patients is essentially metastasis-dependent (Leibel et al. 1994).

However, nodal irradiation in patients with documented positive nodes can have a curative effect. Twenty years ago, Bagshaw reported 9 survivors at 10 years post-irradiation out of 66 patients with pathologically staged positive nodes, supporting the view that nodal invasion is not invariably associated with distant metastases (Bagshaw 1984). An earlier report by the same author correlated disease-free survival rates with the site(s) of nodal involvement (follow-up interval 1–50 months): 32/37 with negative nodes were NED, versus 10/14 with positive pelvic nodes and 3/10 with positive pelvic and periaortic nodes (Bagshaw et al. 1977).

Malignant lymph nodes can be the source of further metastases in patients previously free of systemic dissemination. In a retrospective series of 738 patients treated at the Mallinckrodt Institute of Radiology between 1967 and 1988, the pelvic failure rate correlated inversely with pelvic node irradiation (45 Gy) for T3 stage (P=0.01), but not for T1 or T2 stages (P=0.62 and 0.36, respectively). Moreover, patients with T3 stage and control of the pelvic tumour had fewer distant metastases (Perez et al. 1994).

The approach is not quite the same when deciding on the basis of positive findings (lymph node sampling or enlarged nodes on CT scan), i.e. when there is demonstrated disease vs. on the basis of a probability index in a patient with cN0 staging. The amount of cancer tissue to be sterilised and, therefore, the likelihood of complete eradication of disease by radiotherapy are different. It is difficult to find data in the literature that is relevant to this specific question. Several series report on the survival of patients with proven node metastases (hence, bulky) which had been treated by surgery, radiotherapy, hormonotherapy or any combination of these. In the absence of appropriate controls, the existence and the degree of a benefit have so far not been possible to assess.

A parallel can perhaps be made with breast cancer, another hormone-associated disease: N+ has long been considered a marker of a disseminated disease and the influence of nodal irradiation on metastasis-free survival and overall survival is not known. This is currently being investigated in a large EORTC trial. For many years, radiotherapy was considered a loco-regional adjuvant to surgery with an impact on local control only. Recent studies from Denmark and Canada have shown that besides resulting in better local control, overall survival was also improved by adjuvant radiotherapy. In both studies axillary and internal mammary nodes were irradiated in patients with demonstrated nodal invasion (Overgaard et al. 1997; Ragaz et al. 1997).

It seems that patients with minimal nodal invasion fare better than those with a more massive nodal invasion. In a series of 132 consecutive patients treated by radical prostatectomy and lymphadenectomy, minimal nodal invasion did not significantly alter overall survival (Schmid et al. 1997). In another series of 73 patients with pelvic node metastases, 5-year survival amounted to 15%, 27% and 44% for gross nodal invasion, microscopic invasion involving more than one node and microscopic invasion of a single node, respectively (Smith and Middleton 1985). One can speculate that clinically node negative patients (i.e. a negative CT scan or MRI) are more likely to fall into this latter category.

Conventional radiotherapy has traditionally indicated internal iliac lymphatics as the target (Fletcher 1973). The emergence of a sizeable group of patients with low PSA, low Gleason score prostate cancer has modified this view. Textbooks of the 1970s or 1980s are more relevant for information on locally advanced tumours diagnosed in symptomatic patients.

The use of CT-based planning and BEV display have clearly improved the accuracy of lymphatic CTV definition. In a study by Forman et al. (1993), DVH showed that as much as 30% of lymph nodes only received half of the prescribed dose with the standard 2D box technique design.

In a series of patients with PSA-detected, non-palpable prostate adenocarcinoma, only initial PSA was predictive of the long-term biological control (bNED); the results of multivariate analysis indicated treatment field size (small pelvis vs. prostate) was not significant, although an unexpected trend was observed of worse biological control with large field irradiation (Horwitz et al. 1998).

Recent 3D-CRT trials have reduced the CTV to the prostate and seminal vesicles, without pelvic irradiation. However, the proximal lymphatics are included, but not the further nodal stations. Short-term local control or PSA control seems an acceptable endpoint, but long-term, metastasis-free survival cannot be obtained (Zelefsky et al. 1998).

When lymph nodes are found to be positive (by lymphadenectomy or on pelvic imaging with cytological confirmation), the question arises of whether irradiation should be considered or not. Arguments exist in support of the use pelvic irradiation (Bagshaw 1984; Paulson et al. 1982) or a combination of hormonotherapy and radiotherapy (Buskirk et al. 2001; Zagars et al. 2001)

7.7.1 Randomised Trials

Two randomised trials addressed the issue of nodal irradiation in cases of prostate adenocarcinoma. RTOG 77-06 was a prospective randomised trial of elective nodal irradiation in patients with T1b and T2 tumours, with treatment randomised between irradiation to the prostate alone versus irradiation to the pelvic nodes and the prostate. Patients were eligible if staged N0 by lymphangiography (75%) or pathological examination (25%). The probability of nodal invasion was thus very limited, which probably explains the lack of significant difference in outcome between the two arms of the study.

RTOG protocol 75-06 was a prospective randomised trial involving similar T stage patients with pN+ and T3 with any nodal status, with treatment randomised between pelvic node and prostate irradiation versus para-aortic node plus pelvic node and prostate irradiation.

Both trials showed no advantage for elective nodal irradiation (Asbell et al. 1988; Pilepich et al. 1986). There is a degree of consensus, however, in considering these trials as suboptimal in design (analysis was not performed according to intention to treat, for example). Also, they were carried out a long time ago and their relevance to current practice is limited, both as regards technique and recruitment.

In the Canadian trial investigating the role of total androgen blockade (TAB) combined with radiotherapy, a four-field box technique with field sizes of 8×8 to 10×10 cm was used (Laverdière et al. 1997). Prophylactic iliac node irradiation was not carried out. Patients with clinical T2a, T2b and T3a prostate cancer were included, i.e. subjects with a sizeable risk of lymph node metastases. The endpoint was negative prostate biopsy at 12 and 24 months, i.e. a local control endpoint. Data on long-term survival are not available. It should be noted that a 10×10 cm field does actually cover the proximal lymphatics and can sterilise transit metastases present at that level.

The EORTC 22863 randomised trial compared radiotherapy alone with radiotherapy combined with goserelin. Patients in both groups received 50 Gy to the pelvis followed by 20 Gy to the prostate. 2D planning was used in most cases. Patients with T1-T2 poorly differentiated adenocarcinomas or T3-T4 of any grade were included. Lymph node staging was determined by CT, lymphangiography or lymphadenectomy. Fourteen patients were staged N+ and 366 N0 (37 unknown) (Bolla et al. 1997).

A small Swedish randomised trial investigated treatment by radical radiotherapy with or without orchiectomy. Ninety-one patients were included out of a projected 400 since an interim analysis demonstrated the high frequency of recurrence in the radiotherapy alone arm (stopping rule). Surgical staging of lymph nodes was carried out in all patients; the rate of nodal positivity was 43%. All patients were irradiated on the pelvis to 50 Gy; a prostate boost delivered 64 Gy. Survival was significantly better in the combined therapy group, but, interestingly, the benefit was limited to the pN+ patients. Negative node patients fared better, but there was no advantage in combining orchiectomy with radiotherapy (Granfors et al. 1998).

In the RTOG 85-31 trial patients were randomised to treatment by radical radiotherapy and long-term androgen suppression versus radiotherapy alone in unfavourable prognosis prostate cancer (T1T2 N+ or T3 any N). Twenty-eight percent of the population was staged N+; two-thirds underwent laparoscopic node staging and one-third imaging only. The pelvis was irradiated up to the L5-S1 interspace to a dose of 44–46 Gy. However, some patients were included after prostatectomy, and these subjects did not receive pelvic irradiation (Pilepich et al. 1997).

The companion trial, RTOG 86-10, investigated short-term hormone therapy with external beam radiotherapy versus radiotherapy only in cases of locally advanced prostate carcinoma (bulky T2 or T3) with or without regional lymph node involvement. The pelvis was irradiated up to 44–46 Gy, followed by a boost to the prostate.

All these trials, although not specifically addressing the issue of nodal irradiation, indicate that prophylactic pelvic irradiation has become common practice in several centres whenever the local T stage exceeded T2a. As indicated by their trial number, all these studies were planned in the seventies or early eighties, i.e. before the widespread adoption of PSA testing and the dramatic shift toward early-stage prostate cancer at diagnosis. PSA testing was approved by the Food and

Drug Administration (FDA) for cancer monitoring in 1986, and in 1994 as a means of aiding cancer detection (Hankey et al. 1999).

7.8 Morbidity Associated with Pelvic Lymph Nodes Irradiation

Staging pelvic lymphadenectomy does not modify the tolerance to radiotherapy (Greskovich et al. 1991), except for the risk of scrotal, penile or leg oedema which nearly never occurs with radiotherapy alone: 0.1% vs. 10% (Perez et al. 1994). This observation is consistent with that of Pilepich et al. (1987) who found a positive correlation between the incidence of leg-penile oedema and the extent of pelvic lymphadenectomy.

Rectosigmoid grade 2 and 3 (RTOG-EORTC morbidity scale) amounted to 10% with pelvic node irradiation followed by a prostate boost vs. 3% with prostate irradiation only in a series of 738 patients treated at the Mallinckrodt Institute of Radiology (Perez et al. 1994). Similar observations were reported by Kurup et al. (1984), Mameghan et al. (1990) and Rosen et al. (1985).

Quality of life as assessed by the Profile of Mood States (POMS) and the Medical Outcome Study's 36-question Health Survey Short Form of General Health Status (SF-36), both validated scales, was also found to be impaired by whole pelvis irradiation when compared to small field radiotherapy (Beard et al. 1997). Using the QLQ-30 of the EORTC, we found a similar correlation in a series of patients treated with a fast neutrons approach (Remouchamps et al. 1998).

Pelvic irradiation, therefore, increases the immediate morbidity (diarrhoea, loss of weight) and slightly increases the risk of late rectitis.

7.9 Conclusion

In summary, an analysis of isolated nodal recurrence after radical prostate irradiation or after radical prostatectomy and its influence on the further development of local relapse and metastases is currently lacking. In the absence of such data, the issue of prophylactic nodal irradiation cannot be fully resolved. It therefore remains a matter of clinical judgment and opinion.

References

Alagiri M, Colton MD, Seidmon EJ et al (1997) The staging pelvic lymphadenectomy: implications as an adjunctive procedure for clinically localized prostate cancer. Br J Urol 80:243–246

Asbell SO, Krall JM, Pilepich ME et al (1988) Elective pelvic irradiation in stage A-2, B carcinoma of the prostate: analysis of RTOG 77–06. IJROBP 15:1306–1316

Bagshaw MA (1984) Radiotherapeutic treatment of prostatic carcinoma with pelvic node involvement. Urol Clin North Am 11:297–304

Bagshaw MA, Pistenma DA, Ray GR et al (1977) Evaluation of extended-field radiotherapy for prostatic neoplasms: 1976 progress report. Cancer Treat Rep 61:297–306

Bagshaw MA, Kaplan ID, Cox RC (1993) Prostate cancer. Radiation therapy for localized disease. Cancer 71: 939–952

Beard CJ, Propert KJ, Rieker PP et al (1997) Complications after treatment with external-beam irradiation in early stage prostate cancer patients: a prospective multiinstitutional outcomes study. JCO 15:223–229

Bishoff JT, Reyes A, Thompson IM et al (1995) Pelvic lymphadenectomy can be omitted in selected patients with carcinoma of the prostate: development of a system of patient selection. Urology 45:270–274

Bluestein DL, Bostwick DG, Bergstralh EJ, Oesterling JE (1994) Eliminating the need for bilateral pelvic lymphadenectomy in select patients with prostate cancer. J Urol 151: 1315–1320

Bolla M, Gonzalez D, Warde P et al (1997) Improved survival in patients with locally advanced prostate cancer treated with radiotherapy and goserelin. NEJM 337:295–300

Bostwick DG, Wheeler TM, Blute M et al (1996) Optimized microvessel density analysis improves prediction of cancer stage from prostate needle biopsies. Urology 48:47–57

Buskirk SJ, Pisansky TM, Atkinson EJ et al (2001) Lymph node-positive prostate cancer: evaluation of the results of the combination of androgen deprivation therapy and radiation therapy. Mayo Clin Proc 76:702–706

Campbell SC, Klein EA, Levin HS, Piedmonte MR (1995) Open pelvic lymph node dissection for prostate cancer: a reassessment. Urology 46:352–355

Catalona WJ, Smith DS, Ratliff TL et al (1993) Detection of organ confined prostate cancer is increased through prostate-specific antigen-based screening. JAMA 270:948–954

Clements R, Griffiths GJ, Peeling WB (1992) Staging prostatic cancer. Clin Radiol 46:225–231

D'Amico AV, Whittington R, Malkowicz SB et al (1996) Role of percent positive biopsies and endorectal coil MRI in predicting prognosis in intermediate-risk prostate cancer patients. Cancer J Sci Am 2:343

Danella JF, deKernion JB, Smith RB, Steckel J (1993) The contemporary incidence of lymph node metastases in prostate cancer: implications for laparoscopic lymph node dissection. J Urol 149:1488–1491

Dinges S, Deger S, Koswig S et al (1998) High-dose rate interstitial with external beam irradiation for localised prostate cancer: results of a prospective trial. Radiother Oncol 48: 197–202

Dugan JA, Bostwick DG, Myers RP et al (1996) The definition and preoperative prediction of clinically insignificant prostate cancer. JAMA 275:288–294

Eastham JA, May R, Robertson JL et al (1999) Development of a nomogram that predicts the probability of a positive prostate biopsy in men with an abnormal digital rectal examination and a prostate-specific antigen between 0 and 4 ng/mL. Urology 54:709–713

Engeler CE, Wasserman NF, Zhang G (1992) Preoperative assessment of prostatic carcinoma by computerised tomography. Weaknesses and new perspectives. Urology 40:346–350

Flanigan RC, McKay TC, Olson M et al (1996) Limited efficacy of preoperative computed tomographic scanning for the evaluation of lymph node metastasis in patients before radical prostatectomy. Urology 48:428–432

Fletcher GH (1973) Textbook of radiotherapy. Lea and Febiger, Philadelphia

Forman JD, Lee Y, Roberson P et al (1993) Advantages of CT and Beam eye's view display to confirm the accuracy of pelvic lymph node irradiation in carcinoma of the prostate. Radiology 186:889–892

Gerber GS, Bales GT, Gornik HL et al (1996) Treatment of prostate cancer using external beam radiotherapy afterr laparoscopic pelvic node dissection. Br J Urol 77:870–875

Glajchen N, Shapiro RD Stock RG et al (1996) CT findings after laparoscopic pelvic lymph node dissection and transperineal radioactive seed implantation for prostatic carcinoma. Am J Roentgenol 166:1165–1168

Granfors T, Modig H, Damber JE, Tomic R (1998) Combined orchiectomy and external radiotherapy versus radiotherapy alone for non metastatic prostate cancer with or without pelvic node involvement: a prospective randomised study. J Urol 159:2030–2034

Greskovich FJ, Zagars GK, Sherman NE and Johnson DE (1991) Complications following external beam radiation therapy for prostate cancer: an analysis of patients treated with and without staging pelvic lymphadenectomy. J Urol 146:798–802

Hankey BF, Feuer EJ, Clegg LX et al (1999) Cancer surveillance series: interpreting trends in prostate cancer, part I. Evidence of the effects of screening in recent prostate cancer incidence, mortality and survival rates. JNCI 91: 1017–1024

Hanks GE, Krall JM, Pilepich MV et al (1992) Comparison of pathologic and clinical evaluation of lymph nodes in prostate cancer: implications of RTOG data for patient management and trial design and stratification. IJROBP 23:293–298

Harisinghani MG, Saini S, Slater GJ, Schnall MD, Rifkin MD (1997) MR imaging of pelvic lymph nodes in primary pelvic carcinoma with ultrasmall superparamagnetic iron oxide (Combidex): preliminary observations. J Magn Reson Imaging 7:161–163

Horwitz EM, Hanlon AL, Pinover W, Hanks GE (1998) The treatment of nonpalpable PSA-detected adenocarcinoma of the prostate with 3-dimensional conformal radiation therapy. IJROBP 41:519–523

Huncharek M, Muscat J (1995) Serum prostate-specific antigen as a predictor of radiographic staging studies in newly diagnosed prostate cancer. Cancer Invest 13:31–35

Huncharek M, Muscat J (1996) Serum prostate-specific antigen as a predictor of staging abdominal/pelvic computed tomography in newly diagnosed prostate cancer. Abdominal Imaging 21:364–367

Kattan MW, Cowen ME, Miles BJ (1997) A decision analysis for treatment of clinically localized prostate cancer. J Gen Intern Med 12:299–305

Kleer E, Larson-Keller JJ, Zincke H, Oesterling JE (1993) Ability of preoperative serum prostate-specific antigen value to predict pathologic stage and DNA ploidy. Influence of clinical stage and tumor grade. Urology 41:207–216

Kurup P, Kramer TS, Lee MS et al (1984) External beam irradiation of prostate cancer: experience in 163 patients. Cancer 53:37–43

Lamb HM, Faulds D (1998) Capromab pendetide. A review of its use as an imaging agent in prostate cancer. Drugs 12: 293–304

Laverdière J, Gomez JL, Cusan L et al (1997) Beneficial effect of combination hormonal therapy administered prior and following external beam radiation, therapy in localised prostate cancer. IJROBP 37:247–252

Leibel SA, Fuks Z, Zelefsky MF, Whitmore WF Jr (1994) The effects of local and regional treatment on the metastatic outcome in prostatic carcinoma with pelvic lymph node involvement. IJROBP 28:7–16

Lerner SE, Blute ML, Bergstralh EJ, Bostwick DG, Eickholt JT, Zincke H (1996) Analysis of risk factors for progression in patients with pathologically confined prostate cancers after radical retropubic prostatectomy. J Urol 156:137–143

Levran Z, Gonzalez JA, Diokno AC et al (1995) Are pelvic computed tomography, bone scan and pelvic lymphadenectomy necessary in the staging of prostatic cancer? Br J Urol 75:778–781

Mameghan H, Fisher R, Mameghan J et al (1990) Bowel complications after radiotherapy for carcinoma of the prostate: the volume effect. Int J Radiat Oncol Biol Phys 18:315–320

Mc Neal JE (1968) Regional morphology and pathology of the prostate. Am J Surg Pathol 49:347–357

Mc Neal JE, Redwine EA, Freiha FS et al (1988) Zonal distribution of prostatic adenocarcinoma: correlation with histologic pattern and direction of spread. Am J Surg Pathol 12:898–906

Narayan P, Gajendran V, Taylor SP, Tewari A, Presti JC Jr, Leidich R, Lo R, Palmer K, Shinohara K, Spaulding JT (1995) The role of transrectal ultrasound-guided biopsy-based staging, preoperative serum prostate-specific antigen, and biopsy Gleason score in prediction of final pathologic diagnosis in prostate cancer. Urology 46:205–212

Oesterling JE, Martin SK, Bergstralh EJ, Lowe FC (1993) The use of prostate-specific antigen in staging patients with newly diagnosed prostate cancer. JAMA 269:57–60

Overgaard M, Hansen PS, Overgaard J et al (1997) Postoperative radiotherapy in high-risk premenopausal women with breast cancer who receive adjuvant chemotherapy. Danish Breast Cancer Cooperative Group 82b Trial. N Engl J Med 337:949–955

Parra RO, Andrus CH, Boullier JA (1992) Staging laparoscopic pelvic lymph node dissection. Experience and indications. Arch Surg 127:1294–1297

Partin AW, Walsh PC (1994) The use of prostate specific antigen, clinical stage and Gleason score to predict pathological stage in men with localized prostate cancer. J Urol 152:172–173

Partin AW, Kattan MW, Subong EN et al (1997) Combination of prostate-specific antigen, clinical stage, and Gleason score to predict pathological stage of localized prostate cancer. A multi-institutional update. JAMA 277:1445–1451

Partin AW, Mangold LA, Lamm DM, Walsh PC, Epstein JI,

Pearson JD (2001) Contemporary update of prostate cancer staging nomograms (Partin Tables) for the new millennium. Urology 58:843–848
Paterson R (1948) Treatment of malignant disease by radium and X-rays; a practice of radiotherapy. Williams and Wilkins, Baltimore
Paulson DF, Cline WA Jr, Koefoot RB et al (1982) Extended field radiation therapy versus delayed hormonal therapy in node positive prostatic adenocarcinoma. J Urol 127: 935–937
Perez CA, Lee HK, Georgiou A, Lockett MA (1994) Technical factors affecting morbidity in definitive irradiation for localised carcinoma of the prostate. IJROBP 28:811–819
Perrotti M, Gentle DL, Barada JH et al (1996) Mini-laparotomy pelvic lymph node dissection minimizes morbidity, hospitalization and cost of pelvic lymph node dissection. J Urol 155:986–988
Pilepich MV, Krall JM, Johnson RJ et al (1986) Extended field (periaortic) irradiation in carcinoma of the prostate-analysis of RTOG 75-06 . IJROBP 12:345–351
Pilepich MV, Krall JM, Sause WT et al (1987) Correlation of radiotherapeutic parameters and treatment related morbidity in carcinoma of the prostate: Analysis of RTOG study 75-06. IJROBP 13:351–357
Pilepich MV, Caplan R, Byhardt RW et al (1997) Phase III trial of androgen suppression using Goserelin in unfavourable-prognosis carcinoma of the prostate treated with definitive radiotherapy: report of RTOG 85-31. JCO 15:1013–1021
Pisansky TM, Kahn MJ, Rasp GM, Cha SS, Haddock MG, Bostwick DG (1997) A multiple prognostic index predictive of disease outcome after irradiation for clinically localized prostate carcinoma. Cancer 79:337–344
Poirier P, Cuneo B, Delamere G (1903) The lymphatics. Archibald Constable, Westminster, pp 175–182
Polascik TJ, Oesterling JE, Partin AW (1999) Prostate specific antigen: a decade of discovery – what we have learned and where we are going. J Urol 162:293–306
Powell IJ, Heilbrun LK, Sakr W et al (1997) The predictive value of race as a clinical prognostic factor among patients with clinically localized prostate cancer: a multivariate analysis of positive surgical margins. Urology 49:726–731
Ragaz J, Jackson SM, Le N et al (1997) Adjuvant radiotherapy and chemotherapy in node-positive premenopausal women with breast cancer. N Engl J Med 337:956–962
Rees MA, Resnick MI, Oesterling JE (1997) Use of prostate-specific antigen, Gleason score, and digital rectal examination in staging patients with newly diagnosed prostate cancer. Urol Clin North Am 24:379–388
Remouchamps V, Richard F, Lhoas F et al (1998) Mixed photon-neutron radiotherapy in prostate cancer: a retrospective quality of life study. Radiother Oncol 48:S67
Rietbergen JB, Hoedemaeker RF, Kruger_AE et al (1999) The changing pattern of prostate cancer at the time of diagnosis: characteristics of screen detected prostate cancer in a population based screening study. J Urol 161: 1192–1198
Rosen E, Cassady R, Connolly JR et al (1985) Radiotherapy for prostate carcinoma: the JCRT experience (1968–1978). II. Factors related to tumour control and complications. IJROBP 11:725–730
Rukstalis DB, Gerber GS, Vogelzang NJ et al (1994) Laparoscopic pelvic lymph node dissection: a review of 103 consecutive cases. J Urol 151:670–674
Schmid HP, Mihatsch MJ, Hering F, RutishauserG (1997) Impact of minimal lymph node metastasis on long-term prognosis after radical prostatectomy. Eur Urol 31:11–16
Schröder FH, Kranse R, Rietbergen JB et al (1999) The European Randomized Study of Screening for Prostate Cancer (ERSPC): an update. Members of the ERSPC, Section Rotterdam. Eur Urol 35:539–543
Smith JA Jr, Middleton RG (1985) Implications of volume of nodal metastasis in patients with adenocarcinoma of the prostate. J Urol 133:617–619
Spevack L, Killion LT, West JC et al (1996) Predicting the patient at low risk for lymph node metastasis with localized prostate cancer: an analysis of four statistical models. Int J Radiat Oncol Biol Phys 34:543–547
Testut L, Latarjet A (1931) Traité d'anatomie humaine. Tome cinquième: appareil urogénital–péritoine. Gaston Doin, Paris, pp 264–268
Walsh PC, Mostwin JL (1984) Radical prostatectomy and cystoprostatectomy with preservation of potency. Results using a new nerve-sparing technique. Br J Urol 56:694–697
Zagars GK, Pollack A, von Eschenbach AC (2001) Addition of radiation therapy to androgen ablation improves outcome for subclinically node-positive prostate cancer. Urology 58: 233–239
Zelefsky MJ, Leibel SA, Gaudin PB et al (1998) Dose escalation with three-dimensional conformal radiation therapy affects the outcome in prostate cancer. IJROBP 41:491–500

8 Intensity-Modulated Radiation Therapy for Lymph Node Metastases in Bladder Cancer

M. Milosevic, M. Gospodarowicz, M. Jewett, R. Bristow, T. Haycocks

CONTENTS

8.1 Introduction

Bladder cancer is a common disease, and causes significant morbidity and mortality. It is estimated that there will be 56,500 new cases diagnosed in the United States in 2002, and that 12,600 men and women will die of the disease (Jemal et al. 2002). The majority of tumors are transitional cell carcinomas that arise from the transitional epithelium of the bladder mucosa. Superficial transitional cell carcinomas account for about 75% of all cases, and have a low potential to metastasize. The remaining 25% of tumors invade the muscularis propria of the bladder wall, and frequently spread to the lymph nodes and distant sites, making muscle-invasive bladder cancer a life-threatening disease. Lymph node involvement at diagnosis is associated with a high risk of occult metastatic disease and has an ominous prognosis.

There is extensive experience on the use of radiotherapy (RT) as primary radical treatment for muscle-invasive bladder cancer. The goal of RT is to permanently eradicate the tumor while preserving normal bladder function and minimizing complications. Overall, approximately 70% of patients show complete regression of the disease following treatment (Blandy et al. 1988; Duncan and Quilty 1986; Gospodarowicz et al. 1989; Greven et al. 1990; Jenkins et al. 1988; Smaaland et al. 1991; Vale et al. 1993), and 30–50% of cases display sustained local control (complete disease regression without subsequent recurrence in the bladder; Gospodarowicz et al. 1991; Greven et al. 1990;Jahnson et al. 1991). However, distant metastases develop in more than 50% of patients (Gospodarowicz et al. 1989), and long-term overall survival is in the range of only 25% to 30% (Duncan and Quilty 1986; Fossa et al. 1993; Gospodarowicz et al. 1989; Moonen et al. 1998; Pollack et al. 1994). Chemotherapy is often administered concurrently with RT, and has been shown to enhance pelvic tumor control (Coppin et al. 1996).

These results indicate that while RT is an effective modality in the treatment of bladder cancer, there is an important need to improve the local effectiveness of RT and also treat occult lymph node and distant metastases that are present at initial diagnosis. This underscores the importance of understanding the multiple, inter-related biologic parameters that influence the natural history of bladder cancer, the development of metastases and the response to radiation. In addition, careful attention to radiation dose delivery is necessary in order to optimize the therapeutic ratio. New techniques of intensity-modulated radiation therapy (IMRT), which allow the dynamic variation of radiation beam orientation, size, shape and intensity during treatment, allow optimization of radiation delivery to the tumor with rela-

M. Milosevic, MD; M. Gospodarowicz, MD
Department of Radiation Oncology, University of Toronto, Princess Margaret Hospital, 610 University Avenue, Toronto, Ontario, Canada M5G 2M9
M. Jewett, MD
Department of Surgical Oncology and Urology, University of Toronto, Princess Margaret Hospital, 610 University Avenue, Toronto, Ontario, Canada M5G 2M9
R. Bristow, MD; T. Haycocks
Department of Radiation Oncology, University of Toronto, Princess Margaret Hospital, 610 University Avenue, Toronto, Ontario, Canada M5G 2M9

tive sparing of the surrounding critical normal tissues (Portelance et al. 2001; Roeske et al. 2000). However, the potential of IMRT to yield significant improvements in local tumor control and patient survival is directly linked to the precision with which clinicians are able to delineate the gross tumor volume (GTV) and clinical target volume (CTV), and then monitor and re-define these volumes on a daily basis during fractionated RT to account for variation in patient setup and organ movement. Also, a detailed knowledge of dose–fractionation–volume relationships is needed for critical normal tissues as a starting point for developing IMRT plans. These issues have begun to be addressed in patients with bladder cancer with respect to treatment of the primary tumor (Larsen and Engelholm 1994; Logue et al. 1998; Miralbell et al. 1998; Turner et al. 1997).

The optimal management of lymph nodes in patients with bladder cancer undergoing RT has not been extensively studied. Failure to control pelvic lymph node metastases may be an important cause of disease recurrence following treatment. Clinically normal lymph nodes are often included in the CTV especially in patients who are judged to be at high risk of harboring occult lymph node metastases. Traditionally, large pelvic fields have been used to deliver a dose of 40 to 50 Gy in 1.8 to 2 Gy daily fractions to the whole pelvis, encompassing the primary bladder tumor and lymph nodes as well as a significant volume of normal tissue including the small bowel and rectum. The pelvic dose is limited by the radiation tolerance of these normal tissues and the need to minimize the risk of late radiation complications. While large-field pelvic RT administered in this manner is generally well tolerated, its contribution to improved pelvic control and patient survival is unknown. Subclinical metastases may consist of a single malignant cell, or a nodule near the threshold of radiographic detection containing 10^8 or more cells. There is likely to be significant heterogeneity of intrinsic cellular radiation sensitivity from tumor to tumor, and also within individual tumors. The moderate doses of radiation that can safely be delivered to the whole pelvis may be insufficient to reliably eradicate the larger more radioresistant metastases in the subclinical range even when administered with concurrent chemotherapy (Marks 1990; Okunieff et al. 1995; Withers et al. 1995). Therefore, the pelvic lymph nodes may be inadequately treated with conventional RT in a high proportion of patients.

This review addresses fundamental questions about the management of lymph nodes in patients receiving RT for bladder cancer, including: 1) which patients are at greatest risk of harboring lymph node metastases at diagnosis; 2) which pelvic lymph node groups are most likely to contain metastases; 3) what are the optimal lymph node staging investigations in patients to be treated with radical RT; 4) is there a role for the surgical staging of pelvic lymph nodes prior to RT; and 5) can IMRT be used to enhance the therapeutic ratio for the treatment of pelvic lymph nodes? It is assumed throughout that local control of the primary bladder tumor with preservation of normal bladder function is achievable using modern RT techniques, with or without concurrent chemotherapy.

8.2 Pelvic Lymph Node Anatomy

The lymphatic drainage of the pelvis has been described in standard anatomy and surgical texts (Williams 1995). However, unlike other regions of the body including the head and neck and thorax, there is no generally accepted classification for pelvic lymph nodes that transcends disease- and discipline-specific boundaries. This has contributed to discrepancies in the description of lymph-node drainage for various pelvic organs including the urinary bladder, and makes it difficult to compare reports of pelvic lymph node metastases across studies (Mangan et al. 1986; Panici et al. 1992). The lack of a standard nomenclature has, at least in part, arisen from the technical difficulties associated with accurately identifying, surgically dissecting and pathologically examining pelvic lymph node specimens. For example, the lymph nodes along the pelvic side walls form a continuous interconnected mesh in close relation to the external and internal iliac vessels and their various branches, and do not conform to a discrete categorization system. The surgical field is often confined, and the anatomic limits of each nodal group (to the extent that boundaries exist) are difficult to assess. Detailed pathologic examination of iliac lymph node specimens may be hampered by fibrous or fatty infiltration of nodal tissue and prior inflammation. However, regardless of these problems, a universal classification scheme for pelvic lymph nodes that is translatable from the surgical to radiographic domains is essential if the development of IMRT for lymph node metastases is to proceed in a coordinated and interpretable fashion.

The classification of pelvic lymph nodes that is probably most easily applied in the context of RT planning is one in which the lymph node groups conform to the distribution of the major pelvic arteries. Gray's Anatomy (Williams 1995) describes the abdominal aorta as bifurcating anterior to the fourth lumbar vertebrae into the left and right common iliac arteries. These diverge and descend into the pelvis anterior to the L5–S1 vertebrae. Each common iliac artery bifurcates into an external iliac and internal iliac artery anterior to the sacroiliac joints. The external iliac artery descends along the lateral border of the psoas muscle to the level of the inguinal ligament, where it becomes the femoral artery. The internal iliac artery begins at the bifurcation of the common iliac artery and descends posteriorly into the pelvis. At the upper border of the greater sciatic foramen it divides into anterior and posterior divisions, which give off branches that supply the pelvic organs, perineum, buttocks and sacral canal. Major branches of the anterior division of the internal iliac artery include the obturator artery, superior and inferior vesical arteries and the inferior gluteal artery. Important branches of the posterior trunk include the superior gluteal and the lateral sacral arteries. Arterial supply to the bladder is principally from the superior and inferior vesical arteries, with contributions from the obturator and inferior gluteal arteries. Venous drainage is via a vascular plexus on the inferolateral aspect of the bladder, which terminates in branches of the internal iliac veins.

A classification of pelvic lymph nodes that conforms to this distribution of vessels is shown in Table 8.1. The medial external iliac, obturator and other internal iliac lymph nodes along the pelvic side wall are the primary drainage routes for most of the pelvic organs. There is often a considerable interconnection among the various nodal groups, and connections between the right and left sides of the pelvis.

Table 8.1. Classification of pelvic lymph nodes

Lymph node group	Subgroup	Location
Common iliac	Lateral Anterior Medial	4–6 nodes surrounding the common iliac artery anterior to L5 and the sacroiliac joints
External iliac	Lateral Anterior Medial (principle)	8–10 nodes surrounding the external iliac artery
Internal iliac	Obturator Superior gluteal Inferior gluteal Presacral	Obturator node located posterior to the medial external iliac nodes at the upper border of the acetabulum. Presacral lymph nodes anterior to the sacrum from L5 inferiorly

8.3 Lymphatic Drainage of the Urinary Bladder

The lymphatic drainage of the urinary bladder was originally determined from meticulous surgical and post-mortem dissection (Rouviere 1938). The lymphatics begin as a network of microscopic channels that permeate the lamina propria, muscularis and serosa of the bladder wall. These terminate in collecting ducts that emerge from the bladder near the trigone and along the anterior and posterior walls. The collecting ducts travel superiorly and laterally and terminate in the medial external iliac, obturator and other internal iliac lymph nodes that are situated along the pelvic side wall medial to the acetabulum (Martinez-Monge et al. 1999). Drainage may also occur directly via the anterior and lateral external iliac lymph nodes, common iliac nodes and presacral lymph nodes. Small paravesical lymph nodes are frequently present in close relation to the bladder wall, and intercalating lymph nodes may be found along the course of the collecting ducts between the bladder and the pelvic side wall.

8.4 Pelvic Lymph Node Dissection in Bladder Cancer

Pelvic lymph node dissection is routinely performed as part of radical cystectomy in patients with bladder cancer, and has yielded important information about the prevalence and location of lymph node metastases. The extent and technique of lymphadenectomy vary from center to center, although thorough removal of all lymph nodes lying between the bifurcation of the aorta superiorly, the inguinal ligament inferiorly and the genitofemoral nerve (overlying the psoas muscle) laterally has been advocated (Stein et al. 2001). This encompasses the common iliac, external iliac, and pelvic side wall internal and external iliac lymph nodes. In addition, because the lymph node specimen is often removed en bloc with the cystectomy specimen, the paravesical and intercalating lymph nodes along the course of the collecting ducts may also be included. However, en bloc lymphadenectomy versus separate dissection and submission of the pelvic lymph nodes as groups corresponding to specific anatomical nodal regions is controversial, and a recent report has suggested that separate dissection may lead to a more detailed evaluation of the number of lymph nodes involved by cancer (Bochner et al. 2001). It is necessary to identify a minimum of eight to nine lymph nodes at lymphadenectomy in order to reliably classify a patient with bladder cancer as being pathologically node-negative (Bochner et al. 2001). Typically, dissection of the external and internal iliac nodal groups alone yields between five and 15 lymph nodes, while a more thorough dissection that also includes the distal para-aortic and common iliac nodes yields between 20 and 30 nodes (Bochner et al. 2001; Lerner et al. 1993; Wishnow et al. 1987). Pre-sacral lymph nodes may or may not be removed as part of routine pelvic lymphadenectomy.

The use of sentinel lymph node detection as a guide to the extent of lymphadenectomy has recently been described in patients with bladder cancer (Sherif et al. 2001). The underlying assumptions are: 1) that bladder cancer spreads in a predictable fashion to first involve a specific regional lymph node, the sentinel node, and then other secondary nodes; and 2) that the sentinel node can reliably be identified intra-operatively. The benefit of extensive pelvic lymphadenectomy is likely to be small if the sentinel node is negative, assuming the validation of these assumptions. Sherif et al. (2001) reported the results of sentinel node detection in 13 patients with T1, G3 or T2–T4 bladder cancer. Identification of the sentinel node was based on pre- and intra-operative detection of a radioactive tracer or blue dye that was injected into the bladder muscularis propria around the visible tumor. Sentinel nodes were detected in 11 of the patients (85%). Four patients had lymph node metastases at lymphadenectomy. In all cases, only the sentinel node was involved by tumor There were no cases of pelvic lymph node metastases in the absence of sentinel node improvement. Verification of this technique is needed before the sentinel node can be used routinely to guide lymph node surgery in patients with bladder cancer.

The overall prevalence of pelvic lymph node metastases in patients undergoing radical cystectomy and lymph node dissection for bladder cancer is in the range of 15% to 30%. The depth of bladder wall invasion as reflected in the pathologic T-category is the strongest surgico-pathologic predictor of lymph node involvement. The risk is less than 10% in patients with superficial bladder cancer (pT1; TNM 1997), 15% to 20% in patients with muscle-invasive disease confined to the bladder wall (pT2), and 30% to 50% in the setting of extravesical disease (pT3; Bassi et al. 1999; Frazier et al. 1993; Poulsen et al. 1998; Smith and Whitmore 1981; Stein et al. 2001; Wishnow et al. 1987). The majority of patients with positive lymph nodes at lymphadenectomy have microscopic involvement of only one or two nodes (Lerner et al. 1993; Wishnow et al. 1987), again emphasizing the important contributions of surgical technique and specimen preparation to accurate nodal staging. Wishnow et al. (1987) reported tumor-containing lymph nodes in patients with bladder cancer to vary in size from 0.1–1.7 cm (median: 0.8 cm), with tumor deposits that ranged from 0.05–0.9 cm (median: 0.3 cm). Lerner et al. (1993) showed that only 30% of patients with lymph node metastases from bladder cancer had visible or palpable nodal involvement that was recognizable at the time of surgery. This observation at least in part reflects patient selection: those with gross nodal disease on pre-operative imaging studies are less likely to undergo surgical exploration, and more likely to be treated with RT and/or chemotherapy.

Although the lymphatic drainage of the normal urinary bladder is well defined as outlined in section 8.3, the actual anatomic distribution of lymph node metastases in patients with bladder cancer has been addressed in relatively few studies. Smith and Whitmore (1981) identified lymph node metastases in 134 patients with bladder cancer who underwent radical cystectomy and pelvic lymph node dissection following pre-operative pelvic radiotherapy. The obturator lymph nodes were most commonly involved (74%), followed by the external iliac (65%), hypogastric (internal iliac in the classification of Table 8.1; 17%), peri-vesical (16%) and common iliac (19%) nodes. The distinction between obturator and medial external iliac lymph nodes was difficult and unreliable. Most patients had lymph node metastases at more than one site. None had common iliac nodal involvement in the absence of internal or external iliac disease, implying stepwise cephalad progression of nodal metastases. In another report, 19% of patients with bladder cancer showed pre-sacral lymph node involvement (Lerner and Skinner 2000). There is a limited body of evidence to suggest that, in the setting of a well lateralized bladder tumor, only the ipsilateral pelvic lymph nodes are at increased risk of harboring occult disease (Wishnow et al. 1987). However, further studies are needed to confirm this, given the interconnections that are known to exist between the lymphatics of the left and right sides of the pelvis and the possible influence of prior pelvic surgery or infection on lymphatic pathways.

The results of these studies are summarized in the TNM classification (1997) of bladder tumors, which specifies the regional lymph nodes broadly as those of the true pelvis below the bifurcation of the common iliac vessels (Sobin and Wiitekind 1997). The TNM classification is shown in Table 8.2. Increasing N-category reflects increasing bulk of external and internal iliac lymph node disease independent of nodal laterality in the pelvis in relation to the primary tumor. Common iliac and para-aortic lymph node involvement is classified as distant metastatic disease, and bears an M1 designation.

Table 8.2. TNM (1997) classification of bladder cancer (Sobin and Wiitekind 1997)

Primary tumor (T)	
TX	Primary tumor cannot be assessed
T0	No evidence of primary tumor
Ta	Noninvasive papillary carcinoma
Tis	Carcinoma in situ (CIS)
T1	Tumor invades subepithelial connective tissue
T2	Tumor invades muscle:
T2a	Tumor invades superficial muscle (inner half)
T2b	Tumor invades deep muscle (outer half)
T3	Tumor invades perivesical tissue:
T3a	Microscopically
T3b	Macroscopically (extravesical mass)
T4	Tumor invades any of the following: prostate, uterus, vagina, pelvic wall, abdominal wall
T4a	Tumor invades prostate, uterus, vagina
T4b	Tumor invades pelvic wall and/or abdominal wall
Regional lymph nodes (N)	
NX	Regional lymph nodes cannot be assessed
N0	No regional lymph node metastasis
N1	Metastasis in a single lymph node 2 cm or less in greatest dimension
N2	Metastasis in a single lymph node over 2 cm but not more than 5 cm in greatest dimension, or multiple lymph nodes, none more than 5 cm in greatest dimension
N3	Metastasis in a lymph node over 5 cm in greatest dimension
Distant metastases (M)	
MX	Distant metastases cannot be assessed
M0	No distant metastases
M1	Distant metastases (including common iliac and para-aortic lymph node metastases)
Stage grouping	
Stage 0a	Ta N0 M0
Stage 0is	Tis N0 M0
Stage I	T1 N0 M0
Stage II	T2a N0 M0
	T2b N0 M0
Stage III	T3a N0 M0
	T3b N0 M0
	T4a N0 M0
Stage IV	T4b N0 M0
	Any T; N1, 2, 3; M0
	Any T; any N; M1

8.5 Radiographic Evaluation of Pelvic Lymph Nodes

Lymphadenectomy remains the gold standard for evaluating pelvic lymph nodes in patients with bladder cancer. Nodal status as determined by lymphadenectomy, providing that a sufficient number of nodes is removed and proper attention is given to specimen preparation and histologic examination, yields important prognostic information about distant recurrence and patient survival that can be used to guide subsequent treatment including adjuvant chemotherapy. However, patients who are treated with RT do not usually undergo lymphadenectomy, but instead are staged clinically using examination under anesthesia and radiologic techniques.

Several studies have investigated the accuracy of computed tomography (CT) and magnetic resonance imaging (MRI) at diagnosing pelvic lymph node metastases in patients with bladder cancer and other pelvic tumors. These techniques rely on lymph node enlargement as an indicator of metastases, which can also arise because of pelvic infection or inflammation. In general, the sensitivity of CT or MRI for detecting pelvic lymph node metastases is only about 50% relative to lymphadenectomy, although the specificity is higher and in the range of 90% (Barentsz et al. 1997; Roy et al. 1997). CT and MRI can only reliably detect metastases in lymph nodes that have a short-axis diameter of at least 1 cm (Barentsz et al. 1997; Roy et al. 1997). Lymph nodes of this size may contain a significant tumor burden that is unlikely to be controlled by conventional whole-pelvis RT (Marks 1990; Withers et al. 1995). Lymphangiography has the theoretical advantage over CT and MRI of visualizing not only lymph node size but also internal lymph node architecture, which may be disrupted by small-bulk metastases. However, lymphangiography does not detect microscopic nodal disease and also does not reliably image the internal iliac lymph nodes, which are among the most commonly involved nodes in bladder cancer (Smith and Whitmore 1981). In one study of 60 patients with bladder cancer who underwent lymphangiography prior to pre-operative radiation and cystectomy with lymph-node dissection, the sensitivity of lymphangiography for nodal metastases was only 64% (Bao-Shan and Wallace 1985). Therefore, none of these anatomic imaging techniques is sufficiently accurate to allow important decisions about management to be made in patients with bladder cancer.

Recent reports have suggested that positron-emission tomography (PET) with fluoro-deoxyglucose (FDG) may be a more sensitive indicator of pelvic lymph node metastases (Grigsby et al. 2001; Narayan et al. 2001; Reinhardt et al. 2001). PET with FDG provides a relative indication of tissue glucose metabolism. Many malignant tumors are characterized by increased glucose metabolism relative to normal tissues, and PET therefore provides a means of detecting lymph node metastases based on functional differences rather than on nodal size or architecture. The sensitivity of PET for pelvic lymph node metastases has been reported to be in the range of 80% to 90%, and its specificity in the range of 90% to 100% (Narayan et al. 2001; Reinhardt et al. 2001). PET detects para-aortic lymph node and distant metastases more frequently than CT, and in cervical cancer provides important prognostic information that is not available from other routine staging tests (Grigsby et al. 2001). Nevertheless, the sensitivity of PET for small-bulk pelvic lymph node metastases may be limited, and the interpretation of the test may be confounded by the urinary excretion of FDG (Williams et al. 2001). Heicappell et al. (1999) reported that, among nine patients with pathologically-proven lymph node involvement from prostate or bladder cancer, the smallest detectable metastasis with PET was 0.9 cm in diameter. Three patients with lymph node metastases smaller than 0.5 cm had normal PET studies. It remains unclear whether PET, while superior to CT and MRI, has sufficient resolution and diagnostic accuracy to be used in place of lymphadenectomy in patients with bladder cancer.

8.6 Significance of Lymph Node Metastases in Bladder Cancer

Pelvic lymph node metastases in patients with bladder cancer imply a high risk of occult distant metastases, a high risk of recurrence outside the pelvis following local treatment alone, and a significantly lower survival rate relative to node-negative patients. Several randomized studies of chemotherapy following cystectomy in patients with either locally extensive primary tumors or involved pelvic lymph nodes have shown improved disease-free survival, although frequently no improvement in overall survival has been noted (Freiha et al. 1996; Skinner et al. 1991; Stockle et al. 1995; Studer et al. 1994). This may in part reflect the fact that chemotherapy administered at the time of recurrence was associated with a high likelihood of response particularly in chemotherapy-naive patients, so that the benefit of adjuvant treatment on overall survival was diminished. Nevertheless, all node-positive patients should be considered for chemotherapy following definitive treatment of the primary bladder tumor with either cystectomy or RT, with the aim of delaying tumor progression and minimizing overall morbidity.

It is clear that pelvic lymphadenectomy provides important prognostic information on patients with bladder cancer. In addition, the experience of several institutions suggests a therapeutic advantage of pelvic lymphadenectomy, although this has never been tested in a randomized study. As summarized in Table 8.3, between 15% and 30% of patients with lymph node metastases may be cured with a combination of cystectomy and bilateral pelvic lymph node dissection alone without chemotherapy, particularly those with small-bulk disease confined to the first-echelon pelvic nodes (Bassi et al. 1999; Bretheau and Ponthieu 1996; Frazier et al. 1993; Poulsen et al. 1998; Smith and Whitmore 1981; Stein et al. 2001; Turner et al. 1998; Vieweg et al. 1999; Zincke et al. 1985). The largest study on therapeutic lymphadenectomy in bladder cancer is from the University of Southern California (Lerner et al. 1993; Skinner et al. 1982; Stein et al. 2001). In a recent report of 1,054 patients who underwent radical cystectomy and extended lymphadenectomy between 1971 and 1997, lymph node metastases were identified in 246 cases (Stein et al. 2001). The 10-year recurrence-free and overall survival rates for these patients were 34% and 23% respectively, and were significantly lower than the corresponding numbers for node-negative patients (75% and 49% respectively). Survival was higher in the setting of four or fewer involved nodes (40% vs. 25%), and also when the primary tumor was confined to the bladder (43% vs. 30%). Distant metastases developed in 52% of node-positive patients. The benefit of adjuvant systemic chemotherapy, which was administered to a proportion of the node-positive patients in the latter years of the study, could

Table 8.3. Results of pelvic lymphadenopathy in bladder cancer

Study	No. of node-positive patients	5-year overall survival (%)
Stein et al. (2001)	246	31
Vieweg et al. (1999)	193	38.1[a]
Bassi et al. (1999)	78	14.5
Turner et al. (1998)	66	30
Poulsen et al. (1998)	51	18
Bretheau and Ponthieu (1996)	40	14
Frazier et al. (1993)	59	15
Zincke et al. (1985)	57	10
Smith and Whitmore (1981)	134	7

[a]3-year overall survival

not be assessed in relation to the benefit of lymphadenectomy given the non-randomized nature of the intervention. While this and other studies imply a poor prognosis for node-positive patients, it can be assumed that the results would have been even worse in the absence of aggressive local surgery and systemic treatment. Lymph-node dissection may also contribute to the cure of patients with small-bulk gross pelvic lymph node metastases identified at the time of surgery (Herr and Donat 2001).

While small-bulk pelvic nodal metastases may be managed effectively with lymphadenectomy and adjuvant chemotherapy, more extensive pelvic nodal disease is associated with a very poor prognosis and patients are unlikely to benefit from aggressive surgery. These patients should be treated in the same manner as those with para-aortic or distant metastases, using chemotherapy and palliative RT, as dictated by symptoms and the patient's clinical course.

8.7 Management of Pelvic Lymph Nodes with Radiotherapy

The surgical experience suggests that: 1) an accurate indication of pelvic lymph node status provides important prognostic information and is a valuable indicator of the need for adjuvant systemic chemotherapy; and 2) aggressive treatment of pelvic lymph node metastases enhances the long-term survival in a substantial proportion of patients.

A proposal based on these principles for the management of pelvic lymph nodes in patients receiving RT as primary treatment for bladder cancer is outlined in Fig. 8.1. This approach combines surgical staging of pelvic lymph nodes as an indicator of the need for adjuvant chemotherapy, with aggressive local management of positive nodes using IMRT. Meticulous clinical evaluation of the efficacy and safety of this approach is required, along with optimization of radiation dose-fractionation-volume schedules. However, it has the potential to yield results comparable to aggressive surgery in the context of an overall management strategy that emphasizes both tumor control and preservation of normal bladder function.

Currently available radiographic staging techniques are not sufficiently sensitive to detect occult lymph node metastases, and reliance on these techniques may result in potentially curable patients being under-treated. Surgical evaluation of pelvic lymph nodes is required to reliably detect nodal metastases in patients who have no visible lymphadenopathy on CT or MRI. However, lymph node dissection prior to RT must not significantly increase the risk of complications compared to radiation alone, or delay the start of definitive treatment for the primary bladder tumor. Open trans-peritoneal pelvic lymphadenectomy followed by conventional large-field pelvic RT has been associated with a higher than acceptable rate of serious small bowel complications (Potish and Dusenbery 1990), which may be overcome by using an extra-peritoneal approach to the pelvic lymph nodes (Ballon et al. 1981; Lanciano and Corn 1994; Potish et al. 1984). Laparoscopic pelvic lymph node sampling has been advocated in the management of prostate cancer and other pelvic tumors, and may also be useful in cases of bladder cancer (Poulsen and Krarup 1995): it yields

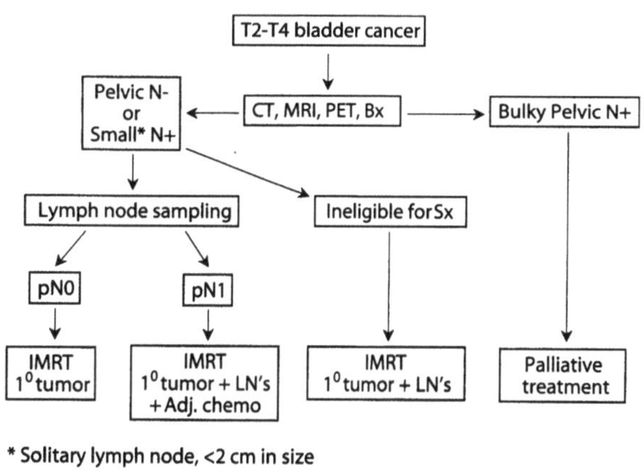

Fig. 8.1. Management of pelvic lymph nodes in patients receiving primary radiotherapy for bladder cancer

an equivalent number of nodes to open sampling procedures with less morbidity and faster patient recovery (Kava et al. 1998; Parkin et al. 2002; Shackley et al. 1999) and is an attractive option in combination with RT. Patients who are pathologically node-negative (pN0), provided that a sufficient number of nodes were removed to reliably establish this designation (Bochner et al. 2001), would receive IMRT to the primary tumor alone with or without concurrent chemotherapy.

Several studies have demonstrated prolonged survival of patients with microscopic lymph node metastases following complete pelvic lymphadenectomy as summarized in Table 8.3, but the relative importance of aggressive local lymph node treatment versus systemic chemotherapy is not known. The experience with breast cancer provides useful information in this regard that can be extrapolated to the management of node-positive patients with bladder cancer: adjuvant nodal irradiation of breast cancer patients with lymphatic metastases identified by axillary dissection has been demonstrated in several studies to improve survival beyond that achievable with systemic adjuvant treatment alone (Overgaard et al. 1999; Ragaz et al. 1997). Based on these results, bladder cancer patients with lymphatic metastases determined at lymph node sampling should be considered for adjuvant nodal irradiation as well as chemotherapy. Targeted high-dose irradiation of pelvic lymph nodes using intensity-modulated techniques to minimize the dose to the small bowel, rectum and other critical normal structures is likely to enhance pelvic control, and possibly also survival without significant toxicity.

The optimal management of patients with small-bulk (solitary, less than 2 cm) pelvic lymphadenopathy determined on CT or MRI is not known. The prognosis of patients with radiographically-evident lymph node metastases is particularly poor, but there is limited evidence to indicate that a small proportion of these patients is curable with aggressive local and systemic treatment (Herr and Donat 2001). Therefore, otherwise healthy patients with internal or external iliac lymph node enlargement and no visible common iliac disease should be considered for lymph node dissection with removal of the enlarged nodes, followed by post-operative intensity-modulated nodal irradiation and adjuvant chemotherapy.

While lymphadenectomy prior to RT is currently the most sensitive and reliable means of determining N-category as a guide to prognosis and the need for adjuvant chemotherapy, many patients with bladder cancer are elderly and have concurrent medical problems that make them ineligible for surgery. A compromise approach in clinical-N0 inoperable patients is to include both the bladder and the pelvic lymph nodes in the CTV in all cases, as is currently common practice, but escalate the dose using IMRT to a level that is compatible with a high probability of tumor control. The greatest limitation of this approach is the lack of a reliable indicator for adjuvant systemic chemotherapy. Regimens like the combination of gemcitabine and cisplatin have proven efficacy in bladder cancer and minimal toxicity, and could be used safely in many of these patients despite the co-morbidities that make them ineligible for surgery. A better understanding of the tumor microenvironmental and molecular factors that predict occult pelvic lymph node involvement and disease recurrence would greatly aid in deciding which patients to treat with chemotherapy, and would reduce the current dependence on detailed surgical staging. Alterations in tumor suppressor genes (p53, retinoblastoma protein), apoptosis-related genes (bcl-2, survivin) and cell-cycle-related markers (Ki-67, E2F-1, MIB-1) have variably been reported to be independent predictors of nodal metastatic spread in patients undergoing cystectomy (Bochner et al. 1997; Rabbani et al. 1999; Swana et al. 1999; Tiguert et al. 2001). However, in a double-blinded study by the National Cancer Institute Bladder Tumor Marker Network, none of these factors was significantly associated with positive lymph node status (Lianes et al. 1998). Active research is ongoing using other nodal-predictive markers including E-cadherin immunoreactivity (Byrne et al. 2001) and plasma levels of interleukin-6 (Andrews et al. 2002). Reverse-transcriptase polymerase chain reaction (RT–PCR) for circulating bladder cancer cells expressing cytokeratin-20 (Gudemann et al. 2000) and other bladder-associated markers requires further prospective testing to determine its usefulness as a tool for predicting occult metastatic spread and the need for adjuvant chemotherapy.

8.8 IMRT Planning

There is little concrete information in the literature to use as a planning guide for the delivery of high-dose IMRT to pelvic lymph nodes in patients with bladder cancer. The evidence from surgical series suggests that the para-vesical, intercalating, pelvic side wall, common iliac and pre-sacral lymph nodes anterior to S1–S2 are all at risk of harboring metastases and therefore need to be included in the CTV. There are sparse data to suggest that well lateralized bladder tumors may preferentially spread to ipsilateral pelvic lymph nodes (Wishnow et al. 1987). However, given the rich left-to-right lymphatic connections in the pelvis, excluding contra-lateral nodes from the CTV may carry a significant risk of missing tumor. Sentinel lymph node evaluation has not yet been developed to the stage where it can provide a reliable indication of the lymph nodes at greatest risk in a particular patient (Sherif et al. 2001). These factors together suggest that all of the pelvic lymph nodes below the level of the mid-common iliac vessels need to be encompassed within the CTV in order to maximize the likelihood of disease control and long-term patient survival, analogous to the surgical experience that supports complete pelvic lymphadenectomy.

Normal pelvic lymph nodes and those with microscopic metastases cannot usually be seen by CT or MRI, and the location of the various pelvic lymph node groups has historically been poorly described in textbooks of radiology and cross-sectional anatomy. This situation is improving, however, in part driven by advances in radiation delivery and the need for more precise delineation of lymph nodes and critical normal structures. Martinez-Monge et al. (1999) have recently published a comprehensive atlas of cross-sectional lymph node anatomy that includes all major lymph node groups in the body including those in the pelvis, and is a useful reference for 3-dimensional RT planning. Nutting et al. (2000) advocates using the internal, external and common iliac vessels with a 1 cm margin as an aid to defining the pelvic lymph node CTV in clinically node-negative patients. Figures 8.2–8.4 outline the lymph node CTV that should be considered when treating patients with bladder cancer at three cranio-caudal levels in the pelvis, and Fig. 8.5 is a 3-dimensional representation of the nodal volume.

The success of IMRT depends not only on the initial definition of primary tumor and nodal volumes, but also on knowledge of day-to-day variation in the 3-dimensional position of these volumes during a course of fractionated radiation. Both patient setup variability and internal organ movement are important factors that if not accounted for, might detract from the therapeutic benefit of dose escalation because of high dose gradients at the edges of the IMRT volumes. Setup variability is likely to be the more significant of these two variables with respect

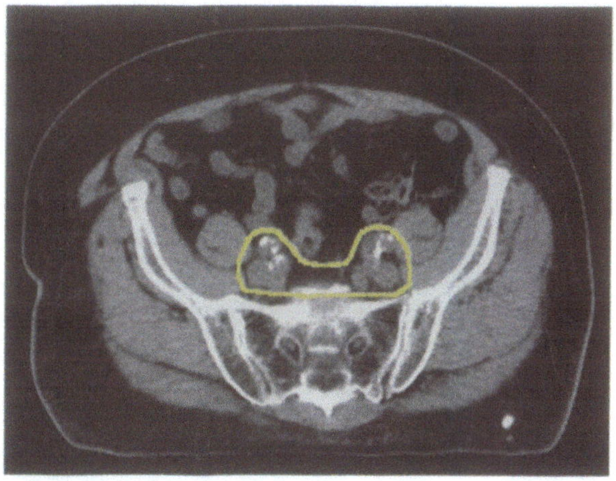

Fig. 8.2. Pelvic lymph node clinical target volume (CTV) at the level of the mid-sacrum

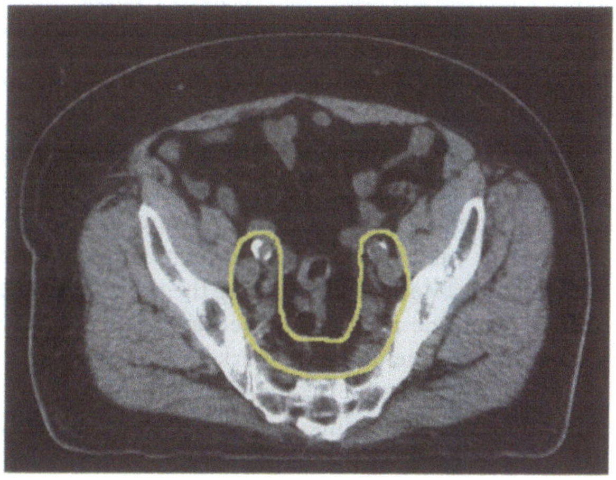

Fig. 8.3. Pelvic lymph node CTV at the inferior aspect of the sacro-iliac joints

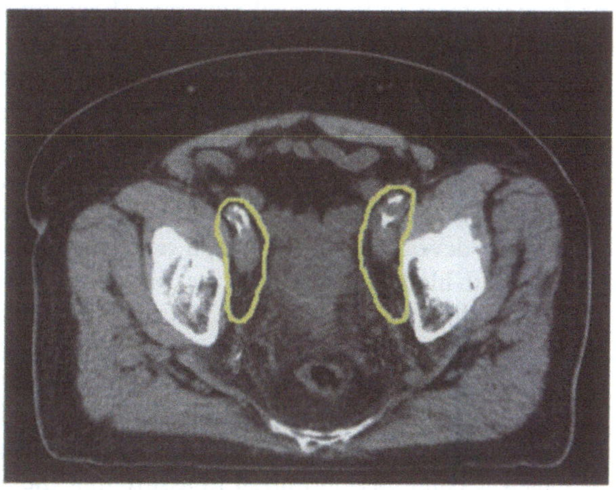

Fig. 8.4. Pelvic lymph node CTV immediately superior to the femoral heads

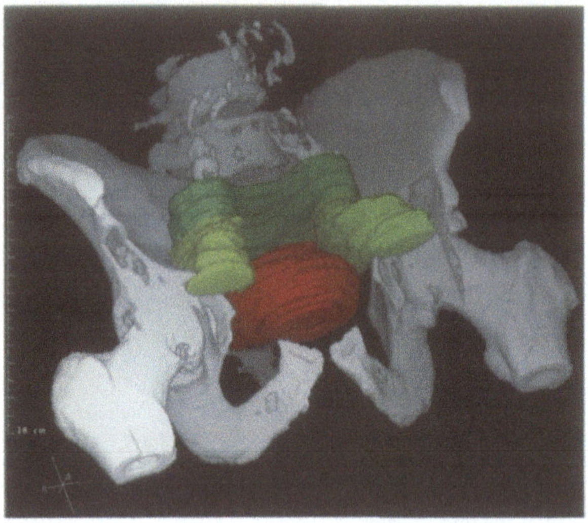

Fig. 8.5. Three-dimensional representation of the bladder tumor CTV (*red*) and pelvic lymph node CTV (*green*)

to pelvic lymph node irradiation, and a variety of techniques and patient immobilization devices have been described to minimize this problem (Malone et al. 2000). The use of IMRT to treat the primary bladder tumor poses more significant challenges because of inter-fraction variation in organ filling and position. Methods of tracking the position of the tumor from one fraction to the next are needed to address this issue. Fiducial markers that are placed cystoscopically in the bladder wall adjacent to the tumor may help in this regard by allowing daily imaging to confirm the target volume immediately prior to treatment.

Traditional whole pelvic radiation doses of 45 to 50 Gy in 1.8 to 2 Gy daily fractions probably offer only a small chance of controlling subclinical lymph node metastases in individual patients. Theoretical studies have suggested that at least 60 Gy is required to achieve a high probability of eradicating occult disease (Marks 1990; Withers et al. 1995), although this will be highly variable depending on factors such as tumor oxygenation and intrinsic radiosensitivity. Nevertheless, this provides an initial target to be used when developing IMRT lymph node plans for patients with bladder cancer. Whether or not it can be achieved will depend on the dose to critical normal tissues and the risk of late radiation complications.

The inverse treatment planning algorithms for IMRT require that tolerance doses for critical normal tissues in close proximity to the CTV be specified. The plan is computer-optimized to assure that these tolerance doses are not exceeded. The ability to escalate dose with IMRT and the overall safety of this approach therefore depends on an accurate knowledge of the dose–volume relationships for the normal tissues concerned. When treating pelvic lymph nodes in patients with bladder cancer, the risk of late radiation toxicity to the rectum and small bowel must be minimized. The dose–volume relationship for the rectum is beginning to be defined from careful evaluation of males receiving conformal RT for prostate cancer. Boersma et al. (1998) found a significantly higher rate of severe rectal bleeding in men who received greater than 65 Gy to at least 50% of the rectal wall, or greater than 70 Gy to at least 30% of the wall. In the Princess Margaret Hospital experience including over 200 patients who received a target absorbed dose (TAD) of 79.8 Gy in 1.9 Gy-daily fractions to the prostate, the risk of RTOG grade 2 or 3 rectal toxicity was 3% when 50% of the rectal wall received 50 Gy or less in 42 fractions. There was no grade 4 or 5 toxicity. There is little concrete information about the dose–volume relationship for the small bowel. Emami et al. (1991), based on a thorough review of the literature, suggested that the entire small bowel would tolerate a radiation dose of 40 Gy in 2 Gy daily fractions, and that one-third of the small bowel volume could safely be treated to 50 Gy. These reports provide first-order estimates of the dose–volume relationships for the bowel, that can be used as a general guide when developing IMRT plans. However, they must be modulated in light of specific patient and treatment-related issues such as prior abdomino-pelvic surgery and the use of concurrent chemotherapy. In general, while awaiting the results of more detailed studies, the radiation dose to the rectum and small bowel in patients with bladder cancer should be kept as low as possible, consistent with delivering a uniform (and if possible escalated) dose to the bladder and regional lymph nodes.

Figure 8.6 shows dose–volume histograms for a 7-field 18 MV coplanar IMRT bladder cancer plan. The CTV included the bladder tumor and the regional lymph nodes, as delineated in Figs. 8.2–8.5. The dose constraints for the bladder tumor and lymph node CTVs were 70 Gy±5% and 60 Gy±5% respectively. The small bowel was contoured as a solid volume and the rectum as a hollow tube defined by the outer and inner walls. The small bowel and rectum dose constraints were 40 Gy to 20% of the volume or less, with a maximum dose of 60 Gy. The dose–volume histograms illustrate the capability of IMRT to deliver escalated doses of radiation to the bladder tumor and regional lymph nodes, and reduced doses to critical normal tissues. The median small bowel and rectal doses were 30 Gy and 23 Gy respectively, and less than 5% of either organ received greater than 55 Gy.

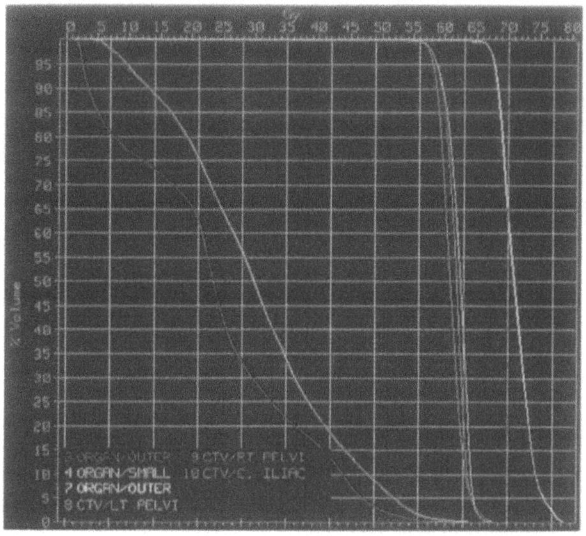

Fig. 8.6. IMRT Dose–volume histograms for bladder tumor (*yellow*), common iliac lymph nodes (*dark blue*), right iliac lymph nodes (*purple*), left iliac lymph nodes (*orange*), small bowel (*light blue*) and rectum (*red*). The prescribed bladder tumor and lymph node doses were 70 Gy and 60 Gy respectively

Overall, IMRT has the potential to revolutionize the practice of RT. It is likely to contribute to higher cure rates with fewer complications in a number of tumors including bladder cancer. The technology for pursuing IMRT studies is currently available in many centers. The safe implementation of this technology requires the combined effort of radiation oncologists, physicists, radiation therapists and nurses. Coordination and communication among these professional groups is essential to assure that important technical and patient-related issues are adequately addressed.

References

Andrews B, Shariat SF, Kim JH et al (2002) Preoperative plasma levels of interleukin-6 and its soluble receptor predict disease recurrence and survival of patients with bladder cancer. J Urol 167:1475–1481

Ballon SC, Berman ML, Lagasse LD et al (1981) Survival after extraperitoneal pelvic and paraaortic lymphadenectomy and radiation therapy in cervical carcinoma. Obstet Gynecol 57:90–95

Bao-Shan J, Wallace S (1985) Lymphatic imaging of solid tumors. In: Clouse ME, Wallace S (eds) Lymphatic imaging. Lymphography, computed tomography and scintigraphy. Williams and Wilkins, Baltimore, pp 290–450

Barentsz JO, Witjes JA, Ruijs JH (1997) What is new in bladder cancer imaging. Urol Clin North Am 24:583–602

Bassi P, Ferrante GD, Piazza N et al (1999) Prognostic factors of outcome after radical cystectomy for bladder cancer: a retrospective study of a homogeneous patient cohort. J Urol 161:1494–1497

Blandy JP, Jenkins BJ, Fowler CG et al (1988) Radical radiotherapy and salvage cystectomy for T2/3 cancer of the bladder. Prog Clin Biol Res 260:447–451

Bochner BH, Esrig D, Groshen S et al (1997) Relationship of tumor angiogenesis and nuclear p53 accumulation in invasive bladder cancer. Clin Cancer Res 3:1615–1622

Bochner BH, Herr HW, Reuter VE (2001) Impact of separate versus en bloc pelvic lymph node dissection on the number of lymph nodes retrieved in cystectomy specimens. J Urol 166:2295–2296

Boersma LJ, van den Brink M, Bruce AM et al (1998) Estimation of the incidence of late bladder and rectum complications after high-dose (70–78 Gy) conformal radiotherapy for prostate cancer, using dose-volume histograms. Int J Radiat Oncol Biol Phys 41:83–92

Bretheau D, Ponthieu A (1996) Results of radical cystectomy and pelvic lymphadenectomy for bladder cancer with pelvic node metastases. Urol Int 57:27–31

Byrne RR, Shariat SF, Brown R et al (2001) E-cadherin immunostaining of bladder transitional cell carcinoma, carcinoma in situ and lymph node metastases with long-term follow-up. J Urol 165:1473–1479

Coppin C, Gospodarowicz M, James K et al (1996) The NCI-Canada trial of concurrent cisplatin and radiotherapy for muscle invasive bladder cancer. J Clin Oncol 14: 2901–2907

Duncan W, Quilty PM (1986) The results of a series of 963 patients with transitional cell carcinoma of the urinary bladder primarily treated by radical megavoltage X-ray therapy. Radiother Oncol 7:299–310

Emami B, Lyman J, Brown A et al (1991) Tolerance of normal tissue to therapeutic radiation. Int J Radiat Oncol Biol Phys 21:109–122

Fossa SD, Waehre H, Aass N et al (1993) Bladder cancer definitive radiation therapy of muscle-invasive bladder cancer. A retrospective analysis of 317 patients. Cancer 72: 3036–3043

Frazier HA, Robertson JE, Dodge RK et al (1993) The value of pathologic factors in predicting cancer-specific survival among patients treated with radical cystectomy for transitional cell carcinoma of the bladder and prostate. Cancer 71:3993–4001

Freiha F, Reese J, Torti FM (1996) A randomized trial of radical cystectomy versus radical cystectomy plus cisplatin, vinblastine and methotrexate chemotherapy for muscle invasive bladder cancer. J Urol 155:495–499

Gospodarowicz MK, Hawkins NV, Rawlings GA et al (1989) Radical radiotherapy for the muscle invasive transitional cell carcinoma of the bladder: Failure analysis. J Urol 142: 1448–1454

Gospodarowicz MK, Rider WD, Keen CW et al (1991) Bladder cancer: long term follow-up results of patients treated with radical radiation. Clin Oncol 3:155–161

Greven KM, Solin LJ, Hanks GE (1990) Prognostic factors in patients with bladder carcinoma treated with definitive irradiation. Cancer 65:908–912

Grigsby PW, Siegel BA, Dehdashti F (2001) Lymph node staging by positron emission tomography in patients with carcinoma of the cervix. J Clin Oncol 19:3745–3749

Gudemann CJ, Weitz J, Kienle P et al (2000) Detection of hematogenous micrometastasis in patients with transitional cell carcinoma. J Urol 164:532–536

Heicappell R, Muller-Mattheis V, Reinhardt M et al (1999) Staging of pelvic lymph nodes in neoplasms of the bladder and prostate by positron emission tomography with 2-[^{18}F]-2-deoxy-D-glucose. Eur Urol 36:582–587

Herr HW, Donat SM (2001) Outcome of patients with grossly node positive bladder cancer after pelvic lymph node dissection and radical cystectomy. J Urol 165:62–64

Jahnson S, Pedersen J, Westman G (1991) Bladder carcinoma – a 20-year review of radical irradiation therapy. Radiother Oncol 22:111–117

Jemal A, Thomas A, Murray T et al (2002) Cancer statistics, 2002. CA Cancer J Clin 52:23–47

Jenkins BJ, Caulfield MJ, Fowler CG et al (1988) Reappraisal of the role of radical radiotherapy and salvage cystectomy in the treatment of invasive (T2/T3) bladder cancer. Br J Urol 62:342–346

Kava BR, Dalbagni G, Conlon KC et al (1998) Results of laparoscopic pelvic lymphadenectomy in patients at high risk for nodal metastases from prostate cancer. Ann Surg Oncol 5:173–180

Lanciano RM, Corn BW (1994) The role of surgical staging for cervical carcinoma. Semin Radiat Oncol 4:46–51

Larsen LE, Engelholm SA (1994) The value of three-dimensional radiotherapy planning in advanced carcinoma of the urinary bladder based on computed tomography. Acta Oncol 33:655–659

Lerner SP, Skinner DG (2000) Radical cystectomy for bladder cancer. In: Vogelzang NJ, Shipley WU, Scardino PT et al (eds) Comprehensive textbook of genitourinary oncology, 2nd edn. Lippincott Williams and Wilkins, Philadelphia, p 1177

Lerner SP, Skinner DG, Lieskovsky G et al (1993) The rationale for en bloc pelvic lymph node dissection for bladder cancer patients with nodal metastases: long-term results. J Urol 149:758–764

Lianes P, Charytonowicz E, Cordon-Cardo C et al (1998) Biomarker study of primary nonmetastatic versus metastatic invasive bladder cancer. National Cancer Institute Bladder Tumor Marker Network. Clin Cancer Res 4:1267–1271

Logue JP, Sharrock CL, Cowan RA et al (1998) Clinical variability of target volume description in conformal radiotherapy planning. Int J Radiat Oncol Biol Phys 41:929–931

Malone S, Szanto J, Perry G et al (2000) A prospective comparison of three systems of patient immobilization for prostate radiotherapy. Int J Radiat Oncol Biol Phys 48: 657–665

Mangan CE, Rubin SC, Rabin DS et al (1986) Lymph node nomenclature in gynecologic oncology. Gynecol Oncol 23:222–226

Marks LB (1990) A standard dose of radiation for "microscopic disease" is not appropriate. Cancer 66:2498–2502

Martinez-Monge R, Fernandes PS, Gupta N et al (1999) Cross-sectional nodal atlas: a tool for the definition of clinical target volumes in three-dimensional radiation therapy planning. Radiology 211:815–828

Miralbell R, Nouet P, Rouzaud M et al (1998) Radiotherapy of bladder cancer: relevance of bladder volume changes in planning boost treatment. Int J Radiat Oncol Biol Phys 41: 741–746

Moonen L, van de Voet H, de Nijs R et al (1998) Muscle-invasive bladder cancer treated with external beam radiotherapy: pretreatment prognostic factors and the predictive value of cystoscopic re-evaluation during treatment. Radiother Oncol 49:149–155

Narayan K, Hicks RJ, Jobling T et al (2001) A comparison of MRI and PET scanning in surgically staged loco-regionally advanced cervical cancer: potential impact on treatment. Int J Gynecol Cancer 11:263–271

Nutting MN, Convery DJ, Cosgrove VP et al (2000) Reduction of small and large bowel irradiation using an optimized intensity-modulated pelvic radiotherapy technique in patients with prostate cancer. Int J Radiat Oncol Biol Phys 48:649–656

Okunieff P, Morgan D, Niemierko A et al (1995) Radiation dose-response of human tumors. Int J Radiat Oncol Biol Phys 32:1227–1237

Overgaard M, Jensen MB, Overgaard J et al (1999) Postoperative radiotherapy in high-risk postmenopausal breast-cancer patients given adjuvant tamoxifen: Danish Breast Cancer Cooperative Group DBCG 82c randomised trial. Lancet 353:1641–1648

Panici PB, Scambia G, Baiocchi G et al (1992) Anatomical study of para-aortic and pelvic lymph nodes in gynecologic malignancies. Obstet Gynecol 79:498–502

Parkin J, Keeley FX, Timoney AG (2002) Laparoscopic lymph node sampling in locally advanced prostate cancer. BJU Int 89:14–17

Pollack A, Zagars GK, Swanson DA (1994) Muscle-invasive bladder cancer treated with external beam radiotherapy: prognostic factors. Int J Radiat Oncol Biol Phys 30:267–277

Portelance L, Chao KS, Grigsby PW et al (2001) Intensity-modulated radiation therapy (IMRT) reduces small bowel, rectum, and bladder doses in patients with cervical cancer receiving para-aortic irradiation. Int J Radiat Oncol Biol Phys 51:1–266

Potish RA, Dusenbery KE (1990) Enteric morbidity of postoperative pelvic external beam and brachytherapy for uterine cancer. Int J Radiat Oncol Biol Phys 18:1005–1010

Potish RA, Twiggs LB, Prem KA et al (1984) The impact of extraperitoneal surgical staging on morbidity and tumor recurrence following radiotherapy for cervical carcaioma. Am J Clin Oncol 7:245–251

Poulsen AL, Horn T, Steven K (1998) Radical cystectomy: extending the limits of pelvic lymph node dissection improves survival for patients with bladder cancer confined to the bladder wall. J Urol 160:2015–2019; discussion 2020

Poulsen J, Krarup T (1995) Pelvic lymphadenectomy (staging) in patients with bladder cancer: laparoscopic versus open approach. Scand J Urol Nephrol Suppl 172:19–21

Rabbani F, Richon VM, Orlow I et al (1999) Prognostic significance of transcription factor E2F-1 in bladder cancer: genotypic and phenotypic characterization. J Natl Cancer Inst 91:874–881

Ragaz J, Jackson SM, Le N et al (1997) Adjuvant radiotherapy and chemotherapy in node-positive premenopausal women with breast cancer. N Engl J Med 337:956–962

Reinhardt MJ, Ehritt-Braun C, Vogelgesang D et al (2001) Metastatic lymph nodes in patients with cervix cancer: detection with MR imaging and FDG PET. Radiology 21: 776–782

Roeske JC, Lujan A, Rotmensch J et al (2000) Intensity-modulated whole pelvic radiation in patients with gyncologic malignancies. Int J Radiat Oncol Biol Phys 48:1613–1621

Rouviere H (1938) Anatomy of the human lymphatic system. Edwards, Ann Arbor
Roy C, Le Bras Y, Mangold L et al (1997) Small pelvic lymph node metastases: evaluation with MR imaging. Clin Radiol 52:437–440
Shackley DC, Irving SO, Brough WA et al (1999) Staging laparoscopic pelvic lymphadenectomy in prostate cancer. BJU Int 83:260–264
Sherif A, de la Torre M, Malmstrom PU et al (2001) Lymphatic mapping and detection of sentinel nodes in patients with bladder cancer. J Urol 166:812–815
Skinner DG, Tift JP, Kaufman JJ (1982) High dose, short course preoperative radiation therapy and immediate single stage radical cystectomy with pelvic node dissection in the management of bladder cancer. J Urol 127: 671–674
Skinner DG, Daniels JR, Russell CA et al (1991) The role of adjuvant chemotherapy following cystectomy for invasive bladder cancer: a prospective comparative trial. J Urol 145:459–464; discussion 464–457
Smaaland R, Akslen L, Tonder B et al (1991) Radical radiation treatment of invasive and locally advanced bladder cancer in elderly patients. Br J Urol 67:61–69
Smith JA, Whitmore WF (1981) Regional lymph node metastases from bladder cancer. J Urol 126:591–593
Sobin LH, Wiitekind CH (1997) TNM classification of malignant tumors, Union Internationale Contre le Cancer, 5th edn. Wiley-Liss, New York
Stein JP, Lieskovsky G, Cote R et al (2001) Radical cystectomy in the treatment of invasive bladder cancer: long-term results in 1,054 patients. J Clin Oncol 19:3 666–675
Stockle M, Meyenburg W, Wellek S et al (1995) Adjuvant polychemotherapy of nonorgan-confined bladder cancer after radical cystectomy revisited: long-term results of a controlled prospective study and further clinical experience. J Urol 153:47–52
Studer UE, Bacchi M, Biedermann C et al (1994) Adjuvant cisplatin chemotherapy following cystectomy for bladder cancer: results of a prospective randomized trial. J Urol 152:81–84
Swana HS, Grossman D, Anthony JN et al (1999) Tumor content of the anti-apoptosis molecule survivin and recurrence of bladder cancer. N Engl J Med 341:452–453
Tiguert R, Bianco FJ, Oskanian P et al (2001) Structural alteration of p53 protein in patients with muscle invasive bladder transitional cell carcinoma. J Urol 166:2155–2160
Turner SL, Swindell SL, Bowl N et al (1997) Bladder movement during radiation therapy for bladder cancer: implications for treatment planning. Int J Radiat Oncol Biol Phys 39:355–360
Turner WH, Markwalder R, Perrig S et al (1998) Meticulous pelvic lymphadenectomy in surgical treatment of the invasive bladder cancer: an option or a must? Eur Urol 33 [Suppl 4]:21–22
Vale JA, A'Hern RP, Liu K et al (1993) Predicting the outcome of radical radiotherapy for invasive bladder cancer. Eur Urol 24:48–51
Vieweg J, Gschwend JE, Herr HW et al (1999) Pelvic lymph node dissection can be curative in patients with node positive bladder cancer. J Urol 161:449–454
Williams AD, Cousins C, Soutter WP et al (2001) Detection of pelvic lymph node metastases in gynecologic malignancies: a comparison of CT, MR imaging, and positron emission tomography. Am J Roentgenol 177:343–348
Williams PL (1995) Gray's anatomy, 38th edn. Churchill Livingstone, New York
Wishnow KI, Johnson DE, Ro JY et al (1987) Incidence, extent and location of unsuspected pelvic lymph node metastases in patients undergoing radical cystectomy for bladder cancer. J Urol 137:408–410
Withers HR, Peters LJ, Taylor JMG (1995) Dose–response relationship for radiation therapy of subclinical disease. Int J Radiat Oncol Biol Phys 31:353–359
Zincke H, Patterson DE, Utz DC et al (1985) Pelvic lymphadenectomy and radical cystectomy for transitional cell carcinoma of the bladder with pelvic lymph node disease. Br J Urol 57:156–159

9 Gynecologic Tumors

K. S. C. Chao, M. Cengiz, T. Herzog

CONTENTS

K. S. C. Chao, MD
Department of Radiation Oncology, Box 97, MD Anderson Cancer Center, 1515 Holcombe Blvd, Houston 77005, USA
M. Cengiz, MD
Department of Radiation Oncology, Hacettepe University Medical School, Ankara, Turkey
T. Herzog, MD
Division of Gynecologic Oncology, Department of Obstetrics and Gynecology, Washington University Medical Center, St. Louis, MO 63110, USA

9.1 Introduction

Primary and adjuvant radiation therapy has contributed significantly to the successful management of gynecologic malignancies. Traditionally, radiation therapy is often performed through either anterior-posterior parallel-opposed fields or a four-field technique consisting of an anterior, a posterior and two lateral portals. Although different authors have varying criteria to classify the severity of side effects, with these conventional techniques severe complications may develop in 8% to 10% of patients. It appears that the incidence of complications requiring surgical management is approximately 5% (Perez 1997).

Besides the complication rate, the use of conventional lateral portals has been reported to result in incomplete coverage of the uterine fundus in 62% of patients. When coverage of the lateral fields was evaluated, although bisecting the S2–3 interspace, 49% of the lateral fields were inadequate to cover the target volume posteriorly (Greer et al. 1990). Furthermore, Bonin et al. (1996) and Pendelbury et al. (1993) have reported inadequate coverage of the external iliac lymph nodes in 45% and 62% of patients respectively when standard irradiation fields were used. Appropriate delineation of the tumor target is a critical factor in the coming decade, when 3D conformal therapy will gradually become the technique of choice.

Although 3D conformal irradiation and intensity-modulated radiotherapy (IMRT) are better tools to precisely deliver the dose to target volumes and protect normal tissues, most radiation oncologists continue to treat their patients with conventional techniques. This is because organ motion of the pelvic structures may defy the conformality provided by this new technology; for example, the uterus and cervix may shift as much as 4 to 5 cm on anterior-posterior projection, depending on whether the bladder and rectum are empty or filled (Greer et al. 1990). In addition, guidance is lacking on lymph node and primary tumor target definition, as this area is as yet largely unexplored for gynecologic malignancies. On the other hand, early results of 3D conformal irradiation to the pelvis for prostate cancer showed fewer gastrointestinal (GI) and genitourinary (GU) complications when compared with conventional techniques despite an escalation of the dose to the prostate. Dosimetric studies on IMRT also showed superior conformality. These encouraging results have revived interest in the potential application of conformal radiation therapy for gynecologic cancers.

Three-dimensional conformal irradiation or IMRT requires a proper knowledge of the volumes to be irradiated and an accurate 3D delineation of these volumes. The objective of this chapter is to provide guidelines for selecting and defining target volumes (nodal regions) for conformal irradiation of gynecologic malignancies.

9.2 Anatomy of Gynecologic Structures

The pelvis is bounded by the sacrum, ischium, ilium and pubic bones. The pelvic inlet is continuous with the abdominal cavity, and its outlet is closed by the piriformis, coccygeus, and levator ani muscles. The true pelvis (pelvis minor) is defined by a plane passing through the pubic crest and the sacral promontory, generally coinciding with the iliopectineal line of the pubic bones. The internal genitalia are located within the true pelvis.

Structures within the pelvis are covered by an expansile endopelvic fascia (often muscular fascia). Together with the vasculature and musculature of the pelvis, these fasciae form supporting ligaments for the pelvic viscera. The fascial tissues are more concentrated where the organs are in close proximity. The pelvic walls and organs are partially covered by the peritoneum. The pelvic cavity is separated into anterior and posterior components by a transversely oriented broad ligament, in the center of which lies the uterus.

The lymph nodes of the pelvic wall, which receive the lymphatics from the perineum, lower extremity, and lower abdominal wall, in addition to the lymphatics from the pelvic viscera (except the sigmoid) have been considered in various groupings by different authors (Gray and Clemente 1985; Harrison and Clouse 1985; Rouviere and Tobias 1938). However, a simple and commonly used clinically functional system divides them into the external iliac, obturator (medial group of external iliac) and internal iliac (hypogastric) lymph nodes. The external iliac nodes include all the lymph glands (lateral, superior, and medial) surrounding the external iliac artery and vein; the obturator nodes include all the nodes in the obturator fossa above and below the obturator nerve, and are commonly considered the most medial group of external iliac nodes; the internal iliac (hypogastric) nodes including the gluteal nodes are medial and inferior to the internal iliac artery. Between the pelvic and aortic nodes lie the lateral and medial common iliac nodes and the nodes inferior to the aortic bifurcation. For the most part the common iliac nodes drain the pelvic wall lymphatics, although direct channels from the adnexa, uterus, and cervix do exist. The nodal groups in the pelvis and paraaortic area are illustrated in Fig. 9.1.

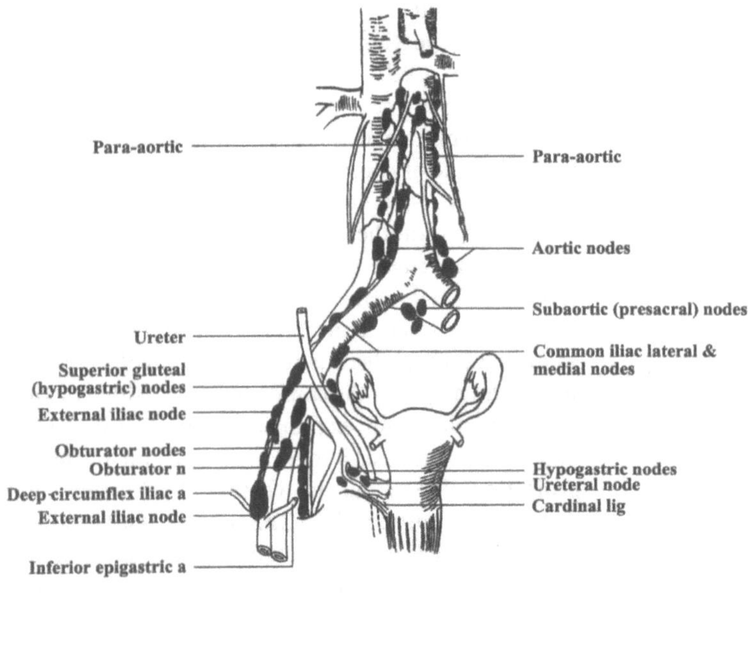

Fig. 9.1. Illustration of a nodal group related to the paraaortic and pelvic region

9.2.1 Vulva

The vulva includes the mons pubis (hair-bearing skin over the pubis), the labia majora, the labia minora, the clitoris and the greater vestibular glands (Bartholin's glands). Most vulvar malignancies are squamous neoplasms, and arise in the labia minora, clitoris, fourchette, perineal body, or the medial aspects of the labia majora. Although very rare, the majority of primary adenocarcinomas arise from Bartholin's glands.

9.2.1.1 Lymphatic Drainage

The lymphatics of the vulva, including the lower one-third of the vagina, drain into the medial group of the superficial inguinal nodes and subsequently to the deep inguinal and external iliac nodes. The lymphatic network of the vulva runs superiorly to the mons pubis area, then turns to drain to the superficial ipsilateral groin lymph nodes. The next area of drainage after the superficial inguinal node group is that of the deep inguinal (femoral) nodes by lymphatic vessels perforating the cribriform fascia (Fig. 9.2). Lymphatic drainage takes place from the lateral sites to the ipsilateral groin. No lymphatic channels are located beyond the labiocrural fold, and crossover drainage to the opposite groin is very rare. It is important to remember that drainage from the midline can be bilateral, and vulvar cancers in the clitoral area can spread directly to the pelvic external iliac nodes. Also very posterior lesions have been reported to drain directly into the sacral nodes. Recent surgical experience has demonstrated that lymphatic drainage from most vulvar sites proceeds initially to a sentinel node located within the superficial inguinal group (Levenback 2000). In the future, sentinel lymph node identification through lymphatic mapping may permit less extensive lymph node dissections and identify anomalous lymph node drainage patterns. Currently, a Gynecologic Oncology Group (GOG) study is evaluating the role of sentinel node mapping in vulvar malignancies with isosulfan blue and lymphoscintigraphy.

9.2.2 Vagina

This muscular canal extends between the vulva and uterus. The uterine cervix pierces its anterior wall. The area of the vaginal lumen that surrounds the uterine cervix is divided into four regions: the anterior fornix, the posterior fornix, the right lateral fornix, and the left lateral fornix. The upper half of the vagina lies within the pelvis between the bladder anteriorly and the rectum posteriorly; the lower half lies within the perineum between the urethra anteriorly and the anal canal posteriorly. The vaginal artery branches from the uterine artery, a branch of the anterior division of the internal iliac artery. Vaginal veins drain into the internal iliac veins.

9.2.2.1 Lymphatic Drainage

The lymphatic drainage of the vagina is complex and unpredictable. The drainage of the upper third

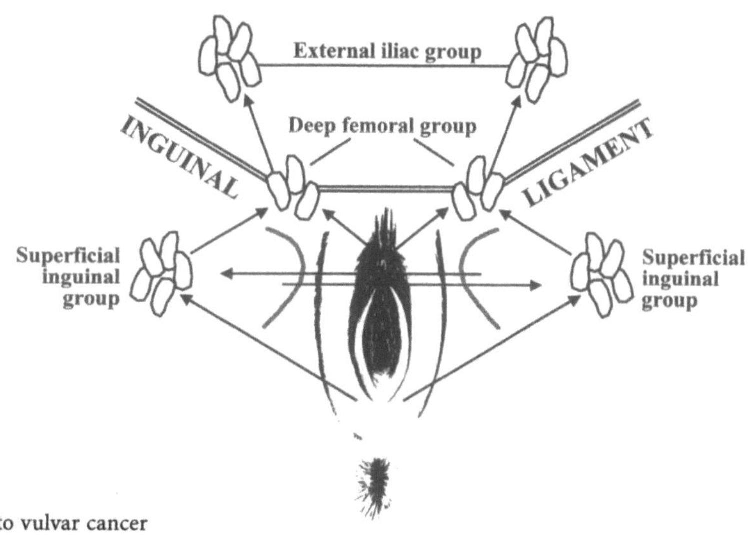

Fig. 9.2. Illustration of a nodal group related to vulvar cancer

of the vagina follows that of the cervix uteri, passing through the cardinal ligaments to the pelvic wall lymph nodes. The lymphatics from the vagina distal to the pelvic floor or urogenital diaphragm may drain into the inguinal nodes as well as upward to the cervix and ultimately into the pelvic nodes. There is also an anterior-posterior division of lymph drainage from the vagina, the anterior lymphatics communicating with the lymphatics of the bladder while the lymphatics from the posterior vagina drain into the inferior gluteal, presacral, and anorectal lymph nodes.

9.2.3 Ovaries and Fallopian Tubes

Each ovary is attached to the back of the broad ligament by the mesovarium. The ovary usually lies near the lateral wall of the pelvis in a depression called the ovarian fossa, bound by the external and internal iliac arteries. The ovarian artery is a branch of the abdominal aorta. Ovarian veins drain into the inferior vena cava on the right and into the left renal vein on the left side. The blood vessels reach the ovary by passing through the lateral part of the broad ligament (also called the infundibular pelvic ligament).

There are two fallopian tubes; each lies within the upper border of the broad ligament. The uterine tube connects the peritoneal cavity in the region of the uterus. The tube can be divided into four parts, from distal to proximal: (1) the infundibulum is the funnel-shaped lateral end with finger-like processes, known as fimbriae, over the ovary; (2) the ampulla is the widest part of the tube; (3) the isthmus is the narrowest part of the tube and lies just lateral to the uterus; and (4) the intramural part is the segment that pierces the uterine wall. The uterine artery from the internal iliac artery and the ovarian artery from the abdominal aorta are the main branches that supply these structures.

9.2.3.1 Lymphatic Drainage

The main lymph channels draining the ovary are from the plexus in the mesovarium, which also has tributaries from the uterine tube and uterine fundus. The lymphatics then follow the ovarian vessels out of the pelvis to the level of the lower pole of the kidney, at which point they turn medially to join the paraaortic lymphatics. On the left side, the ovarian lymphatics also communicate with lymph nodes at the level of the renal vessels. It is clear from clinical experience that the pelvic and inguinal node groups can also be sites of ovarian or tubal cancer, either as a result of direct lymphatic connections or via the lymphatics of the peritoneal cavity.

9.2.4 Uterus and Cervix

The uterus is divided into the fundus, body, and cervix. The fundus lies above the entrance of the uterine tubes. The uterus may be anteverted, midpositioned, or retroverted. These terms describe the positioning of the uterus on the long axis of the vagina. The body of the uterus lies below the entrance of the uterine tubes. It then narrows and continues to become the cervix. The cervix pierces the anterior wall of the vagina. The cavity of the cervix, the cervical canal, communicates with the cavity of the body through the internal os, and with that of the vagina through the external os. The pelvic diaphragm consists of the levator ani and the coccygeus muscles and their fascia, which form the pelvic floor. The perineal body consists of fibromuscular tissue that is located in the perineum between the vagina and the anal canal; it is supported by the levator ani muscles. The transverse cervical (cardinal) ligaments attach the cervix and upper part of the vagina to the lateral pelvic walls. The pubocervical ligaments attach the cervix to the pubic bones. The sacrocervical ligaments attach the cervix and upper part of the vagina to the lower end of the sacrum. Broad ligaments consisting of two-layered folds of peritoneum extend across the pelvic cavity from the lateral margins of the uterus to the lateral pelvic walls. Each broad ligament contains the uterine tube, the round ligaments of the ovary and the uterus, the uterine and ovarian blood vessels, lymphatics, and nerves. The uterine artery arises from the anterior division of the internal iliac artery and the ovarian artery. The veins correspond to the arteries.

9.2.4.1 Lymphatic Drainage of the Uterus (Body and Fundus)

From the fundus of the uterus, the lymphatics drain along the upper broad ligament and tube with communications to the subovarian plexus and then to the aortic nodes via the infundibulopelvic ligament. The lymphatic drainage of the corpus is primarily via broad ligament lymphatics that follow the uterine vessels to the ureteral node, the external iliac nodes (especially the interiliac or medial external iliac), and the obturator lymph nodes.

9.2.4.2
Lymphatic Drainage of the Cervix

The cervical lymphatics follow the uterine artery after crossing either over or under the ureter and the cardinal ligament to the pelvic wall lymph nodes, including the external iliac (especially the interiliac), obturator, and hypogastric (inferior and superior gluteal, sacral) node groups. The lymphatics passing through the uppermost part of the cardinal ligament give off branches to the ureteric node, which lies just lateral to the junction where the uterine artery crosses over the ureter. From the posterior cervix, lymphatic channels also extend through the rectal pillars or the uterosacral ligaments to the rectal lymph nodes. These presacral nodes are situated in the region anterior to the sacrum and the coccyx, and posterior to the rectum (Park et al. 1994).

9.3
Clinical and Pathologic Features that Determine Lymph Node Metastasis

9.3.1
Vulva

It was estimated that approximately 3,600 women in the United States would develop vulvar cancer in the year 2001 (Greenlee 2001). Inguinal node metastasis from vulvar cancer can be predicted by the presence of certain parameters including a lesion diameter >2 cm, poorly differentiated histology, lymph-vascular space involvement, and increasing tumor thickness. The depth of invasion seems to be the most important determinant of lymph node metastasis. Invasion of 5 mm or more has a lymph node metastasis rate of 25% or higher. Tumors with 3 mm invasion have a lymph node metastasis rate of about 10%. Tumors with a depth of invasion of 1 mm or less can be considered superficial and carry little or no risk of lymph node metastasis. The incidence of inguinal lymph node metastasis is a function of the depth of tumor invasion, tumor size, and tumor extension, as summarized in Table 9.1.

Clinically, features contributing to nodal metastases include the following: (1) the superficial inguinal nodes are the most frequent site of lymphatic metastasis; (2) in-transit metastases within the vulvar skin are exceedingly rare, suggesting that most initial lymphatic metastases represent an embolic phenomenon; (3) metastasis to the contralateral groin or deep pelvic nodes is very unusual in the absence of ipsilateral groin metastases; and (4) nodal involvement generally proceeds in a stepwise fashion from the superficial inguinal to the deep inguinal and then to the pelvic nodes unless the lesion is very anterior or posterior in location.

Table 9.1. Summary of the incidence of lymph node involvement as a function of primary tumor size and extent of tumor invasion in vulvar cancer (Donaldson et al. 1981; Hacker 1990; Hoffman et al. 1988; Krupp and Bohm 1978; Parker et al. 1975; Rutledge et al. 1970)

Depth of invasion or tumor size	No. of patients	No. (%) of patients with positive lymph nodes
Depth of invasion		
<1 mm	120	0
1.1–2 mm	121	8 (6.6%)
2.1–3 mm	97	8 (8.2%)
3.1–4 mm	50	11 (22%)
4.1–5 mm	40	10 (25%)
Size of tumor		
>5 mm	32	12 9 (37.5%)
>2 cm	168	77 (45.8%)
Tumor extending beyond vulva	70	38 (54.3%)

9.3.2
Vagina

Primary vaginal tumors are a rare entity, representing 1% to 2% of all gynecologic malignancies, mostly of squamous epithelial histology. It was estimated that approximately 2,100 women in United States would develop vaginal cancer in the year 2001 (Greenlee 2001). These tumors occur most commonly on the posterior wall of the upper third of the vagina. In an extensive literature review, Plentl and Friedman (1971) found that 51.7% of primary vaginal cancers occurred in the upper third of the vagina, and 57.6% on the posterior wall. The incidence of positive pelvic nodes at diagnosis varies with tumor stage and location of the primary tumor. The involvement of inguinal lymph nodes is common when the tumor is located in the lower third of the vagina. The incidence of clinically positive inguinal nodes at the time of diagnosis ranges from 5.3% to 20% (Table 9.2). In the series of Stock et al. (1995), out of 100 patients with stage I and II disease, 59 subjects underwent surgery, 29 of whom had pelvic lymph

Table 9.2. Clinically positive pelvic nodes at diagnosis of carcinoma of the vagina

Author	No. of cases	No. of clinically positive lymp nodes	% of clinically positive lymph nodes
Brown et al. (1971)	76	5	6.6
Perez et al. (1973)	113	6	5.3
Whelton and Kottmeier (1962)	117	8	6.8
Chyle et al. (1996)	301	14 (pelvic)	5.0
		10 (inguinal)	3.0
Plentl and Friedman 1971	679	141	20.8

Modified from Perez and Garipagaoglu (1998)

Table 9.3. Influence of lymph node status on survival in FIGO stage IB cervical cancer

Author	Negative nodes		Positive nodes	
	No. patients	5-year survival (%)	No. patients	5-year survival (%)
Kolstad (1968)	397	91	101	48
Masubuchi et al. (1969)	282	92	14	57
Burch and Chalfant (1970)	115	87	23	56
Hsu et al. (1972)	234	88	37	40
Rampone et al. (1973)	456	93	81	63
Piver and Chung (1975)	106	91	39	55
Morley and Seski (1976)	125	96	18	56

Table 9.4. Incidence of lymph node group involvement in carcinoma of the uterine cervix

Site	No. of lymph nodes	Percentage
Paracervical	3	2
Obturator	65	20
External iliac	154	47
Hypogastric	24	7
Common iliac	46	14
Periaortic	31	10

node dissections. Ten out of 29 (34%) patients had positive lymph nodes. Chyle et al. (1996) reported a retrospective analysis of 301 patients from the M.D. Anderson Cancer Center. They noted that nodal recurrence is closely related to local tumor control. They found a 10-year actuarial pelvic nodal failure rate of 28% and an inguinal failure rate of 16% in patients who developed local recurrence, in contrast to 4% and 2% respectively in the group without local recurrence ($P<0.001$).

9.3.3 Uterine Cervix

Cervical cancer is the third leading cause of gynecologic cancer in the United States; it was estimated that approximately 12,900 women would develop cancer of the uterine cervix in the year 2001 (Greenlee 2001). Carcinoma of the cervix may spread to the paracervical and parametrial lymphatics, metastasizing to the obturator lymph nodes, to the hypogastric lymph nodes and to the external iliac nodes. Tumor metastases to the common iliac or paraaortic lymph nodes may also be present. Surgical series have long demonstrated the importance of nodal metastases as a prognostic indicator (Table 9.3). The incidence of metastasis to the pelvic and paraaortic lymph nodes is listed in Table 9.4. Among patients with early-stage disease, the risk of nodal involvement increases in proportion to the size of the primary tumor (Table 9.5). The incidence of lymph node metastasis to the pelvic lymph nodes is also related to the depth of invasion. Dissemination usually follows an orderly sequence. Although cervical cancer may metastasize outside the pelvic area, metastasis to the paraaortic nodes without pelvic node involvement is an unusual occurrence (Henriksen 1949). In line with this early observation, Sakuragi et al. (1999) recently reported a surgical series of 208 patients with stage IB, IIA, and IIB cervical carcinoma who underwent radical

Table 9.5. Correlation between size of primary tumor and lymph node metastases in stage IB and IIA cervical cancer (Piver and Chung 1975)

Size (cm)	Stage IB			Stage IIA		
	No. of patients	No. with metastases	Percentage	No. of patients	No. with metastases	Percentage
≤1	22	4	18.1	11	3	27.2
2–3	72	16	22.1	27	5	18.5
4–5	45	16	35.5	44	19	43.1
≥6	6	3	50.0	13	5	38.4

hysterectomy and systematic pelvic and paraaortic lymph node dissection. Fifty-three patients (25.5%) had lymph node metastases. The obturator lymph nodes were most frequently involved, with a rate of 18.8% (39/208). Forty-nine out of 53 node-positive patients had lymph node metastases in the obturator, internal iliac, or common iliac lymph nodes. A multiple logistic regression analysis revealed that deep cervical stromal and lymphovascular space invasion were related to paraaortic lymph node metastasis. It was also shown that tumor metastasis into the bilateral pelvic and common iliac lymph nodes was significantly related to paraaortic lymph node metastasis. The authors suggested that paraaortic lymph node metastasis appears to occur secondarily to widespread pelvic node metastasis.

In addition to the pelvic lymph nodes, there are lymph nodes distributed throughout the parametrium. Girardi et al. (1989) studied 359 specimens from radical hysterectomies: 132 clinical stage IB, eight stage IIA, and 219 stage IIB. They identified parametrial lymph nodes in 280 patients (78%), 63 (22.5%) of which showed malignant lymph node involvement. The incidence of positive nodes was 11.4% in stage IB and 21.5% in stage IIB. Lymph node involvement was found in the medial parametrium (44.4%), lateral parametrium (38%), or in both areas (17.5%). There was close a correlation between involvement of the parametrial lymph nodes and the iliac lymph nodes; in the patients with negative parametrial nodes, only 26% had positive iliac lymph nodes, but 81% of patients with positive parametrial lymph nodes also had metastatic involvement of the pelvic lymph nodes.

9.3.4 Uterus

Endometrial adenocarcinoma is the most common gynecologic malignancy in the United States; it was estimated that approximately 38,300 women would develop cancer of the uterine corpus in year 2001 (Greenlee 2001). This adenocarcinoma arises in the epithelial lining of the endometrial cavity, mostly in the sixth and seventh decades of life. The procedures for surgical staging of endometrial cancer include exploratory laparotomy, washings for cytology, total abdominal hysterectomy, bilateral salpingo-oophorectomy, and an assessment of the pelvic and paraaortic lymph nodes. The number of lymph nodes that need to be dissected to detect the presence of nodal metastases is a subject of considerable debate. However, existing data suggest that selective dissection of grossly enlarged lymph node(s) may not be sufficient to reflect the true extent of tumor metastasis. Girardi et al. (1989) showed that 37% of metastatic lymph nodes were less than 2 mm, and 50% were less than 1 cm in size. Creasman et al. (1987) from the GOG surgical staging study revealed that less than 10% of patients with nodal metastases had grossly positive nodes. Imaging techniques, visualization, and palpation are inadequate to accurately predict lymph node involvement. Techniques for evaluating the true status of the pelvic and paraaortic lymph nodes in clinical stage I patients were described by Chuang et al. (1995). They advised limited assessment of lymph nodes by sampling from the retroperitoneal nodal groups. This sampling classification divides lymph node groups into left and right paraaortic, common iliac, external iliac, hypogastric, and obturator nodes. The patterns of lymphatic spread depend on the location of the tumor. The lower and middle portions of the uterus drain laterally to the parametrium and the paracervical and the obturator lymph nodes. The upper corpus and fundus drain to the common iliac and the paraaortic lymph nodes. A third pathway is along the round ligament to the inguinal nodes.

In a GOG study of 621 patients with clinical stage I and occult stage II cancers, 70 subjects (11%) had metastases to the pelvic and paraaortic nodes. There was a 3.5% (n=22) incidence of both pelvic and aortic node metastases, a 6% (n=36) incidence of pelvic lymph node metastases without associated aortic node metastases, and only 2 patients presented with aortic node metastases in the absence of pelvic node metastases. The highest rate of paraaortic node metastases (32%) occurred when pelvic nodes were involved. There was an increased risk of lymph node metastases among patients with deep myometrial invasion, poor-grade tumors, lymphatic vessel invasion and advanced stage of disease. The frequency of pelvic and paraaortic nodal metastases with respect to other pathologic risk factors is shown in Table 9.6. Patients with positive nodes have a poorer outcome. The 5-year recurrence-free survival rates of patients with negative pelvic and aortic nodes, positive pelvic nodes and negative aortic nodes, and positive aortic nodes were 85%, 70% and 36%, respectively. There have been recent reports citing increased survival for patients with endometrial cancer who have undergone complete lymphadenectomy in comparison to lymph node sampling (Kilgore et al. 1995).

9.3.5 Ovarian and Fallopian Tube Carcinoma

Ovarian cancer is the second leading cause of gynecologic cancer in the United States; it was estimated that approximately 23,400 women would develop ovarian cancer in year 2001 (GREENLEE 2001). Epithelial tumors arising from the surface epithelium of the ovarium are the most common form. The mortality rate exceeds that of cervical and endometrial carcinoma combined. The fallopian tube is the least common site of origin for malignant neoplasms of the female genital tract, although the epithelial area is much larger than that of the ovary. Fewer than 2,000 cases have been reported in the literature worldwide, representing less than 1% of all gynecologic neoplasms.

Table 9.6. Frequency of nodal metastases according to various risk factors for endometrial carcinoma

Risk factor	No. of patients	Pelvic (no., %)	Aortic (no., %)
Histology			
Endometrioid adenocarcinoma	599	56 (9%)	30 (5%)
Others	22	2 (9%)	4 (18%)
Grade			
Grade I	180	5 (3%)	3 (2%)
Grade II	288	25 (9%)	14 (5%)
Grade III	153	28 (18%)	17 (11%)
Muscle invasion			
Endometrial	87	1 (1%)	1 (1%)
Superficial	279	15 (5%)	8 (3%)
Middle	116	7 (6%)	1 (1%)
Deep	139	35 (25%)	24 (17%)
Tumor location			
Fundus	524	42 (8%)	20 (4%)
Isthmus-cervix	97	16 (16%)	14 (14%)
Lymphovascular space invasion			
Negative	528	37 (7%)	19 (9%)
Positive	93	21 (27%)	15 (19%)
Other extrauterine metastases			
Negative	586	0 (7%)	26 (4%)
Positive	35	18 (51%)	8 (23%)
Peritoneal cytology			
Negative	537	8 (7%)	20 (4%)
Positive	75	19 (25%)	4 (19%)

9.4 Radiologic Evaluation of Gynecologic Malignancies

9.4.1 Imaging Modalities to Detect Lymph Node Metastasis

Lymphangiography was considered to be the best option for detecting paraaortic nodal metastasis in an early GOG study. The GOG investigated the clinical–pathologic correlation of paraaortic lymph node involvement by computed tomography (CT), lymphangiogram (LAG), and ultrasound (US) in patients with stage IIB, III, and IVA cervical carcinoma. Of the 264 patients evaluated, positive paraaortic nodes occurred in 21% of stage IIB, 31% of stage III, and 13% of stage IVA cancers. LAG sensitivity was 79%, with a specificity of 73%. The sensitivity of CT and US was 34% and 19%, respectively, with specificities of 96% and 99%, respectively (HELLER et al. 1990). However, the advantage of LAG was not so obvious in detecting metastatic pelvic lymph nodes. SWART et al. (1989) reported the radiologic–pathologic correlation in 54 patients with FIGO stage Ib–IIa operable cervical cancer. Only 29% of patients with pathologically proven lymph node metastases had lymphographic evidence at the site of these metastases. BOIE et al. (1989) studied 89 stage Ib cervical carcinoma patients. LAG results were compared with histopathologic examinations of the corresponding lymph nodes. The positive predictive value of the LAG was only 13%, and the negative predictive value was 98%. Because the procedure is invasive and interpretation may be subjective, the LAG is viewed as less preferable for the diagnosis of lymph node metastases in cervical cancer. Recent refinement in CT and magnetic resonance imaging (MRI) techniques has led to the reconsideration of whether noninvasive imaging modalities could be of comparable or better diagnostic value in detecting nodal metastases in cervical cancer. In a meta-analysis, Scheidler et al. concluded that LAG, CT, and MRI perform equivalently in the detection of lymph node metastases from cervical cancer. As CT and MRI are less invasive than LAG and can also assess local tumor extent, they should be considered the preferred adjuncts to clinical evaluation of invasive cervical cancer (SCHEIDLER et al. 1997). Although the patterns of tumor spread may vary between cervical cancer and other gynecologic malignancies, the aforementioned information regarding radiologic detection of nodal metastases should also be applicable in the clinical management of other gynecologic cancers.

Although MRI may be better than CT in demarcating a primary tumor, with recent advances in CT technology the accuracy of detecting metastatic lymph nodes is equivalent. In addition, CT offers convenient and rapid imaging of the pelvis and abdomen as compared with MRI. Table 9.7 briefly summarizes the sensitivity, specificity, and accuracy of CT and MRI. Detection of lymph node metastases by CT or MRI is based on the size of the lymph node. The most reliable criterion is the minimal axial diameter (MIAD) of the lymph node measured from transverse scans. When the MIAD is over 10 mm, metastatic involvement is probable. With this criterion, a positive predictive value of 82% and a negative predictive value of 94% have been reported with MRI (Kim et al. 1994; Vinnicombe et al. 1995). The false-positive rate may be decreased when the anatomic location of the lymph node is taken into consideration, because internal iliac and obturator nodes with a diameter of 8 to 10 mm may contain metastases. Peripheral enhancement usually means a necrotic lymph node metastasis despite its size. Neither CT nor MRI can distinguish lymph node enlargement due to reactive hyperplasia from metastatic disease, nor detect small tumor deposits in normal-sized nodes. Lymphography can demonstrate tumor deposits in lymph nodes of normal size. Because large nodes totally replaced by tumor may fail to opacify, and the internal iliac and presacral nodes are only occasionally seen, lymphography has little advantage today (Scheidler et al. 1997).

Table 9.7. Comparison of CT and MRI for the detection of lymph node metastases from cervical cancer

Modality	MIAD criteria (mm)	Sensitivity (%)	Specificity (%)	Accuracy (%)
MRI (Kim et al. 1994)	10	62.2	97.9	93.0
MRI (Yang et al. 2000)	10	70.6	89.8	85.5
3-mm slice CT (Fukuda et al. 1999)	3	54.5	96.7	79.7
Helical CT (Yang et al. 2000)	10	64.7	96.6	89.5

9.4.2 Ovarian Carcinoma

Laparotomy identifies the primary site of the disease, determines tumor spread and histologic features, while allowing complete staging for early stage disease and debulking of the tumor for advanced stages. No imaging method can replace surgery, because microscopic or small peritoneal, omental, and bowel implants are difficult to detect radiologically. CT and MRI do not differ in accuracy of tumor staging but they are better than sonography, although sonography remains the modality of choice in characterizing adnexal masses.

CT is more practical than MRI in the staging of ovarian malignancies, because the entire abdomen can be scanned within a reasonable time frame to avoid the influence of organ motion during the protracted imaging process that commonly occurs with MRI. The entire abdomen should be evaluated because ovarian cancer spreads via seeding tumor implants throughout the abdominal cavity, often to the subphrenic region. Retroperitoneal lymph node metastasis is also frequent. Psammomatous calcifications can easily be seen on CT images, but most nodes are not calcified. With the new generation of CT and MRI scanners, implants smaller than 5 mm may be detected, but intravenous contrast enhancement is essential. Implants in the omentum, pelvic peritoneum, peritoneum covering the colon or small bowel, and uterine and ovarian ligaments may be most difficult to identify (Kawamoto et al. 1999).

9.4.3 Cervical Carcinoma

The overall accuracy of CT in the staging of cervical cancer is reported to be 66% to 69%; it is not superior to clinical staging (accuracy of 66% to 79%). However, MRI is a much better tool for pretreatment staging of cervical carcinoma, because it demarcates tumor extension well. Tumor volume and the depth of cervical stromal invasion can be measured, except for cases that are limited to microinvasion. Response to treatment and operability can be assessed accurately with MRI. Invasion of the vaginal wall can also be evaluated (Yu et al. 1997).

The greatest benefits of MRI are related to a better assessment of the parametrial extension of the tumor and the noninvasive monitoring of tumor response during a course of irradiation. Bimanual pelvic examination under general anesthesia is not accurate in assessing parametrial tumor extension (Hricak et al. 1996; Mayr et al. 1997). Underestimation commonly occurs. Parametrial tumor extension can be excluded with great certainty by MRI (negative predictive value of 89% to 99%). The problem with MRI is a very high false-positive rate (positive predictive value of 43% to 81%) in differentiating stage IB and IIB disease, which has major therapeutic implications. Parametrial extension is difficult to exclude when there is full-thickness stromal invasion, and microscopic invasion cannot be detected with MRI. The use of an endorectal surface coil has reduced the false-positive rate (Yu et al. 1998). The value of CT in the examination of stage I to IIIA tumors is minimal, because tumor volume and vaginal and parametrial growth cannot be assessed adequately. The accuracy of CT and MRI does not differ noticeably when more advanced cervical cancers (stages IIIB to IVB) are evaluated. Invasion of the bladder and rectum is best seen on sagittal MRI. Because ureteral obstruction and hydronephrosis can be seen on CT and MRI, excretory urography can be eliminated. Both modalities are effective for the detection of upper abdominal disease.

9.4.4 Endometrial Carcinoma

The accuracy of CT and MRI in staging endometrial carcinoma is reported to be 84% to 89% and 85% to 92%, respectively. Both are more accurate than clinical staging (49% to 73%). Although CT can differentiate deep from superficial myometrial invasion, it is not accurate. MRI is preferable for pretreatment imaging of endometrial carcinoma, because it accurately predicts the depth of myometrial invasion (positive predictive value of 50% to 80%, and negative predictive value of 72% to 88%) and cervical involvement can be seen on sagittal images (Frei et al. 2000). The evaluation of myometrial invasion is equally accurate with transvaginal ultrasound and MRI, but the latter has the advantage of imaging the entire pelvis and lower abdomen. MRI is limited in differentiating tumors confined entirely to the endometrium from those invading the inner half of the myometrium. However, this shortcoming has little clinical impact because tumors with both radiologic characteristics have a low risk of nodal metastases.

9.4.5 Other Malignant Tumors

Carcinomas of the fallopian tube, vagina, and vulva and gestational trophoblastic disease are relatively rare malignancies. If imaging is necessary, MRI is generally the most effective method to assess local tumor growth.

9.5 Selection of Target Volume

Although 3D conformal therapy has gradually gained popularity in the radiation oncology community, there are few data describing the details of target volume conformality and its impact on therapeutic outcome for gynecologic malignancies. In this section, the recommended target volume is based on the patterns of failure from published clinical studies in which most patients were treated with conventional beam arrangements. Examples of lymph node delineation at different anatomical levels for paraaortic, common iliac, external iliac, internal iliac, and inguinal lymph nodes are shown in Figs. 9.3–9.6. The summary of nodal target determination is also presented in Table 9.8.

9.5.1 Carcinoma of the Vulva

The target volume in patients undergoing radiation therapy for groin node involvement detected at the time of surgery, particularly if more than one lymph node is positive, should include both the groin area and the pelvic lymph nodes. In the absence of pathologically confirmed pelvic lymph node involvement or if there is no clinical evidence of pelvic lymph node involvement, involvement of only the caudal part of the external iliac lymph nodes up to the mid-level of the sacroiliac joint is sufficient. If there is involvement of pelvic lymph nodes or if groin nodes are extensively involved, all the external iliac lymph nodes should be treated. In the groin, lateral lymph nodes extending to the anterior iliac spine should be included within the treatment volume. If there is extensive nodal involvement (more than microscopic, subcapsular embolization), anterior femoral lymph nodes that are located in the upper medial thigh should also be included due to the possibility of contamination of lymph nodes by retrograde lymphatic spread. If the primary tumor has spread across the labiocrural fold, the treatment volume should include the lymph nodes of the upper medial thigh. Some patients with pathologically negative groin nodes may require irradiation to the primary tumor site. In these circumstances, the treatment volume should not include the lymphatic region because this will only cause an increased risk of lymphedema. If there is invasion of the overlying skin, 5 cm of margin should be used due to the risk of dermal lymphatic involvement. If preoperative radiation therapy is to

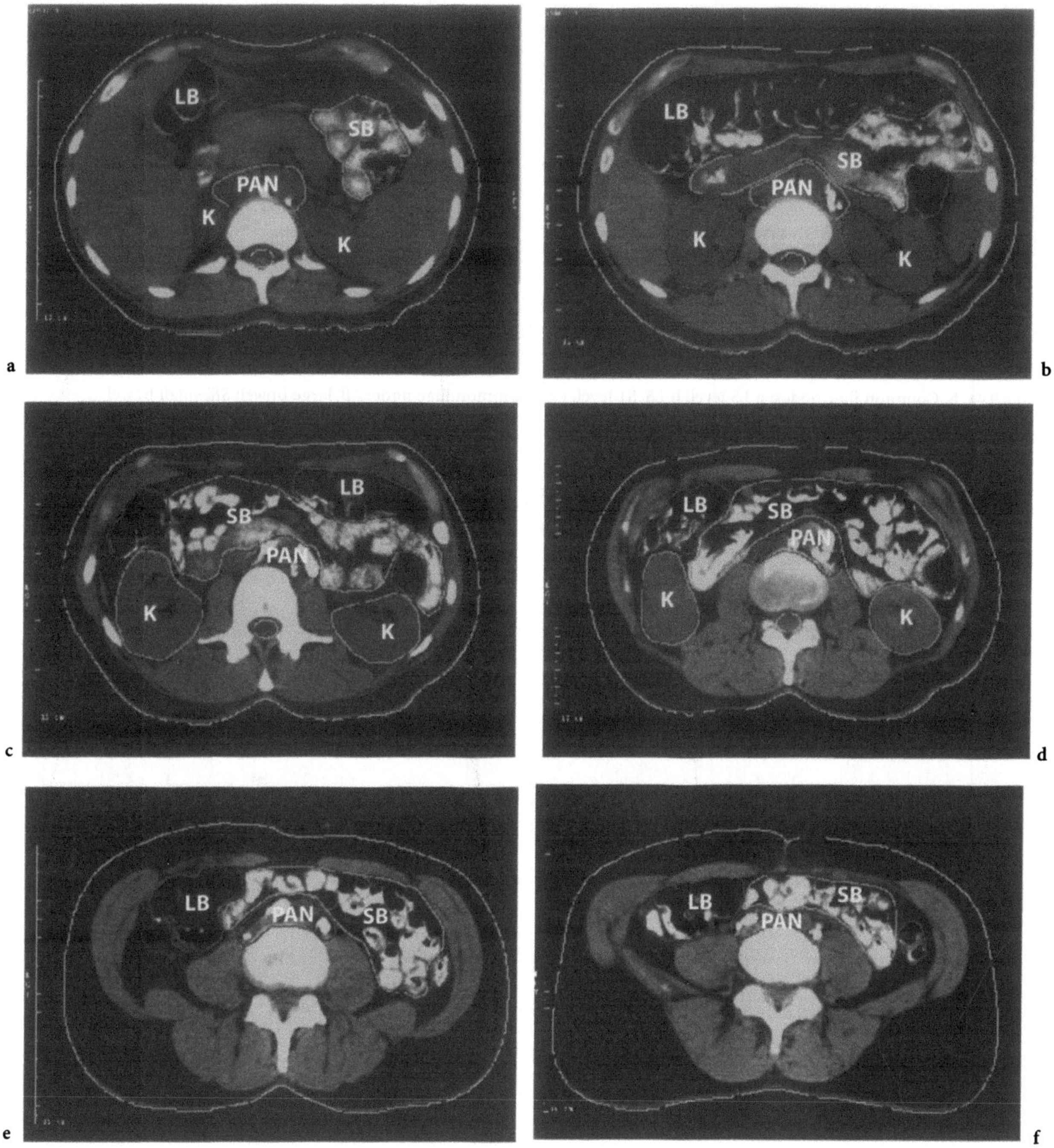

Fig. 9.3a–f. Paraaortic nodes: **a** T12 level; **b** L1 level; **c** L2 level; **d** L3 level; **e** L4 level; **f** L4–5 level. *PAN*, paraaortic node; *K*, kidney; *LB*, large bowel; *SB*, small bowel

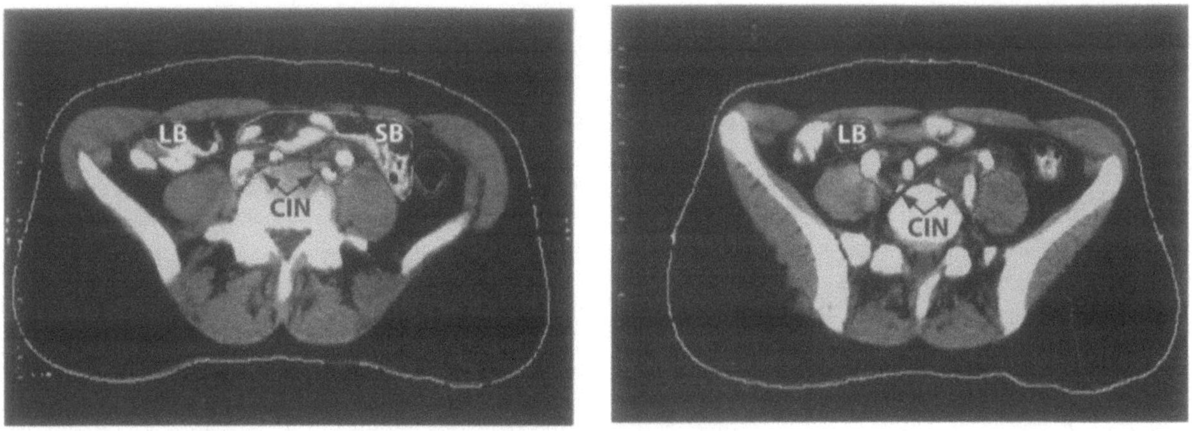

a b

Fig. 9.4a, b. Common iliac nodes: **a** L5 level; **b** L5, S1 level. *CIN*, common iliac node; *LB*, large bowel; *SB*, small bowel

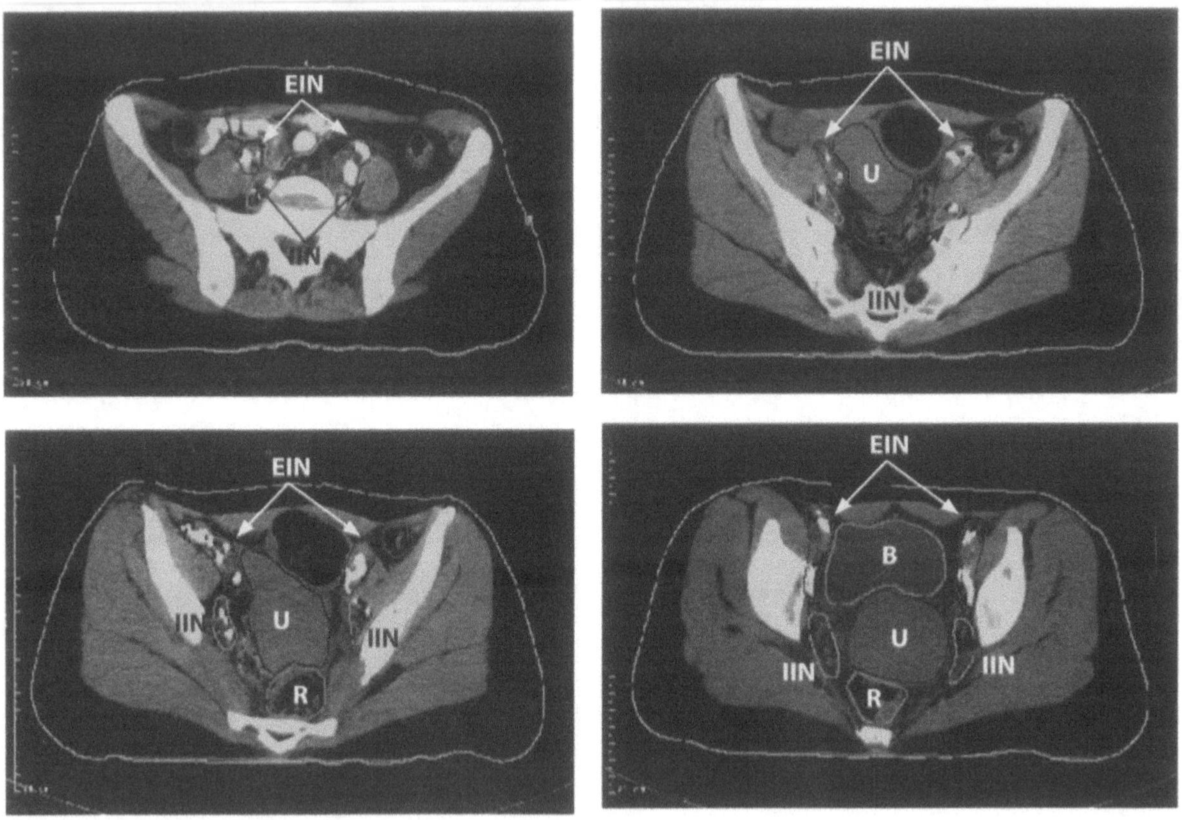

a b c d

Fig. 9.5a–d. External and internal iliac nodes: **a** S1 level; **b, c** S2–3 level; **d** S3 level. *B*, bladder; *EIN*, external iliac node; *IIN*, internal iliac node; *U*, uterus (cervix); *R*, rectum

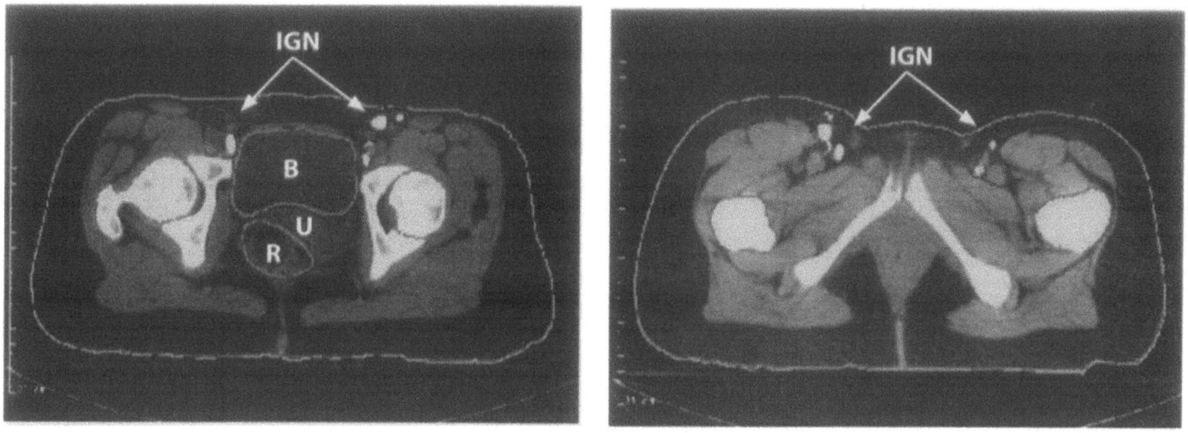

a b

Fig. 9.6a, b. Inguinal nodes: **a** cephalic; **b** caudal. *IGN*, inguinal node; *B*, bladder; *U*, uterus (cervix); *R*, rectum

Table 9.8. Summary of nodal target determination in gynecological malignancies

Disease status	PAN	CIN	IIN	EIN	IGN
Vulvar cancer					
>One IGN positive	–	–	+	+	+
Pelvic node positive	–	+	+	+	+
Vaginal cancer					
Stage I	–	–	–	–	–
Stage II–IV	–	+	+	+	+[a]
Pelvic node positive	+	+	+	+	+[a]
Cervical cancer					
Pelvic node negative	–	+	+	+	–[b]
Pelvic node positive	+	+	+	+	–[b]
Endometrial cancer					
>Stage IB grade 3 or IC, II	–	+	+	+	–
Stage IIIB	+[c]	+	+	+	–

PAN, paraaortic node; *CIN*, common iliac node; *EIN*, external iliac node; *IIN*, internal iliac node; *IGN*, inguinal node
[a] When the mid or lower third of the vagina is involved
[b] Includes IGN when the lower third of the vagina is involved
[c] When PAN or CIN are involved

be used for T3, T4 primary tumors, assessment of the groin and suspicious lymph nodes by fine-needle aspiration (FNA) should be considered to assist in determining the target volume and dose.

9.5.2 Carcinoma of the Vagina

Most authors prefer to treat vaginal intraepithelial neoplasia or stage I vaginal cancer with brachytherapy alone. Based on surgical evaluation, the risk of nodal involvement in stage I is about 6% (1/17 patients). Thus, in this group of patients there is no need for lymphatic irradiation. Treatment of only the primary tumor volume is sufficient; however, risk of nodal involvement increases to 26% (8/36) in stage II patients. Treatment of local lymphatics in addition to the primary tumor is inevitable. The target volume depends on the location of the primary tumor within the vagina and whether pretreatment assessments have clinically or histopathologically documented nodal metastases. Regardless of the extent of the primary lesion, most authors recommend treating the whole vagina by external-beam radiation therapy and boost with brachytherapy.

Diagnostic evaluations of the regional lymph nodes are important for identification of suspicious lymph nodes and treatment planning. FNA under CT guidance is recommended for suspicious lymph nodes. For tumors confined to the upper third of the vagina, treatment volume should encompass the external and internal iliac nodes, in addition to the parametrial lymph nodes up to the bifurcations of the common iliac arteries. If involvement of the pelvic lymph nodes has been histologically demonstrated, the common iliac lymph nodes should also be included in the treatment volume up to the level of the aortic bifurcation. When vaginal cancer involves the middle or caudal third of the vagina, the inguinofemoral nodes should be treated in addition to the pelvic lymph nodes. Similar rules to those used for vulvar cancer with the inclusion of inguinofemoral nodes should also be applied for vaginal cancers. Patients with advanced tumors (stages III and IV) should have disease extent verified by cystoscopy and proctosigmoidoscopy before treatment. Basically, target volume determination is the same for stage II; in almost all cases it includes both pelvic and inguinofemoral lymph nodes. To delineate tumor volume and lymphatics and for follow-up purposes, it is better to include pretreatment MRI.

9.5.3 Cervical Cancer

Patients who have carcinoma in situ or stage IA1 can be treated with brachytherapy alone without regional lymphatic irradiation. However, for tumors with >3 mm depth of invasion, the risk of lymph node metastases is sufficient to justify external-beam irradiation. In patients with stage IB lesions or higher-stage disease, the whole uterus, bilateral parametria, presacral nodes, internal and external iliac nodes, uterosacral ligaments, and other paracervical tissues should be included even if not grossly involved. Prophylactic irradiation of the paraaortic nodes has not been shown to be beneficial when concurrent cisplatin-based chemotherapy is included (Morris et al. 1999). In patients treated with radical hysterectomy and lymph node dissection, if at least two of the following risk factors for recurrence in the pathologic specimen are present, postoperative irradiation to the nodal targets in the pelvis should be performed: (1) more than one-third stromal invasion; (2) lymphovascular space invasion; and (3) large tumor diameter. GOG-92 demonstrated a statistically significant reduction in the overall recurrence rate in the irradiation arm (15% versus 28%; Sedlis et al. 1999). Furthermore, when at least one of the following pathologic features is present after radical hysterectomy with lymph node dissection (positive pelvic lymph nodes, positive surgical margins, microscopic involvement of the parametrium), postoperative chemoirradiation is recommended. GOG-109 has shown a statistically significant improvement in 4-year progression-free (63% versus 80%) and overall survival (71% versus 81%) in favor of chemoirradiation versus radiation therapy alone (Peters et al. 2000).

Posterior vaginal or uterosacral space involvement increases the risk of perirectal node metastases (Chao et al. 1998). Elective irradiation of inguinal lymph nodes is necessary if the distal half of the vagina is involved. If there are one or more discontiguous foci in the vagina that represent retrograde spread through the lymphatics of the vaginal wall, the whole vagina should be included within the target volume.

9.5.4 Endometrial Cancer

Patients with disease limited to the endometrium have a very low risk for relapse. In general, for surgical stage IA grades 1 and 2 disease, adjuvant radiation therapy is not recommended. For stage IA grade 3 and stage IB grades 1 and 2 disease, vaginal brachytherapy alone is recommended. Lymphatic irradiation is not needed. In stage IB grade 3 disease, and for all grades of stage IC, typically these high-risk patients undergo total abdominal hysterectomy and bilateral salpingo-oophorectomy (TAH–BSO) only; irradiation of the pelvic lymph nodes and primary tumor bed is recommended. In patients with stage II tumors, regardless of the extent of surgery, postoperatively the pelvic lymph nodes and tumor bed should be included in the target volume. Patients with adnexal metastases or pelvic lymph node involvement and pathologically negative paraaortic lymph nodes should receive radiation therapy to the target volume, including at least the upper one-half to two-thirds of the length of the vagina, uterus, and parametria with pelvic lymph nodes. For stage IIIB disease, the entire length of the vagina should be included in the target volume. If there is involvement of the paraaortic lymph nodes, the abdominal paraaortic lymph node chain should be treated.

Although primary surgery followed by radiation therapy is standard treatment, patients with a high risk of complications for surgery can be effectively treated by primary irradiation. For early stages with grade 1 disease, intracavitary radiation therapy without lymphatic irradiation may be sufficient. However, large uterine size with large tumor volume and high grades are considered to be indications for external radiation therapy to the uterine tumor and pelvic lymph nodes.

9.5.5 Conclusion

Three-dimensional conformal radiation therapy may reduce the dose to normal tissues, but should be used with caution because erroneous selection or demarcation of paraaortic, pelvic and inguinal lymphatics may result in tumor recurrence. The information provided in this chapter should not be viewed as definitive but as a reference, since no clinical data are yet available for validation. Future development and refinement of functional imaging techniques may provide the physicians with better tools to delineate macro- and microscopic disease in the primary tumor and lymph nodes. Together with intensity modulated radiation therapy, patients with gynecologic malignancies will be able to receive high-precision irradiation with maximal normal tissue sparing.

References

Boie H, Jakobsen A, Petersen J et al (1989) Diagnostic value of lymphography in cervical cancer stage Ib. Eur J Cancer 10:393–395

Bonin SR, Lanciano RM, Corn BW et al (1996) Bony landmarks are not an adequate substitute for lymphangiography in defining pelvic lymph node location for the treatment of cervical cancer with radiotherapy. Int J Radiat Oncol Biol Phys 34:167–172

Brown GR, Fletcher GH, Rutledge FN (1971) Irradiation of "in situ" and invasive squamous cell carcinoma of the vagina. Cancer 28:1278–1283

Burch J, Chalfant R (1970) Preoperative radium irradiation and radical hysterectomy in the treatment of cancer of the cervix. Am J Obstet Gynecol 106:1054–1064

Chao KSC, Williamson J, Grigsby PW et al (1998) Uterosacral space involvement in locally advanced carcinoma of the uterine cervix. Int J Radiat Oncol Biol Phys 40:397–403

Chuang L, Burke TW, Tornos C et al (1995) Staging laparotomy for endometrial carcinoma: assessment of retroperitoneal lymph nodes. Gynecol Oncol 58:189–193

Chyle V, Zagars GK, Wheeler JA et al (1996) Definitive radiotherapy for carcinoma of the vagina: outcome and prognostic factors. Int J Radiat Oncol Biology Phys 35:891–905

Creasman WT, Morrow CP, Bundy BN et al (1987) Surgical pathologic spread patterns of endometrial cancer. Gynecol Oncol Group Study Cancer 60 [Suppl]:2035–2041

Donaldson ES, Powell DE, Hanseon MB et al (1981) Prognostic parameters in invasive vulvar cancer. Gynecol Oncol 11: 184–190

Frei KA, Kinkel K, Bonel HM et al (2000) Prediction of deep myometrial invasion in patients with endometrial cancer: clinical utility of contrast-enhanced MR imaging – a meta-analysis and Bayesian analysis. Radiology 216:444–449

Fukuda H, Nakagawa T, Shibuya H (1999) Metastases to pelvic lymph nodes from carcinoma in the pelvic cavity: diagnosis using thin-section CT. Clin Radiol 54:237–242

Girardi F, Lichtenegger W, Tamussino K et al (1989) The importance of parametrial lymph nodes in the treatment of cervical cancer. Gynecol Oncol 34:206–211

Gray H, Clemente ED (1985) The lymphatic system. Gray's anatomy, 30th edn. Lea and Febiger, Philadelphia, pp 896–917

Greenlee RT (2001) Cancer statistics, 2001. CA Cancer J Clin 51:15–36

Greer BE, Koh WJ, Figge DC et al (1990) Gynecologic radiotherapy fields defined by intraoperative measurements. Gynecol Oncol 38:421–424

Hacker NF (1990) Current treatment of small vulvar cancers. Oncology 4:21–25

Harrison DA, Clouse ME (1985) Normal anatomy. Lymphatic imaging, 2nd edn. Williams and Wilkins, Baltimore, pp 15–94

Heller PB, Malfetano JH, Bundy BN et al (1990) Clinical-pathologic study of stage IIB, III, and IVA carcinoma of the cervix: extended diagnostic evaluation for paraaortic node metastasis – a Gynecologic Oncology Group study. Gynecol Oncol 38:425–430

Henriksen E (1949) The lymphatic spread of carcinoma of the cervix and the body of the uterus. Am J Obstet Gynecol 58:924–942

Hoffman MS, Roberts WS, Ruffolo EH (1988) Basal cell carcinoma of the vulva with inguinal lymph node metastases. Gynecol Oncol 29:113–119

Hricak H, Powell CB, Yu KK et al (1996) Invasive cervical carcinoma: role of MR imaging in pretreatment work-up – cost minimization and diagnostic efficacy analysis. Radiology 1982:403–409

Hsu C, Cheng Y, Su S (1972) Prognosis of uterine cervical cancer with extensive lymph node metastases: special emphasis on the value of pelvic lymphadenectomy in the surgical treatment of uterine cervical cancer. Am J Obstet Gynecol 114: 954–962

Kawamoto S, Urban BA, Fishman EK (1999) CT of epithelial ovarian tumors. Radiographics 19:S85–S102

Kilgore LC, Partridge EE, Alvarez RD et al (1995) Adenocarcinoma of the endometrium: survival comparisons of patients with and without pelvic node sampling. Gynecol Oncol 56:29–33

Kim SH, Kim SC, Choi BI et al (1994) Uterine cervical carcinoma: evaluation of pelvic lymph node metastasis with MR imaging. Radiology 190:807–811

Kolstad P (1968) Lymph node metastases in cancer of the cervix stage 1b. Aust NZ J Obstet Gynaecol 8:107–116

Krupp PJ, Bohm JW (1978) Lymph gland metastases in invasive squamous carcinoma of the vulva. Am J Obstet Gynecol 130:943–952

Levenback C (2000) Intraoperative lymphatic mapping and sentinel node identification: gynecologic applications. Rec Res Cancer Res 157:150–158

Masubuchi K, Tenjin Y, Kubo H et al (1969) Five-year cure rate for carcinoma of the cervix uteri with special reference to the comparison of surgical and radiation therapy. Am J Obstet Gynecol 103:566–573

Mayr NA, Yuh WT, Zheng J et al (1997) Tumor size evaluated by pelvic examination compared with 3-D quantitative analysis in the prediction of outcome for cervcial cancer. Int J Radiat Oncol Biol Phys 39:395–404

Morley GW, Seski JC (1976) Radical pelvic surgery versus radiation therapy for stage I carcinoma of the cervix (exclusive of microinvasion). Am J Obstet Gynecol 126:785–798

Morris M, Eifel PJ, Lu J et al (1999) Pelvic radiation with concurrent chemotherapy compared with pelvic and paraaortic radiation for high-risk cervical cancer. N Engl J Med 340:1137–1143

Park JM, Charnsangavej C, Yoshimitsu K et al (1994) Pathways of nodal metastasis from pelvic tumors: CT demonstration. Radiographics 14:1309–1321

Parker RT, Duncan I, Rampone J et al (1975) Operative management of early invasive epidermoid carcinoma of the vulva, Am J Obstet Gynecol 123:349–355

Pendlebury SC, Cahill S, Crandon AJ et al (1993) Role of bipedal lymphangiogram in radiation treatment planning for cervix cancer. Int J Radiat Oncol Biol Phys 27: 959–962

Perez CA (1997) Uterine cervix. Principles and practice of

radiation oncology, 3rd edn. Lippincott-Raven, Philadephia, pp 1733–1834
Perez CA, Garipagaoglu M (1998) Vagina. In: Perez CA, Brady LW (eds) Principles and practice of radiation oncology. Lippincott-Raven, Philadelphia, pp 1891–1914
Perez CA, Arneson AN, Galakatos A et al (1973) Malignant tumors of the vagina. Cancer 31:36–44
Peters WA, Liu PY, Barrett RJ et al (2000) Concurrent chemotherapy and pelvic radiation therapy compared with pelvic radiation therapy alone as adjuvant therapy after radical surgery in high-risk early-stage cancer of the cervix. J Clin Oncol 18:1606–1613
Piver M, Chung W (1975) Prognostic significance of cervical lesion size and pelvic node metastases in cervical carcinoma. Obstet Gynecol 46:507–510
Plentl AA, Friedman EA (1971) Lymphatic system of the female genitalia. The morphologic basis of oncologic diagnosis and therapy. Saunders, Philadelphia
Rampone JF, Klem V, Kolstad P (1973) Combined treatment of stage IB carcinoma of the cervix. Obstet Gynecol 41: 163–167
Rouviere H, Tobias MJ (1938) Lymphatic system of the abdomen and pelvis. Anatomy of the human lymphatic system. Edwards, Ann Arbor, pp 158–237
Rutledge F, Smith JP, Franklin EW (1970) Cacinoma of the vulva. Am J Obstet Gynecol 106:1117–1130
Sakuragi N, Satoh C, Takeda N et al (1999) Incidence and distribution pattern of pelvic and paraaortic lymph node metastasis in patients with stages IB, IIA, and IIB cervical carcinoma treated with radical hysterectomy. Cancer 85: 1547–1554
Scheidler J, Hricak H, Yu KK et al (1997) Radiological evaluation of lymph node metastases in patients with cervical cancer. A meta-analysis. J Am Med Assoc 278:1096–1101
Sedlis A, Bundy BN, Rotman MZ et al (1999) A randomized trial of pelvic radiation therapy versus no further therapy in selected patients with IB carcinoma of the cervix after radical hysterectomy and pelvic lymphadenectomy: a Gynecologic Oncology Group Study. Gynecol Oncol 73: 177–183
Stock RG, Chen AS, Seski J (1995) A 30-year experience in the management of primary carcinoma of the vagina: analysis of prognostic factors and treatment modalities. Gynecol Oncol 56:45–52
Swart E, Bouma J, Schuur K (1989) The clinical value of lymphography in cervical cancer, FIGO-stage Ib–IIa. Eur J Cancer 10:85–90
Vinnicombe SJ, Norman AR, Nicolson V et al (1995) Normal pelvic lymph nodes: evaluation with CT after bipedal lymphangiography. Radiology 194:349–355
Whelton RH, Kottmeier HL (1962) Primary carcinoma of the vagina: a study of a Radiumhemmet series of 145 cases. Acta Obstet Gynecol Scand 41:22–40
Yang WT, Lam WWM, Cheung TH et al (2000) Comparison of dynamic helical CT and dynamic MR imaging in the evaluation of pelvic lymph. Am J Radiol 175:759–766
Yu KK, Forstner R, Hricak H (1997) Cervical carcinoma: role of imaging. Abdom Imaging 22:208–215
Yu KK, Hricak H, Subak LL et al (1998) Preoperative staging of cervical carcinoma: phased array coil fast spin-echo versus body coil spin-echo T2-weighted MR imaging. Am J Roentgenol Radium Ther Nucl Med 171: 707–711

10 Rectal and Anal Cancers in Conformal Radiotherapy Planning: Selection and Delineation of Lymph Node Areas

L. L. Gunderson, M. G. Haddock, P. A. Gervaz, H. Nelson

CONTENTS

10.1 Introduction

This chapter discusses indications for and results of lymphatic treatment for lower gastrointestinal (GI) malignancies (large bowel and anus) and the use of conformal irradiation techniques to accomplish this. The rationale for including nodes will be based on patterns of relapse in autopsy, reoperation, and clinical analyses, since randomized trials have not been performed to test the inclusion of nodes in irradiation fields.

Involvement of nodes detected by imaging techniques is usually demonstrated by computed tomographic (CT) evidence of nodal enlargement at either initial workup or subsequent follow-up. Although a lymphangiogram (LAG) can demonstrate filling defects in normal-sized nodes, this technique is rarely utilized as a diagnostic tool for large bowel or anal cancers. Transluminal ultrasound is currently used diagnostically to evaluate node involvement in rectal

L. L. Gunderson, MD, MS
Professor of Oncology, Mayo Medical School, Chair and Consultant in Radiation Oncology, Mayo Clinic Scottsdale, 13400 East Shea Blvd , Scottsdale, AZ 85259, USA
M. G. Haddock, MD
Assistant Professor of Oncology, Mayo Medical School, Consultant in Radiation Oncology, Mayo Clinic, Desk SR Charlton Building, Rochester, MN 55905, USA
P. A. Gervaz, MD
Fellow in Colorectal Surgery, Mayo Clinic and Mayo Medical School, Rochester, MN 55905, USA
J. A. Martenson, MD
Associate Professor of Oncology, Mayo Medical School; Consultant in Radiation Oncology, Mayo Clinic, Rochester, MN 55905, USA
H. Nelson, MD,
Professor and Chair of Colorectal Surgery, Mayo Clinic and Medical School, Rochester, MN 55905, USA

cancers. With either CT or transluminal ultrasound, the accuracy of predicting nodal involvement is £50% unless needle biopsy is performed of enlarged or suspicious nodes. The only procedure with an accuracy of +90% is surgical exploration with resection or biopsy. Autopsy or reoperative series provide the best data concerning nodal patterns of relapse after initial treatment.

10.2 Classification of Node Levels – Anatomy

10.2.1 Rectal Cancer

Lymphatic and venous drainage of lesions limited to the rectum depends on the level of the lesion. The upper rectum drains into the inferior mesenteric system via the superior hemorrhoidal vessels, and the middle and lower rectum can, in addition, drain directly to the internal iliac and presacral nodes. Lesions that extend to the anal canal can spread to the inguinal nodes.

If the primary rectal cancer extends beyond the rectal wall to involve adjacent organs or structures, nodal drainage is via the lymphatics of the involved organ (prostate, posterior vaginal wall, uterus, bladder) or structure (presacrum, pelvic side wall). With anterior extension and adjacent organ involvement, the external iliac nodes become at risk. If the lower third of the vagina is involved, the inguinal nodes are also at risk. With posterior extension, the internal iliac system becomes at risk, independent of the level of the rectal lesion.

10.2.2 Anal Cancer

For evaluation of both tumor spread and ultimate prognosis, anal lesions are commonly divided into those of the anal canal versus the perineal aspect of the anus, also known as the anal margin. Anal canal lesions more frequently exhibit invasion of the adjacent perianal tissues and can also involve the sphincter muscles or adjacent organs.

Lymphatics of the anal canal drain either to the superficial inguinal nodes or to the nodes of the lower rectum (internal iliac and inferior mesenteric). Lesions on the external margin drain primarily to the superficial inguinal nodes.

10.3 Distribution and Incidence of Regional Nodes – Pathways of Spread and Incidence of Relapse After Surgery Alone

10.3.1 Rectal Cancer

10.3.1.1 Pathways of Spread

Rectal cancers can spread by the four standard mechanisms of direct extension, lymphatic spread, hematogenous spread, and surgical implantation – but peritoneal spread is also possible. Peritoneal spread is rare with rectal lesions because most of the rectum is below the peritoneal reflection. Extension within the bowel wall is a rare occurrence, and usually only involves short distances. Because primary venous and lymphatic channels originate in the submucosal layers of the bowel, lesions limited to the mucosa are at little risk for either lymphatic or venous dissemination.

Lymph node involvement is found in nearly 50% of patients in most series, and patterns of spread are usually orderly and predictable. Occasional skip metastases or abnormal spread can occur, but in the past this was considered to be due to lymphatic blockage (Grinnell 1966). Gabriel et al. (1935) found nodal involvement in 62 of 100 consecutive cases of rectal cancer, but skip metastasis was present in only one case. Grinnell (1966) analyzed 913 cases and found atypical nodal metastases in 34 instances in 28 patients. Most patients with atypical metastases had advanced nodal involvement, and none survived 5 years after operation. Dukes (1943) analyzed 1,500 cases and found distal spread to lymph nodes in only 6.9%. In only 2% of cases was such spread greater than 0.62 cm below the inferior margin of the rectal lesion.

Although the major spread through lymphatic channels is in a cephalad direction, lateral and distal (caudad) spread can also occur. Enquist and Block (1966) attempted to map lymphatic pathways in females utilizing dye injections at approximately 5-, 10-, and 15-cm levels above the anal verge. With injections at the 5-cm level, distal spread with staining of the pelvic diaphragm was observed. At the 10- and 15-cm levels, some lateral spread was found but no distal spread was seen. Slanetz et al. (1972) utilized the findings of a number of studies to define the critical level regarding the direction of lymphatic flow as being approximately at the 8-cm level. Above

8 cm only cephalad flow was found, but below 8 cm some lateral and distal flow also occurred.

As noted above, atypical or skip nodal metastases were previously considered to be both rare and related to lymphatic blockage. However, when sentinel node biopsy sampling techniques are utilized more routinely for rectal cancers, alternate or abnormal patterns of nodal spread may either become more clearly defined or at least become diagnosed more easily.

Suha et al. (2000) recently published data on a series of 86 patients with colorectal cancer in which sentinel lymph node (SLN) mapping was performed in an attempt to enhance the identification of micrometastases. At the time of surgery, peritumoral injection of isosulfan blue was used to demonstrate the location of SLNs. A standard resection was then performed, and the first to fourth nodes which entrapped the isosulfan blue were considered to be SLNs. The pathologic evaluation included serial sections of the SLNs (at 2- to 3-mm intervals) with the aim of obtaining 10 microsections per SLN. For non-SLN nodes, the usual pathologic evaluation is the review of 1–2 microsections per node. In the Suha et al. series, SLNs were identified in 85 of 86 patients. In 53 of 56 patients (95%) in whom SLNs were negative for cancer, all remaining nodes sampled were also without metastases. In the 29 of 85 patients (34%) with histologically positive SLNs, non-SLN nodes were found to contain metastases in 14 of 29 subjects. In the remaining 15 patients (18% of 85 patients at risk), the SLNs were the only nodes identified to contain micrometastases. Therefore, the SLN mapping procedure may have improved staging in 18% of the patients in the series.

As noted by Ota (2000) in an editorial review of this publication, only a randomized trial comparing blue dye intraoperative node mapping versus no mapping can establish the claim of improved node mapping. The American College of Surgeons Oncology Group is developing such a protocol.

10.3.1.2
Incidence of Relapse – Tumor Bed or Nodal

The risk of local-regional relapse (tumor bed or nodal) after complete surgical resection relates to the degree of primary tumor extension beyond the rectal wall as well as to nodal involvement. The incidence of lesions with involved nodes but with the tumor confined to the wall (TNM T_{1-2}, N_{1-2}; modified Astler–Coller C_1) varies from 20% to 40%, which is approximately the same as for lesions without nodal involvement but with extension beyond the wall (T_{3-4}, N_0; MAC B_{2-3}) where the risk is 20% to 35%. Lesions that have both nodal involvement and extension beyond the wall (T_{3-4}, N_{1-2}; MAC C_{2-3}), have nearly an additive risk, varying from 40% to 65% in clinical series to 70% in a reoperative series.

Nodal versus pelvic relapse was coded in the University of Minnesota re-operative series (Gunderson and Sosin 1974), in which 52 of 75 patients at risk developed relapse (tumor bed, 33; perineum, 12; nodal, 20; wound implant, 4 patients). This distinction is difficult to identify in clinical analyses, however. Therefore, the term pelvic relapse or pelvic recurrence is commonly used to include both tumor bed and pelvic nodal relapses. Even in the reoperative series, some of the relapses coded as lateral or posterior pelvis were undoubtedly due to relapse within the lymphatics or replaced internal iliac nodes rather than tumor bed relapse. In a Massachusetts General Hospital (MGH) series, the incidence of both total and pelvic relapse in the 'node-negative' group of patients increased with each degree of tumor extension beyond the wall (Rich et al. 1983). In patients with nodal involvement, the degree of extrarectal extension also appears to be an independent factor influencing the risk of local recurrence.

10.3.1.3
Incidence and Patterns of Nodal Relapse – University of Minnesota Reoperative Series

Local failure alone or plus regional lymph node relapse (LF-RF) was a major problem in the reoperative series, being the sole relapse site in 25 patients (48%) and occurring as any component of relapse in 48 patients (92%; Table 10.1; Gunderson and Sosin 1974). In comparison, only four patients (8%) had only distant metastases (DM).

An exact breakdown of the area of local failure and/or regional lymph node spread is found in Table 10.2.

Table 10.1. Local and/or regional failure (relapse; *LF-RF*) in the University of Minnesota rectal reoperative series of 75 patients. From Gunderson and Sosin (1974) with permission

Area of relapse	Single area LF-RF		Any component LF-RF	
	No.	%	No.	%
Pelvis	19	(40)	33	(69)
Perineum	2	(4)	12	(25)
Lymph node	10	(21)	20	(42)
Wound implant	1	(2)	4	(8)

LF-RF found as the only failure in 25 patients and in combination with other relapse in 23 out of a total of 48 patients.

Table 10.2. Lymph node relapse: only LF–RF, University of Minnesota rectal reoperative series. From GUNDERSON and SOSIN (1974) with permission

Findings at initial surgery			Area of LN relapse			
MAC stage[a]	Level of primary[b]	LN no. area	Iliac	Aortic	Other	Description
C_2	8 cm	5/8 regional		Y		L. sided paravertebral mass to diaphragm
C_3	17 cm	3/20 adjacent			Y	Unknown- grossly + int. iliac but diagnosis not made until later serial section
C_2	At pect.	1/10 regional	Y			Common iliac near aortic bifurcation
C_1 or C_2	At pect.	1/unknown			Y	L. inguinal
C_2	15 cm	1/55		Y		Upper level unknown
C_2	At pect.	15/68 with specimen 1/1 ureter	Y		Y	R. ext. iliac just proximal to ing. ligament; R. obturator
C_2	6 cm	All positive including iliac & aortic	Y	Y		Bilateral ext. iliac; junction common and bifurcation; aortic as high as renal veins
C_2 (m)	10 cm	4/26		Y		To celiac axis with involvement of aorta
C_2	12 cm	7/9 mesenteric 3/4 inferior mesenteric			Y	Nodal mass in mesentery of colostomy
C_2	5–6 cm	Unknown mesenteric & pericolic		Y	Y	Aortic bifurcation to celiac axis; sacral promontory

Total of 10 patients: 4, only failure; 6 in combination with distant metastases (DM); Y, yes

[a] Staged according to modified Astler–Coller (*MAC*) method. All C_2 lesions were classified on both a microscopic (m) and a gross (g) basis, unless noted as C_2 (m)

[b] Centimeters (cm) above pectinate (pect.) line on pathologic specimen-inferior extent

No difference in patterns of local-regional relapse was found between the 25 patients in which it was the sole relapse site and the 23 patients in which it occurred in combination with other sites of relapse. The highest incidence of local-regional relapse was within the pelvic soft tissues and residual organs. The exact sites of relapse within the pelvis were as follows (70 sites in 33 patients): anterior: 21; posterior: 25; lateral: 13; pelvic floor: 10; uncertain: 1. The exact superior extent of these relapses was difficult to ascertain. Evidence of perineal relapse without other components of pelvic failure was rare. Relapse involving either the abdominal or perineal incision (wound implant) was a rare occurrence. No anastomotic recurrences were found in the small number of patients with anterior resection. The diagrammatic representation of these relapses, shown in Fig. 10.1, is a rough approximation by area and is not meant to be exact.

Lymph node relapses were also common. Ten patients had lymph node relapse without other evidence of local or regional involvement. Table 10.3 lists the extent of the initial pathology and the subsequent area of lymph node involvement. There were three cases of only aortic lymph node, one aortic and iliac, and one aortic and sacral promontory relapse. Upper levels of aortic involvement were as follows: celiac axis: 2; diaphragm: 1; renal veins: 1; and unknown: 1. The original lesion was at the pectinate line in the single

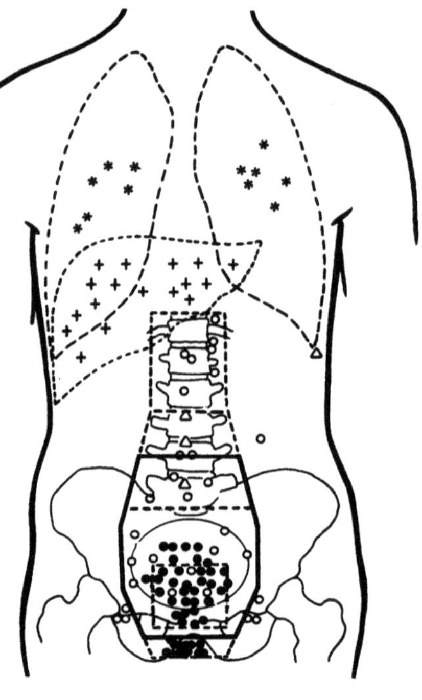

Fig. 10.1. Rectal cancer: patterns of relapse in University of Minnesota rectal reoperation series, with superimposed irradiation fields to pelvis alone or including perineum. From GUNDERSON and SOSIN (1974) with permission

patient with relapse in the inguinal nodes and in one of the two patients with external iliac nodes.

Ten additional patients had lymph node involvement in combination with pelvic or perineal relapse. Aortic nodes were involved in five cases. Three patients had inguinal lymph node involvement; two experienced perineal relapse and one had a surgical implant in the abdominal wound. The rate of nodal relapse is considered to be an underestimate, however, since some of the relapses coded as lateral or posterior pelvis were undoubtedly due to relapse within the lymphatics, or replaced iliac nodes rather than tumor bed relapse.

Table 10.3 shows the relationship between the extent of the initial disease and the incidence and patterns of subsequent relapse. Overall patterns of relapse were basically similar, but most relapses (42 of 52) occurred in patients whose primary lesion extended through the entire rectal wall. Nearly 50% of these patients had only local relapse and/or regional lymph node involvement (20 of 42), and 49 patients (95%) had some component of involvement. Four patients with lymph nodes involved and the primary lesion confined to the rectal wall (T_{1-2}, N_{1-2}) developed later local and/or regional failure; three of the four had more than three nodes (N_2 stage) initially involved.

10.3.1.4
Impact of Adjuvant Treatment on Local-Regional Relapse

Both pre- and postoperative adjuvant irradiation (in doses equivalent to or +39.6 Gy in 1.8-Gy fractions) have resulted in a statistically significant reduction in local-regional recurrence when compared with surgery alone in randomized trials (Gunderson 1999). In the randomized trials, no distinction has been made between tumor bed and nodal relapse; the impact of nodal irradiation on either disease control or survival is impossible to detect in either randomized trials or single institution analyses. Little interest exists in randomizing the extent of irradiation fields in high-risk patients (T_4N_0, $T_{3-4}N_{1-2}$), since pelvic irradiation is generally well tolerated alone or in conjunction with chemotherapy. However, in intermediate-risk patients (T_3N_0, $T_{1-2}N_1$), it may be reasonable to evaluate irradiation field extent in an attempt to improve tolerance.

10.3.2
Anal Cancers

10.3.2.1
Pathways of Spread

Perirectal or inferior mesenteric node involvement at the time of initial resection has varied from 28% to 64%, and inguinal node involvement from 13% to 25%. In a Mayo Clinic analysis by Boman et al. (1984), the incidence of nodal involvement at diagnosis was +30%, with a lesion size of >2 cm independent of histology, and with grade 3 or 4 non-keratinizing basaloid tumors of any size.

Table 10.3. Extent of disease versus patterns of relapse; University of Minnesota reoperative series. From Gunderson and Sosin (1974) with permission

Extent of initial disease	Total no. of patients	Total no. with relapse	Patterns of relapse[a]			
			LF-RF alone	LF-RF component	DM alone	DM component
Within bowel wall	18	5				
LN+(C_1)	17	5	2	4	1	3
LN–(B_1)	1	0	–	–	–	–
Through bowel wall	49[b]	42	20 (48%)	40 (95%)	2 (5%)	21 (50%)
LN+($C_{2,3}$)	40	34	15 (44%)	33 (97%)	1 (3%)	18 (53%)
LN–($B_{2,3}$)	6	5	3	4	1	2
LN ? (B_2 vs. C_2)	3	3	2	3	0	1
Unknown extent	5	5	3	4	1	2
LN+(C_1 vs. C_2)	4	4	2	3	1	2
LN unknown	1	1	1	1	0	0

Fifty-two patients with evidence of relapse after initial treatment. *LF-RF*: local-regional failure
[a] Peritoneal seeding was so rare that it was not included for analysis in this table
[b] Two additional patients with unknown disease status

10.3.2.2
Incidence and Patterns of Local-Regional Relapse – Surgery Alone

Although abdominoperineal resection has been replaced with irradiation and chemotherapy as the standard treatment for anal cancer, some excellent data exist on relapse patterns after surgery alone. In the BOMAN analysis (1984), local-regional relapse was shown to be the predominant relapse pattern in 106 evaluable patients with abdominoperineal resection (Table 10.4). Of the 38 evaluable patients who relapsed, 84% had a local-regional component of relapse, and 29% had a distant component. The risk of local relapse was related to the degree of local invasion and nodal involvement. Fifteen of 38 patients (39%) had an inguinal node component of relapse. Seven patients underwent inguinal node dissection for clinically apparent involvement at the time of initial abdominoperineal resection. The 5-year relapse-free survival amounted to 71% (five out of seven cases) in these patients.

10.3.2.3
Incidence and Patterns of Local-Regional Relapse – Radiation Alone or Radiation Plus Chemotherapy

Separate analyses by Princess Margaret Hospital (PMH; CUMMINGS et al. 1991; Table 10.5), University of Kansas (NIGH et al. 1991), RTOG (SISCHY et al. 1989) and MGH (CONSTANTINOU et al. 1997) investigators support the need to evaluate both irradiation dose levels as well as the type and duration of chemotherapy in an attempt to improve both local and distant control of disease. The pelvic relapse rate (anal primary plus pelvic and inguinal nodes) in these series ranged from 20% to 30% at dose levels of approximately 40 to 50 Gy plus chemotherapy (1.8–2.0 Gy fractions in the US analyses, and 2.0 to 2.5 Gy in the PMH trial). In the PMH analysis, the most optimal combination of irradiation plus 5-fluorouracil-mitomycin C (5-FU–MMC) still resulted in a 19% pelvic relapse rate (13 of 69 cases) and a 17% systemic relapse rate (12 of 69 cases; Table 10.5). A nodal component of relapse was found in five patients (7%), which may be falsely low since intrapelvic node relapse is difficult to diagnose without reoperation or autopsy. In the RTOG trial 83–14 in which irradiation to 40.8 Gy was combined with 5-FU–MMC, the 3-year colostomy-free survival rate was 63% (SISCHY et al. 1989). Pelvic relapse occurred in 24 of 77 patients or 31% (5-year actuarial rate of 32%), and systemic failure in 12 of 77 patients or 16% of cases (5-year actuarial rate of 19%).

Primary tumor control may increase as a function of irradiation dose level. In pooled data on 57 patients from five Kansas City institutions, 77% of the patients received chemotherapy with irradiation by 5-FU with MMC or cisplatin (CDDP) (NIGH et al. 1991). Local control (LC) was achieved in 81% of cases; all local relapses occurred within 1.5 years of treatment, and salvage was achieved in eight of 11 patients for an eventual LC of 95%. LC by irradiation dose level was as follows: £45 Gy, 64%; 45 to 55 Gy, 72%; >55 Gy, 92% (P=0.05). On the basis of Cox multivariate analysis, a radiation therapy (RT) dose of >55 Gy was the only variable associated with improved LC.

In a separate analysis from MGH by CONSTANTINOU et al. (1997), irradiation dose level appeared to impact on both LC and survival. For patients with a dose of +54 Gy in 1.8-Gy fractions, LC was achieved in 77% of patients versus 61% in patients with a dose of <54 Gy (P=0. 04). Five-year survival rate was respectively 84% versus 47% (P=0.02).

Irradiation field design has been shown to have a probable impact on nodal control. In early trials by PAPILLON et al. (1983), no attempt was made to include the pelvic nodes and the incidence of documented nodal relapse was 24%. This was reduced to 3.6% after irradiation fields were appropriately altered to include

Table 10.4. Cancer of the anus: stage versus survival and patterns of relapse after abdominoperineal resection (Mayo). Modified from BOMAN et al. (1984)

Mayo stage	Extent of disease	Incidence % (n=114)	5-year survival		Patterns of initial relapse (component)			
					Local		Distant	
			No.	%	No.	%	No.	%
A	Mucosa and submucosa	4	4/4	100	0	–	0	–
B_1	Internal sphincter	24	20/26	77	2	8	2	8
B_2	External sphincter	13	10/13	77	3	23	0	–
B_3	Beyond sphincters	29	15/31	48	14	48	2	7
C	Nodes involved	36	19/40	48	13	36	7	19

Table 10.5. Cancer of the anus: survival and patterns of relapse with irradiation and chemotherapy. Modified from CUMMINGS et al. (1991)

Treatment	Relapse component (at any time)								5-year survival, % (cause-specific)	
	Primary		Nodal		Distant		Total			
	No.	%	No.	%	No.	%	No.	%		
Continuous EBRT										
EBRT	25	44	11	19	10	18	28/57	49	68	
EBRT, 5-FU, Mito	2	13	0	–	1	6	3/16	19		p0.14
Split-course EBRT									76	
EBRT, 5-FU, Mito	8	15	5	9	11	21	17/53	32		p0.02
EBRT, 5-FU	26	40	5	8	8	12	31/65	48	64	

EBRT, external beam irradiation; mito, mitomycin C

the pelvic nodes. Elective inguinal irradiation appears to decrease the risk of subsequent inguinal failure (risk of 11% to 24% without irradiation versus 0% to 5% with irradiation). In a PMH analysis by CUMMINGS et al. (1991), the risk was 18% versus 3%, and in PAPILLON's series (1983) 13% versus 0%.

10.4 Guidelines for Selection of Target Volumes and Radiation Field Design

10.4.1 Rectal Cancer

When both surgery and irradiation are indicated in an adjuvant setting for rectal cancer, differences of opinion exist regarding the preferred sequence. A theoretical advantage of preoperative irradiation is the potentially damaging effect on cells that may become spread locally or distantly at the time of resection. The major advantage of postoperative irradiation is the ability to avoid treating patients who have metastatic disease that could not be diagnosed before surgical exploration or those at low risk for local relapse. Only those patients at high risk for local relapse on the basis of operative and pathologic findings are irradiated. For clinically mobile rectal lesions, both preoperative and postoperative irradiation are reasonable options, as improved imaging can now define patients at high risk for relapse [i.e., endoscopic ultrasound (EUS) which includes thin needle biopsy of suspicious nodes].

For rectal cancers, the aim is to include within the irradiation field the primary tumor and/or tumor bed with 3 to 5-cm margins as well as nodal areas that either are not removed by the surgeon or cannot be removed without manipulation (Table 10.6). In most institutions, internal iliac and presacral nodes are not standardly dissected during surgery for rectal cancer because of limited gain, thus these nodes should probably be included in the initial irradiation volume. External iliac nodes are not a primary nodal drainage site and should not be included, unless pelvic organs with major external iliac drainage

Table 10.6. Rectal cancer: general guidelines of impact of T and N stage on irradiation treatment volumes

TN stage	Organ or site of adherence or invasion	Tumor or tumor bed volumes	Nodal volumes
T1–3N1–2	Not applicable	Rectum/rectal bed[b]	Internal iliac, pre-sacral
T4N0	Anterior or posterior	Rectum/rectal bed plus organ/structure involved	Internal iliac, pre-sacral; optional: external/common iliac if anterior adherence
T4N1–2 (anterior adherence or invasion)	Prostate, bladder, uterus, vagina (proximal 2/3)[a]	Rectum/rectal bed plus organ/structure involved	Internal iliac, pre-sacral, External/common iliac[a]
T4N1–2 (posterior/lateral adherence or invasion)	Presacrum or pelvic side-walls	Rectum/rectal bed plus organ/structure involved	Internal iliac, pre-sacral

[a] Include inguinal nodes if distal vagina or anus is involved by direct extension of primary or recurrent tumor
[b] Primary tumor plus 3–5 cm margin

are involved by direct extension (i.e. involvement of bladder, prostate, cervix, or vagina). Inguinal nodes should be included in the irradiation field only if the lesion extends to involve the anal canal or distal one-third of the posterior vaginal wall.

Most tumor bed relapses after complete surgical resection are in the posterior one-half to two-thirds of the true pelvis, and the internal iliac and presacral nodes have a posterior location relative to the external iliac nodes (Fig. 10.2). Lateral treatment fields can logically be combined with anterior-posterior (AP/PA) fields to reduce the dose to anteriorly located normal structures, including the small bowel.

Field arrangements depend on the location of the primary tumor, presence or absence of adjacent organ involvement, and area and number of nodes involved, but some generalizations can be made (see Fig. 10.2). The width of AP/PA ports (see Figs. 10.2a and 10.3a) should cover the pelvic inlet with a margin around the targeted iliac nodes. Lateral margins extending 1 to 2 cm beyond the widest point of the bony pelvis are usually sufficient, depending on treatment energy and penumbra. The superior margin should usually be at least 1.5 cm above the level of the sacral promontory (occasionally mid-L5 to L4, depending on the superior extent of the lesion). The superior field margin may depend on the extent of inferior mesenteric and/or iliac nodal involvement, which is usually not known preoperatively (infrequently, periaortic nodes are included to the level of T_{12} or T_{11} if proximal nodes are pathologically involved). The inferior extent of the field is also somewhat variable. For both preoperative irradiation and postoperative irradiation after anterior resection, the usual procedure is inclusion of the obturator foramina. This field is occasionally more extensive than necessary for upper

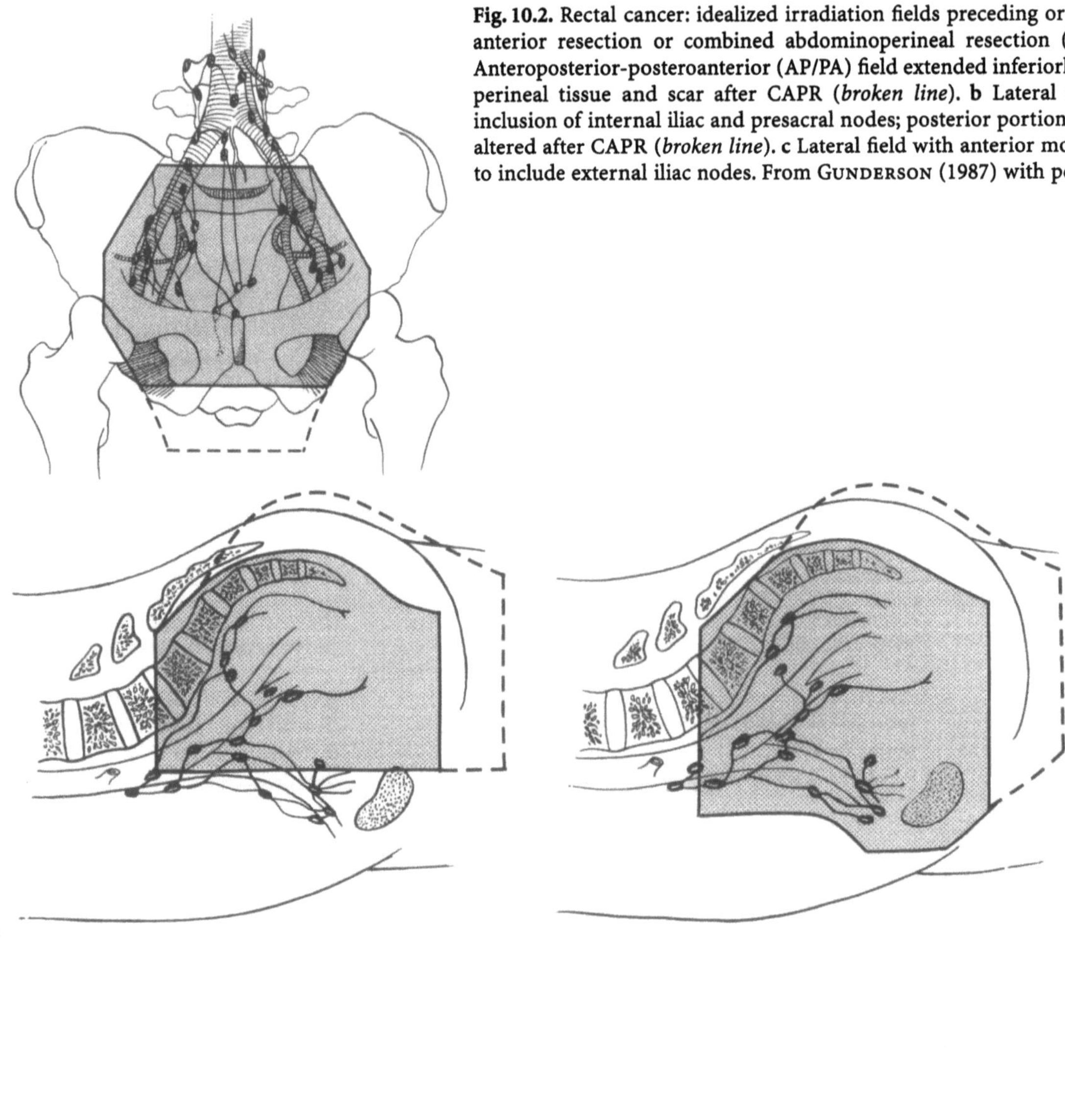

Fig. 10.2. Rectal cancer: idealized irradiation fields preceding or following anterior resection or combined abdominoperineal resection (CAPR). **a** Anteroposterior-posteroanterior (AP/PA) field extended inferiorly to cover perineal tissue and scar after CAPR (*broken line*). **b** Lateral field with inclusion of internal iliac and presacral nodes; posterior portion of field is altered after CAPR (*broken line*). **c** Lateral field with anterior modification to include external iliac nodes. From GUNDERSON (1987) with permission

a

b

c

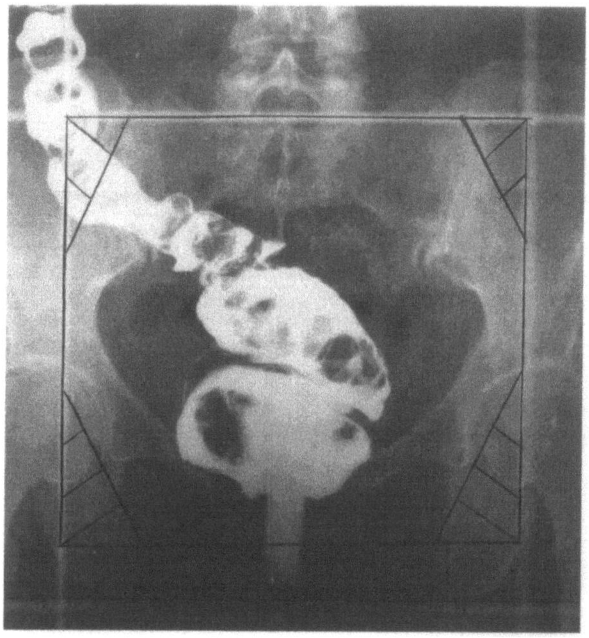
a

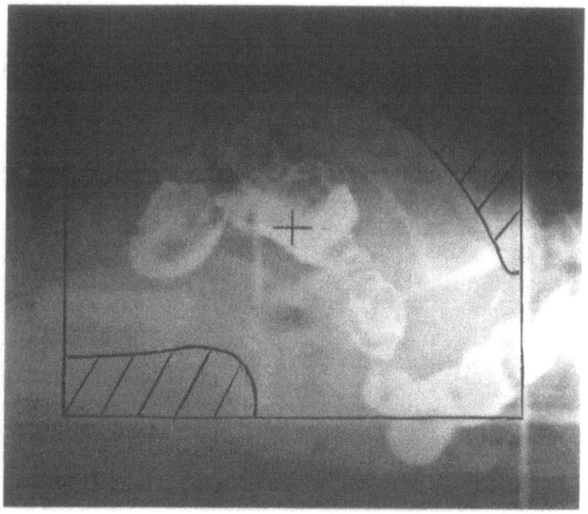
b

Fig. 10.3. Rectal cancer: postoperative irradiation with four-field technique after anterior resection of rectum and reanastomosis. **a** Posteroanterior-anteroposterior field; **b** lateral field. Patient is simulated in prone position with contrast material in rectum, tampon with contrast material in vagina, and lead shot on anal verge. From Gunderson and Martenson (1991) with permission

rectal cancers, but may be too limited for distal rectal cancers. The minimal field extent should usually be 3 to 5 cm below the gross tumor (preoperative) or 1.5 to 2 cm below the most inferior extent of dissection or mobilization of the distal limb (postoperative), which ideally would be marked with surgical clips. Coverage of the perineum after abdominoperineal resection is discussed in a separate section.

When using lateral fields (see Figs. 10.2b, c, and 10.3b), treatment in the prone position allows visualization of the sacrum and more positional shift in the small bowel. The posterior field margin is vital, because the rectum and perirectal tissues (tumor plus target volume) lie just anterior to the sacrum and coccyx. Accordingly, the posterior field margin should be a minimum of 1.5 to 2 cm behind the anterior bony sacral margin to allow for some daily patient movement. Individually shaped blocks can be used to spare posterior muscle and soft tissues. The anterior margin can be shaped to reduce the amount of irradiation to the femoral head and bladder inferiorly, or when the external iliac lymph nodes need to be included to decrease the amount of small bowel superiorly and anteriorly. Anteriorly, the lower one-third of the rectum abuts the posterior vaginal wall and prostate, and these structures should be included. In female patients, inclusion of the vagina can be verified at simulation if a contrast-soaked gauze pad or tampon is placed therein during treatment planning (Fig. 10.3b).

After abdominoperineal resection, the perineum, with its anteroposterior and inferolateral aspects of operative dissection, should be included in the tumor-bed-nodal irradiation volumes, otherwise marginal relapse may occur. In an MGH series, the incidence of perineal relapse following surgery alone was 8.5% (6 of 71 patients at risk) (Rich et al. 1983), and in the patients receiving postoperative irradiation, the incidence was only 2% (1 of 60 patients at risk; a marginal recurrence because of inappropriate lateral fields; Hoskins et al. 1985). In a Mayo Clinic series of rectal cancer patients treated with postoperative irradiation (Schild et al. 1989), the incidence of a perineal component of relapse was less than 2% after anterior resection (perineum not irradiated) or abdominoperineal resection with adequate inclusion of the perineum (to +40 Gy), but was about 20% when the perineum was not adequately irradiated after abdominoperineal resection ($P<0.05$). Lead shot or wire should be used to mark the entire extent of the perineal scar for CT simulation or when localization films are obtained (Fig. 10.4). The inferior (caudad) and posterior field edges should be 1.5–2 cm beyond the scar as marked. Inferolaterally, the margin should be at the level of the lateral aspect of the ischial tuberosities. The perineum usually can be treated to a dose level of 45 Gy in 25 fractions over 5 weeks, with acceptable acute and chronic tolerance.

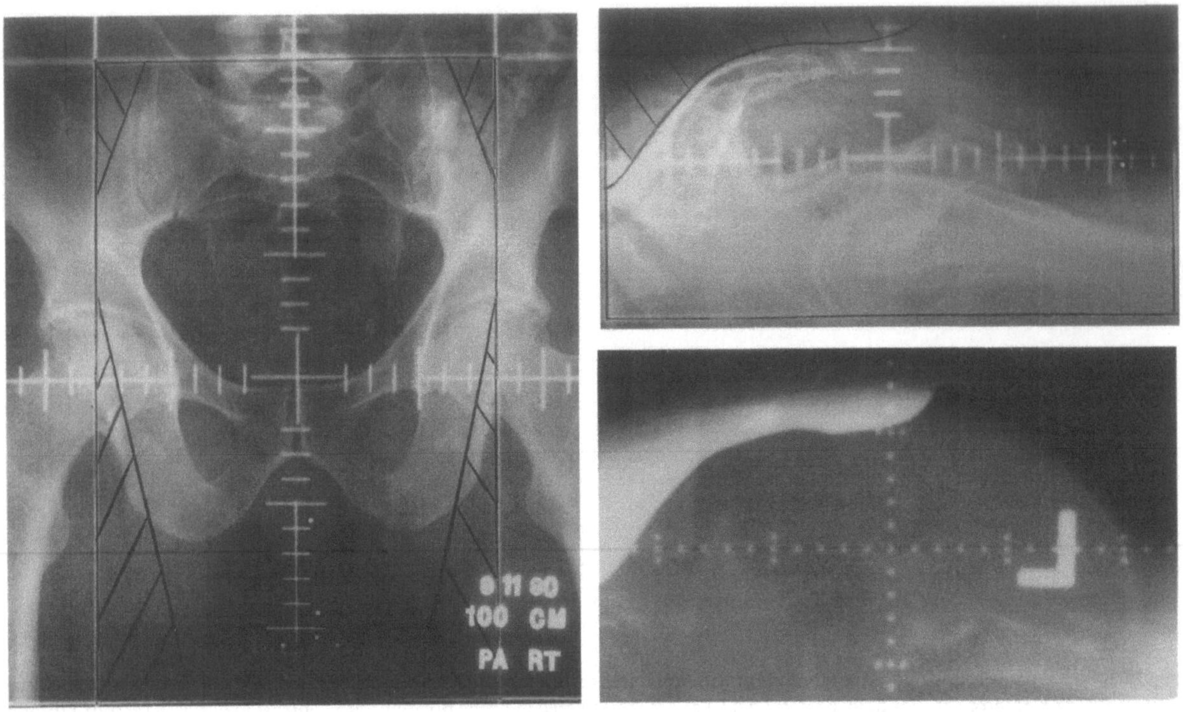

a b c

Fig. 10.4. Rectal cancer: postoperative four-field technique after CAPR. **a** and **b** Lead shot marks entire length of perineal scar on posteroanterior (**a**) and lateral (**b**) views. Posterior extent of scar is often more posterior than the sacrum, necessitating posterior fall off, as seen on port film (**c**). From GUNDERSON and MARTENSON (1991) with permission

10.4.2 Anal Cancer

Currently, most single institution and group studies design fields to include the primary lesion as well as major nodal groups (inguinal and pelvic) to 30 to 36 Gy in 1.8- to 2.0-Gy fractions when irradiation is combined with concomitant chemotherapy, or 45 Gy in 25 fractions for irradiation alone schemas (Table 10.7). The majority of investigators utilize parallel-opposed fields to these dose levels, with the superior field extent varying by series from the level of the sacral promontory to the bottom of the sacroiliac joint (Fig. 10.5). If the superior field extent is at the sacral promontory level and a nodal dose of 45 Gy is planned, lateral fields could be considered for a component of treatment in order to reduce the dose to the small bowel. When the superior extent is at the bottom of the sacroiliac joint, lateral fields would be of little value except for boost fields to the primary lesion.

10.5 Guidelines for 3-D Delineation of Lymph Node Areas Based on Imaging – CT or Lymphangiogram

10.5.1 Rectal Cancer

As noted in Sect. 10.4.1, if a cancer of the rectum does not extend to involve adjacent structures, the lymph node areas that should be considered as target volume include the perirectal, internal iliac and presacral nodes (Fig. 10.2b). The internal iliac and presacral nodal areas can be defined either pre- or postoperatively with a pelvic CT using both oral and intravenous (IV) contrast (Fig. 10.6a). Transrectal endoscopic ultrasound (EUS) can be used preoperatively to determine whether malignant perirectal nodes appear to be involved. Needle biopsies can be selectively performed at the time of EUS to document malignant involvement, which may guide decisions

Table 10.7. Anal cancer: general guidelines of impact of T and N stage on irradiation treatment volumes (in patients with either anal canal cancers or anal margin cancers invading the anal canal)

TN stage	Organ or site of adherence or invasion	Tumor volumes	Nodal volumes
T1–3N0–2	Not applicable	Anal canal and verge, distal rectum[b]	Inguinal, external iliac, internal iliac, presacral, inferior mesenteric; optional: common iliac[a]
T4N0	Anterior or posterior	As for T1–3N0–2 plus organ/structure involved	As for T1–3N0–2
T4N1–2 (anterior adherence or invasion)	Prostate, bladder, uterus, vagina	Anal canal and verge, distal rectum plus ant. organ/structure involved	As for T1–3N0–2
T4N1–2 (posterior/lateral adherence or invasion)	Presacrum or pelvic side-walls	Anal canal and verge, distal rectum plus post. or lat. structure involved	As for T1–3N0–2

ant., anterior; post., posterior; lat., lateral

[a] Optional common iliac node inclusion dependent on physician preference of superior extent of irradiation field. If the sacral promontory is chosen for the initial superior field extent, common iliac nodes should be included to 30.6 Gy

[b] Primary tumor plus 3–5 cm margin

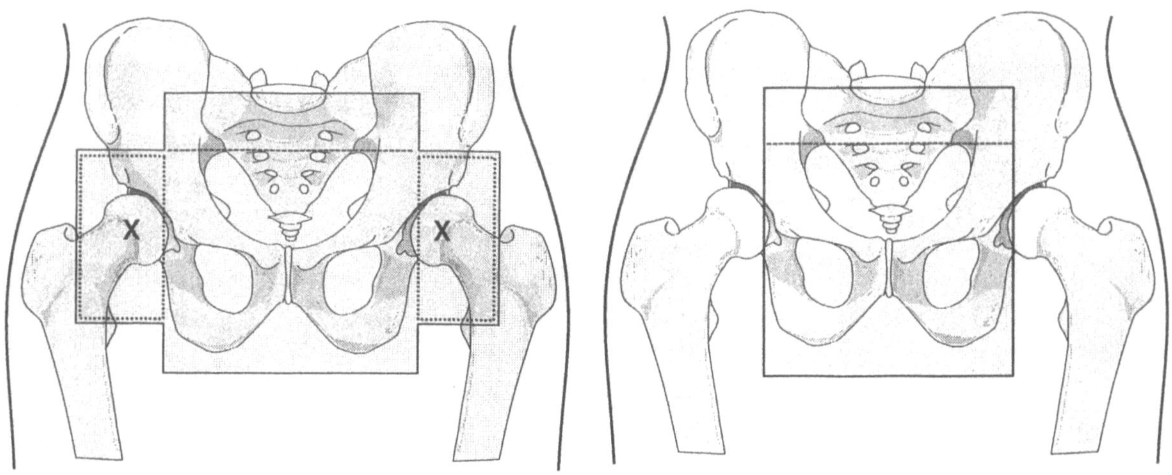

a b

Fig. 10.5. Anal cancer: idealized AP/PA irradiation fields. **a** AP field includes primary tumor plus pelvic and inguinal nodes. Lateral inguinal nodes are brought to prescribed dose with the aid of electron boost fields (*interrupted lines*). **b** PA field includes primary tumor plus pelvic nodes and medial inguinal nodes. From Gunderson et al (1994) with permission

about the sequencing of chemoirradiation and surgical resection.

When rectal cancers extend beyond the rectal wall, they may be adherent to or invade organs with lymphatic drainage to the external iliac nodes (Fig. 10.2c; Table 10.6). These nodes can best be delineated using either LAG or pelvic CT scans (Fig. 10.6b; oral and IV contrast). Since LAG usage is diminished or unavailable in most institutions, pelvic CT is the best and most uniform method of 3-D delineation of the external iliac nodes when they are at risk, and should be included within either the preoperative or postoperative irradiation fields (Fig. 10.6c–g).

Prophylactic nodal areas at risk are usually treated to 45 Gy in 25 fractions of 1.8 Gy with multiple field techniques before irradiation fields are reduced in size. Conformal CT planning is used for both the initial fields and subsequent boost fields. For T_4 lesions it is common to use shrinking field techniques to carry boost 1 to 50.4 Gy (PA and lateral boost of 3×1.8 Gy) and boost 2 to 54 Gy (paired lateral fields for two fractions of 1.8 Gy).

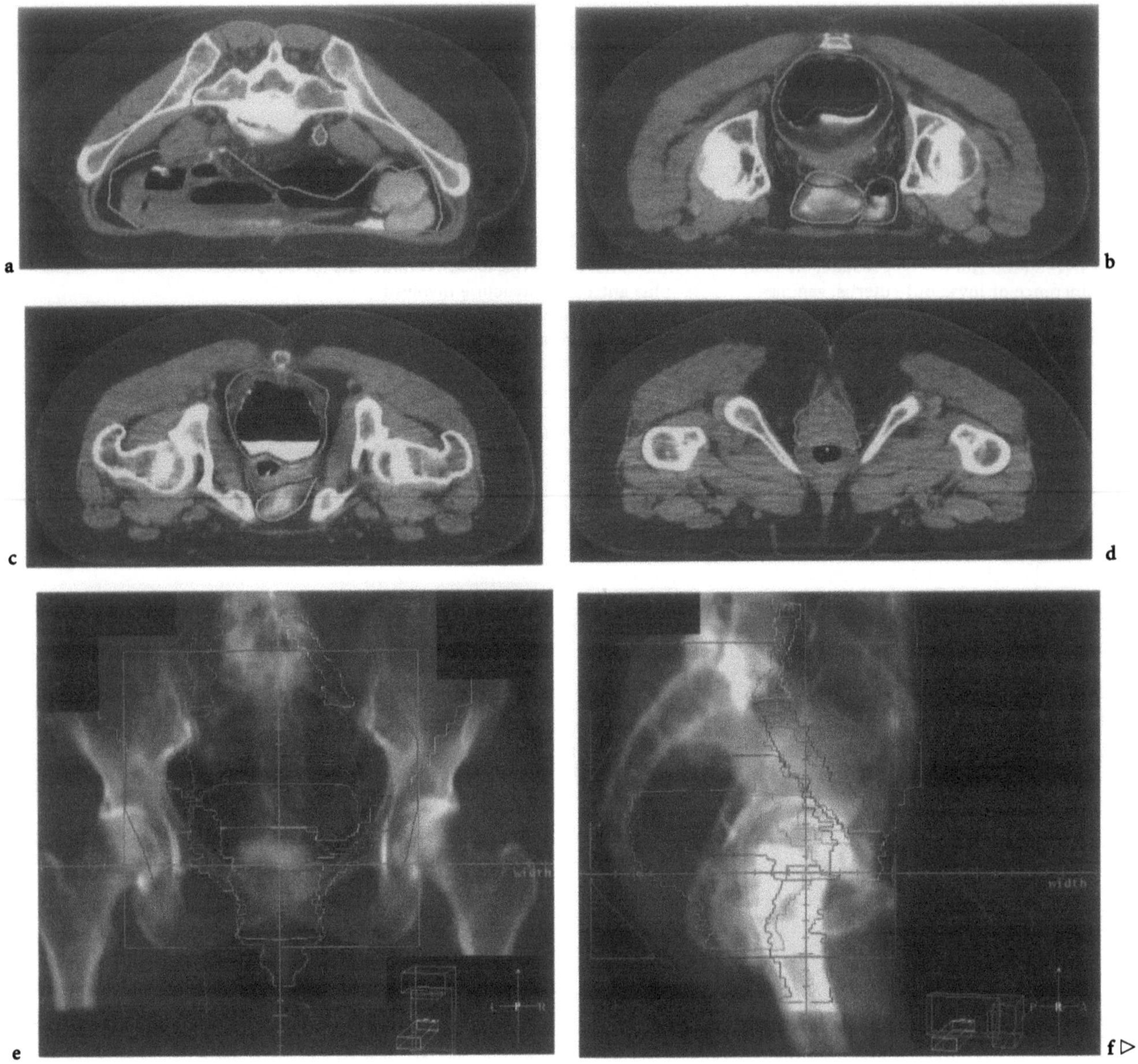

10.5.2 Anal Cancer

Lymphangiograms can be useful in designing the nodal portion of shaped blocks for both AP/PA and lateral fields (Fig. 10.7). In order to decrease the dose to the head and neck of the femur, inguinal nodes can be excluded from the PA field and an anterior electron boost can be used to supplement the dose given to those nodes with the anterior photon field. In patients with uninvolved nodes who are treated with irradiation plus 5-FU–MMC, the inguinal and presacral nodal groups are excluded after a dose of 30 to 36 Gy. The primary lesion plus lower pelvic nodes are then carried to a higher dose with multiple field techniques including lateral fields.

For institutions in which LAGs are unavailable, CT simulation or conformal field design based on CT imaging is the most accurate method of delineation of inguinal and iliac nodes. Delineation of these nodal regions with CT simulation, and construction of fields based on such is shown in Fig. 10.8.

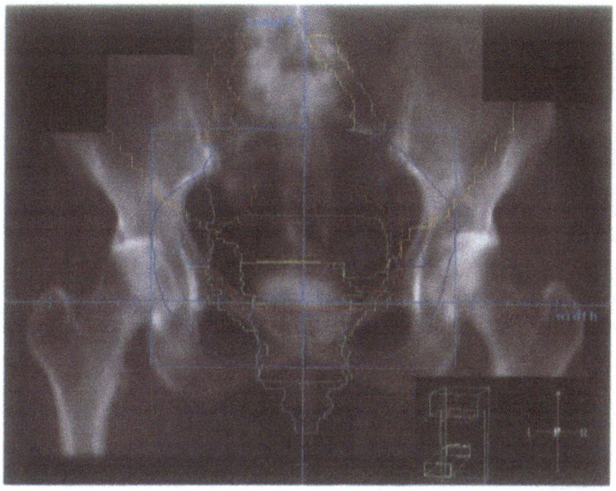

g

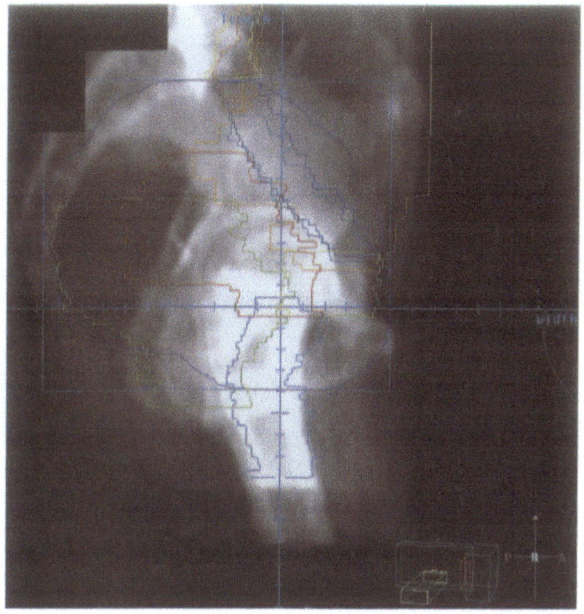

h

Fig. 10.6. Rectal cancer: 3-D delineation of pelvic lymph nodes at risk for lymphatic spread from either primary or locally recurrent rectal cancer and planning of irradiation fields with the aid of digital radiograph reconstruction (DRR). The patient shown in this figure developed a pelvic relapse of a large bowel cancer at the level of the anastomosis that was primarily extraluminal, invaded the apex of the vagina (prior hysterectomy) and abutted the base of the bladder. **a** CT image 32 demonstrates (*left: red-orange; right: yellow*) common iliac vessels along with anterior small bowel loops (*orange*). **b** External iliac nodes are delineated on CT image 65 (*right: dark blue; left: blue-green*); other structures demonstrated include the inferior aspect of the small bowel (*orange*) and the relationship of the recurrent tumor (gross tumor volume: *red*) to the rectal ampulla (*green*) and bladder (*yellow-green*). **c** CT image 74 demonstrates the relationship of recurrent tumor (*red*) to vagina (*blue*), bladder and rectum. **d** CT image 88 shows the distal rectum and vagina. **e, f** Pelvic irradiation fields of PA/AP (PA DRR shown) and paired laterals (right lateral DRR shown) treated to 45 Gy in 25 fractions over 5 weeks. **g, h** Boost field no. 1: PA/AP and paired laterals; 3×1.8 Gy for a total of 50.4 Gy

10.6 Conclusions

Imaged-based 3-D conformal irradiation fields are useful in treating rectal cancer patients. Adjuvant (rectal) or curative (anal) irradiation dose levels can usually be achieved with acceptable morbidity.

For rectal cancer patients, pelvic CT with oral and IV contrast is the most useful imaging modality in delineating both nodal and primary tumor location in 3-D fashion. Prior to resection, transrectal EUS and pelvic magnetic resonance imaging (MRI) can supply additional valuable information for preoperative irradiation treatment planning. For T_4 lesions in which the external iliac nodes are at risk, LAGs yield the most accurate information with regard to both lymphatic channel and nodal location, and can be very useful when available. In the CT simulation era, however, it is likely that LAG-based treatment planning will become obsolete.

Anal cancers are treated with primary chemoirradiation as opposed to adjuvant chemoirradiation, thus allowing the availability of all imaging techniques for irradiation treatment planning. Pelvic CT with IV and oral contrast remains the most useful imaging modality.

For both anal and rectal cancers, the use of dose volume histograms may prove useful in attempting to improve the therapeutic ratio of local control to the tolerance of pelvic structures. After a dose level of 45 Gy in 25 fractions of 1.8 Gy over 5 weeks, use of 3-D planning including evaluation of non-coplanar beams may result in a reduction of field size that allows adequate margins around the tumor (preoperative rectal or primary anal) or tumor bed (postoperative rectal irradiation), yet decreases the volume of bladder and sphincter muscle that is treated to the higher dose levels.

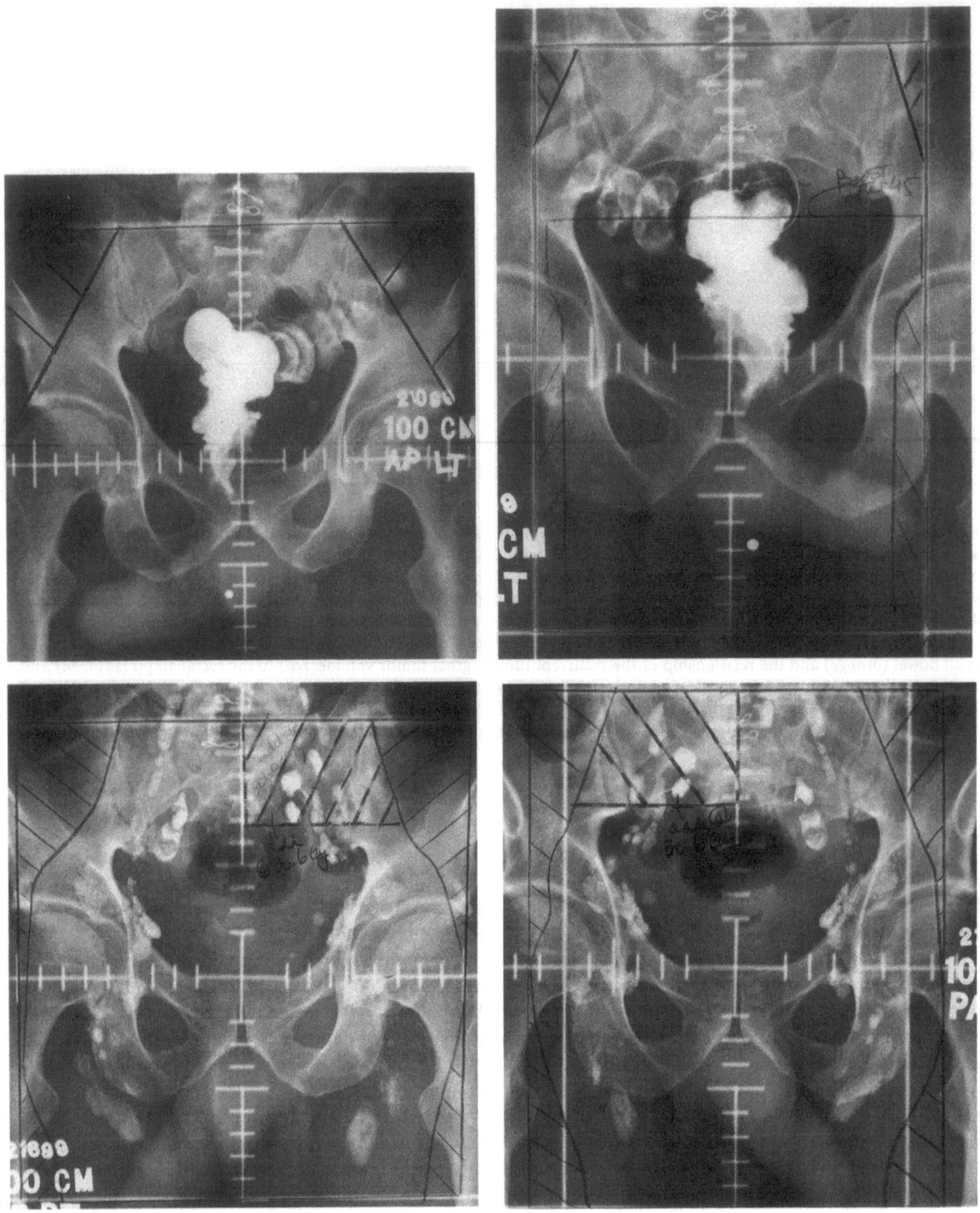

a b c d ▷

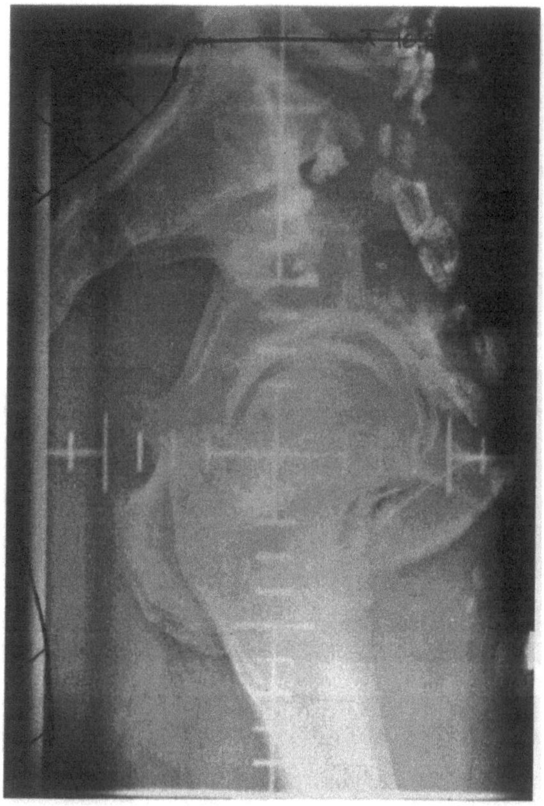

e

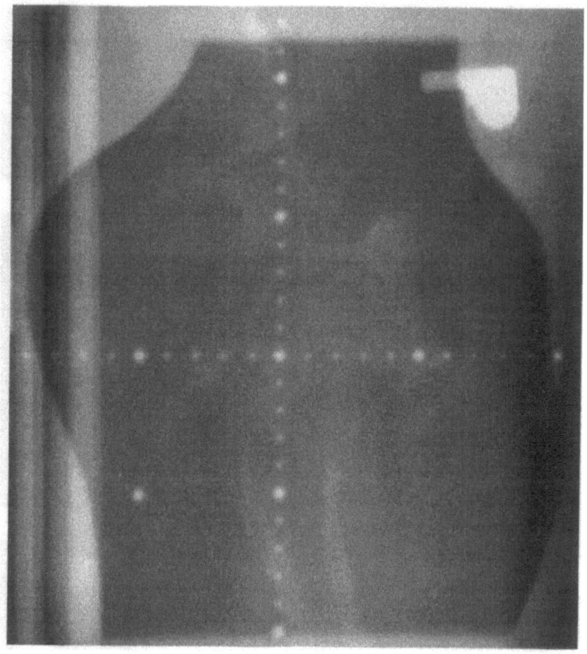

f

Fig. 10.7. Anal cancer: irradiation field design with and without LAG assistance. **a, b** AP and PA field design with anorectal contrast prior to LAG. Had these fields been maintained, an AP electron field would have been designed to supplement lateral inguinal dose (see Fig. 10.5a). **c–e** Modification of AP and PA fields and development of the lateral field after LAG was carried out to demonstrate actual location of nodes. Note filling defect approximately 1.0 cm in diameter in right common iliac node at the inferior level of the sacroiliac (SI) joint (the involved node would have been bisected in institutions that design fields with superior field extent at the bottom of the SI joint). The involved node was kept within boost field no. 1 to the level of 45 Gy in 25 fractions (block added to left common iliac region after 30.6 Gy). **f** Port film of the initial lateral field that demonstrates exact field boundaries (difficult to interpret from simulation image). From Gunderson et al. (2001) with permission

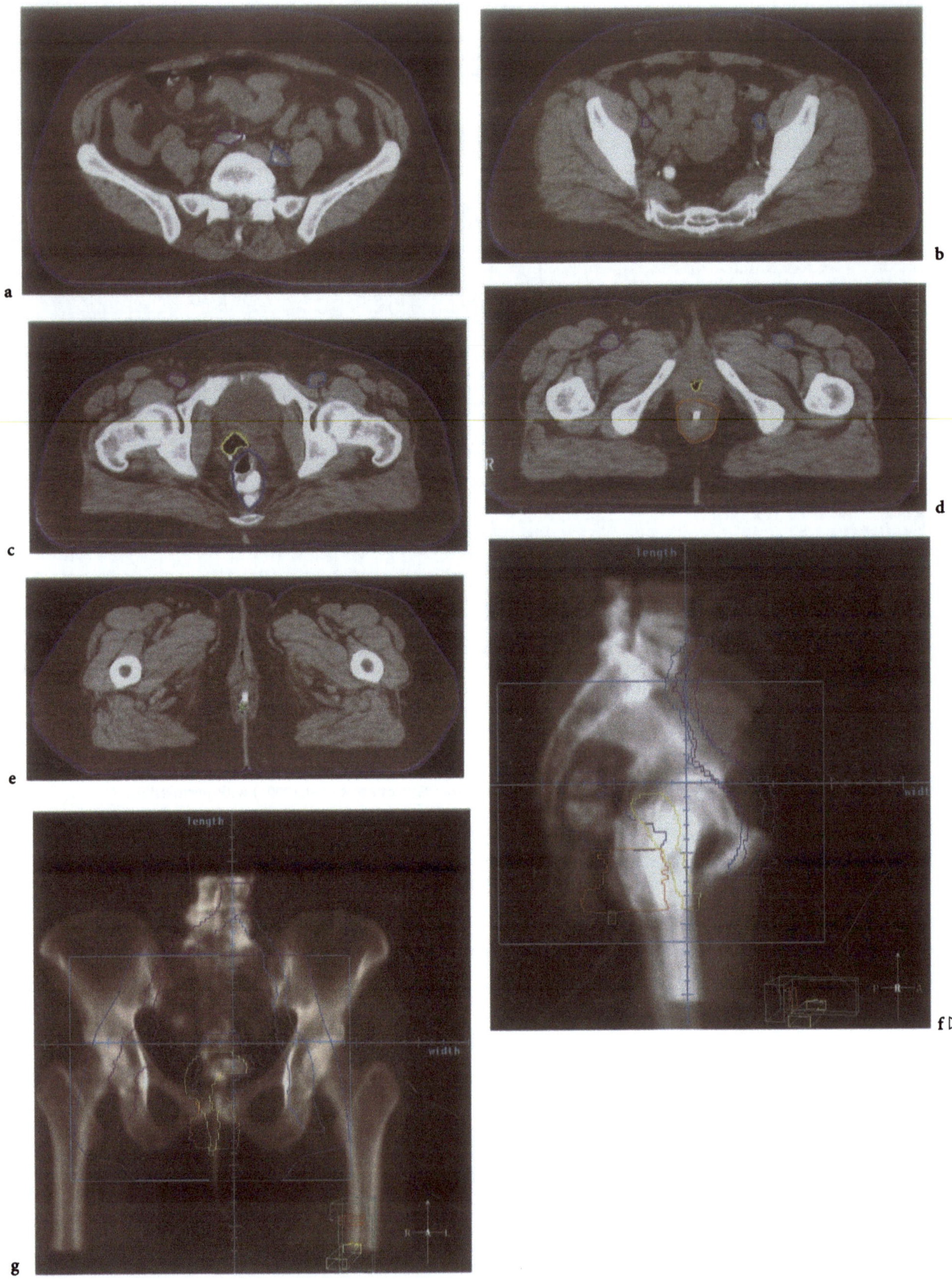
a
b
c
d
e
f ▷
g
length
width

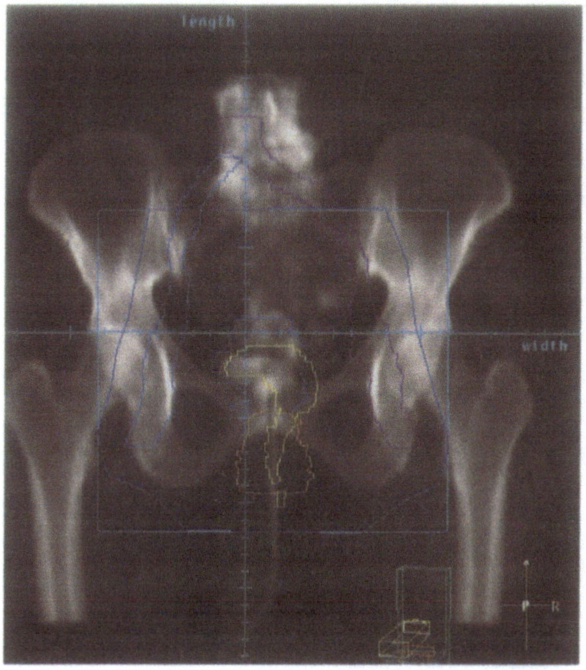

h

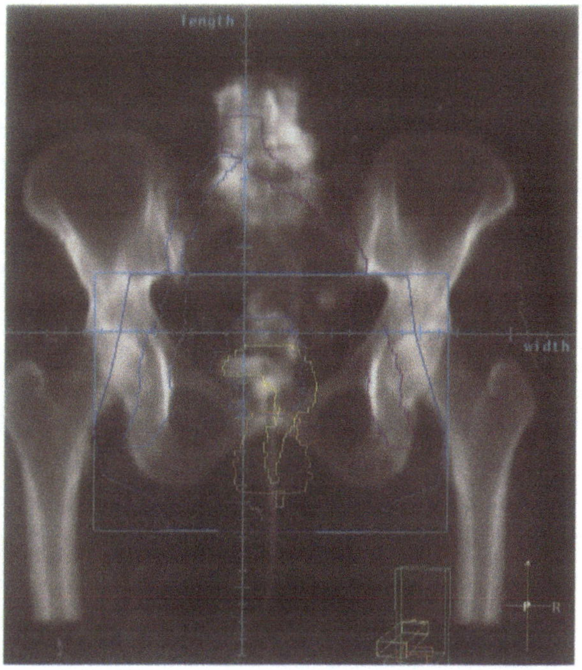

i

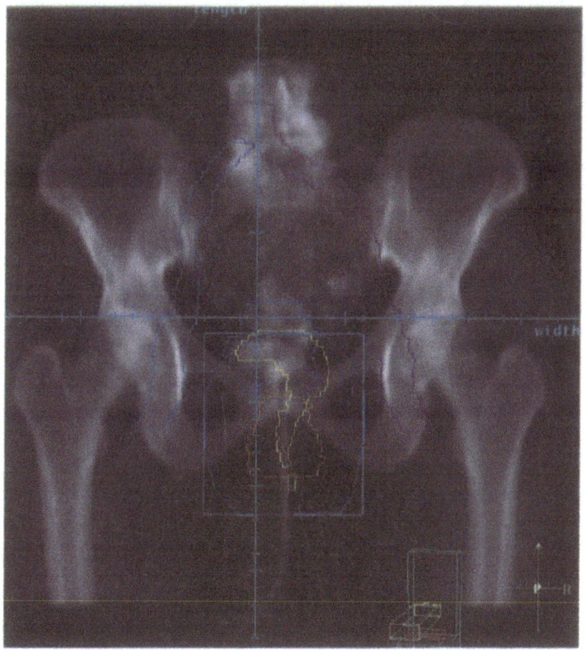

j

Fig. 10.8. Anal cancer: 3-D delineation of nodal areas at risk and primary tumor using CT simulation (**a–e**) and design of irradiation fields with the aid of DRR images (**f–j**). **a** CT image 21: common iliac vessels at the level of upper SI joint (*left: blue; right: purple*). **b** CT image 42 at the level of the inferior aspect of the SI joint where the common iliac vessels have divided into external iliac (*left: blue; right: purple*) and internal iliac (not denoted) **c** CT image 62: vagina (*yellow*) and rectum (*dark blue*) are shown. **d** CT image 74: at the level of mid-anal cancer (GTV: *red-orange*). **e** CT image 82: at the level of the anal verge (*green*), inferior level of the vagina and left and right inguinal regions (*left: blue; right: purple*). **f** Lateral DRR of structures delineated on CT simulation sections. **g, h** Initial AP and PA irradiation fields were designed to include both the external iliac and inguinal regions (nodes plus primary tumor) and treated to 30.6 Gy in 1.8-Gy fractions. Separate anterior electron boost fields were not necessary, since divergence from the PA field was sufficient to include the inguinal vessels/nodes (also shown in Fig. 10.7 with the aid of LAG). **i** In a boost pelvic field, the superior field extent was reduced to the inferior aspect of the SI joint and carried to 36 Gy with AP and PA fields (PA shown). **j** The final boost field to the anal primary lesion plus margin was carried to 45 Gy with AP and PA fields (PA shown)

References

Boman BM, Moertel CG, O'Connell MJ et al (1984) Carcinoma of the anal canal. A clinical and pathologic study of 188 cases. Cancer 54:114–125

Constantinou EC, Daly W, Fung CY et al (1997) Time-dose considerations in the treatment of anal cancer. Int J Radiat Oncol Biol Phys 39:651–657

Cummings BJ, Keane TH, O'Sullivan MB et al (1991) Epidermoid anal cancer: treatment by radiation alone or by radiation and 5-fluorouracil with and without mitomycin C. Int J Radiat Oncol Biol Phys 21:1115–1125

Dukes CE (1943) The surgical pathology of rectal cancer. Proc R Soc Med 37:131–144

Enquist IF, Block IR (1966) Rectal cancer in the female – selection of proper operation based upon anatomic studies of rectal lymphatics. Prog Clin Cancer 2:73–85

Gabriel WB, Dukes C, Bussey HJR (1935) Lymphatic spread in cancer of the rectum. Br J Surg 23:395–413

Grinnell RS (1966) Lymphatic block with atypical and retrograde lymphatic metastasis and spread in carcinoma of the colon and rectum. Ann Surg 163:272–280

Gunderson LL (1987) Colorectal cancer. In: Perez C, Brady L (eds) Principles and practice of radiation oncology, 1st edn. Lippincott, Philadelphia, pp 813–829

Gunderson LL (1999) Indications for and results of combined modality treatment of colorectal cancer. Franz Buschke Lecture – UCSF 17th annual course. Acta Oncol 38:7–21

Gunderson LL, Martenson JA (1991) Cancers of the colon and rectum. In: Levitt S, Khan F, Potish R (eds) Technological basis of radiation therapy, 2nd edn. Lea and Febiger, Philadelphia, pp 342–350

Gunderson LL, Sosin H (1974) Areas of failure found at reoperation (second or symptomatic look) following 'curative surgery' for adenocarcinoma of the rectum: clinicopathologic correlation and implications for adjuvant therapy. Cancer 34:1278–1292

Gunderson LL, Martenson JA, Smalley SR, Garton GR (1994) Lower gastrointestinal cancer: rationale, results and techniques of treatment. Front Radiat Ther Oncol 28:140–154

Gunderson LL, Haddock MG, Burch P et al (2001) Anal cancer. Section in alimentary cancer. In: Rubin P (ed) Clinical oncology, 8th edn. Saunders, Philadelphia, pp 747–761

Hoskins RB, Gunderson LL, Dosoretz D et al (1985) Adjuvant postoperative radiotherapy in carcinoma of the rectum and rectosigmoid. Cancer 55:61–71

Martenson JA, Gunderson LL (1993) Radiation therapy without chemotherapy in the management of cancer of the anal canal. Cancer 71:1736–1740

Nigh SS, Smalley SR, Elman AT et al (1991) Conservative therapy for anal carcinoma: an analysis of prognostic factors. ASTRO proceedings. Int J Radiat Oncol Biol Phys 21:224

Ota DN (2000) Is intraoperative lymph node mapping and sentinel lymph node biopsy for colorectal carcinoma necessary? Ann Surg Oncol 7:82–84

Papillon J, Mayer M, Montbarbon JF et al (1983) A new approach to the management of epidermoid carcinoma of the anal canal. Cancer 51:1830–1837

Rich T, Gunderson LL, Galdabini J et al (1983) Clinical and pathologic factors influencing local failure after curative resection of carcinoma of the rectum and rectosigmoid. Cancer 52:1317–1329

Schild SE, Martenson JA, Gunderson LL et al (1989) Postoperative adjuvant therapy of rectal cancer: an analysis of disease control, survival, and prognostic factors. Int J Radiat Oncol Biol Phys 17:52–62

Sischy B, Doggett RLS, Krall JM et al (1989) Definitive irradiation and chemotherapy for radiosensitization in management of anal carcinoma: interim report on RTOG 83-14. Natl Cancer Inst 81:850–856

Slanetz CA, Herter FP, Grinnell RS (1972) Anterior resection versus abdominoperineal resection for cancer of the rectum and rectosigmoid. Ann J Surg 123:110–117

Suha S, Wiese D, Badin J et al (2000) Technical details of sentinel lymph node mapping in colorectal cancer and its impact on staging. Ann Surg Oncol 7:120–124

11 Target Description for Radiotherapy of Soft Tissue Sarcoma

B. O'Sullivan, J. Wunder, P. W. T. Pisters

CONTENTS

11.1 Introduction

One of the most common yet difficult issues in the treatment of soft tissue sarcoma (STS) is the choice of the radiotherapy (RT) target volume. The existence of a zone of uncertain size and location that may contain subclinical disease in proximity to the presenting site of the primary tumor presents a frequent dilemma. The size and extent of the putative 'risk zone' depends on a number of factors, and taking this into account will affect the target volume chosen for RT. Also, perhaps more than for most cancers, the pathway to appropriate treatment may already have been declared by events that have taken place prior to referral. For example, the type of biopsy that may have already been performed, or a prior inappropriate excision may jeopardize the form and outcome of local treatment thereafter (Mankin et al. 1996). In addition, the choice of target volume may also be influenced by the type of reconstruction chosen following tumor resection. In fact numerous factors may impact on the local management of STS with RT and surgery, a more complete account of which is available (O'Sullivan et al. 1999).

This discussion will focus on practical issues faced by the sarcoma specialist (especially surgeons and radiation oncologists), whose task is to determine the optimal management of the tissues at risk of harboring local disease or regional lymph node involvement. Most of our comments will address RT treatment planning with contemporary computerized tomographic (CT) planning, assuming the

B. O'Sullivan, MD, FRCPC
Department of Radiation Oncology, Princess Margaret Hospital, University Health Network, University of Toronto, Toronto, Canada
J. Wunder, MD, FRCSC
Department of Surgical Oncology, Princess Margaret Hospital, University Health Network, University of Toronto, Toronto, Canada *and* University Musculoskeletal Oncology Unit, Mount Sinai Hospital, University of Toronto, Toronto, Canada
P. W. T. Pisters, MD, FACS
Department of Surgery, University of Texas M.D. Anderson Cancer Center, Houston, Texas, USA

availability of CT simulation and the capabilities provided by virtual fluoroscopy and simulation, digitally reconstructed radiographs (DRR) and beam eye views (BEV), and three-dimensional surface rendering of images as shown in sample cases.

Throughout, it is emphasized that multidisciplinary assessment is of paramount importance and should be accompanied by a comprehensive review of imaging and pathology studies, in addition to the clinical issues in the individual case. The latter include a detailed appraisal of relevant anatomic issues, most optimally addressed in the clinic or at a multidisciplinary tumor conference before any treatment intervention takes place. It is also notable that the target tissues for RT planning are also those for surgical planning if RT is not being used. In fact the approach taken by the radiation oncologist should be practically and conceptually identical to the planning considerations taken into account by surgeons treating the same disease. For STS, RT is generally used to permit more conservative tissue resections and therefore less extensive operations than would have ordinarily been the case. This concept will be repeated in the deliberations surrounding decisions about which tissues need to be treated either with RT or surgery.

11.2 Overview of RT STS Planning

11.2.1 Evidence About RT Coverage in STS

No formal verification or assessment of target volumes has been introduced in the management of STS, at least using contemporary hypothesis-solving techniques such as comparative clinical trials. At the same time the unprecedented improvements in treatment planning and delivery that have recently become available are likely to be used in STS planning where individualized approaches have always been desirable. These improvements have been made possible by technical innovation in digital imaging processing and fusion techniques, as well as dose calculation software and exceptional new hardware for treatment delivery and quality assurance. For this reason, some of the principles and concepts outlined in this chapter should be regarded as provisional since further implementation of techniques regarding the treatment of STS is likely in the near future. Among the notable advances are conformal beam approaches and intensity modulated radiotherapy (IMRT) which can be expected to lend themselves to specific aspects of the management of STS subsites because of the clear advantages provided by reduction and shaping of target volumes and minimizing radiation dose (Jones et al. 2002; O'Sullivan et al. 1999, 2002a).

11.2.2 Primary Tumor Coverage

Until very recently, planning has almost exclusively employed wide field approaches that have remained unchanged for decades (Tepper et al. 1982). Advances in imaging techniques and the knowledge of outcome in some disease paradigms where different volumes are used [e.g. the use of brachytherapy (BRT) where RT volumes have tended to be significantly smaller than those with external beam techniques] (Pisters et al. 1996), challenge us to revise our concepts about what should be the appropriate target volume in STS RT planning. This is important because evidence is emerging from recent controlled data that the outcome may be different depending on volumes and doses of RT used in STS RT delivery (O'Sullivan et al. 2002a). Additional technical innovations, including the availability of magnetic resonance (MR) simulation in the near future should further facilitate changes in RT targeting because of the superior capability of MR imaging (MRI) in demonstrating soft tissue anatomy, including target (i.e. diseased) and normal tissues. At the same time, the challenge will remain that of developing new approaches appropriately, with attention to ensuring that disease control is not compromised if traditional RT target volumes are reduced and refined. Preferably these developments should take place in a prospective controlled manner.

11.2.3 Lymph Node Coverage

An important consideration in defining target volumes for RT is the unusually low risk of regional node involvement for most histologic subtypes of STS. Because of this, the chapter will not emphasize lymph node management in the same way as many non-sarcoma disease descriptions where the risk of nodal disease is much higher. However, the principles of anatomic delineation of potential lymph node involvement would be expected to follow those of other diseases. In addition, despite their rarity, the large range of possibilities for regional lymphatic involvement extends far beyond the scope of this text due to the great variation in anatomic heterogeneity presented by STS. Nonetheless, examples of lymph node delineation will take into account issues of histologic specificity, principles of anatomic pathways of lymph node involvement, or established descriptions of lymph zones at risk which have already been documented for some anatomic regions such as the head and neck (GREGOIRE et al. 2000; NOWAK et al. 1999; WIJERS et al. 1999).

11.3 Target Delineation: Outlining the Principles

11.3.1 Indications for Combined Treatment

RT is ordinarily used in combination with surgical approaches intended to achieve conservative resections in STS (O'SULLIVAN et al. 1999). The alternative would require amputation or functionally debilitating surgery in the case of limb lesions, or substantial ablation with structural, functional or cosmetic deficits in other anatomic sites (STOTTER et al. 1990). However, it should be recognized that superficial lesions and smaller 'contained' lesions confined to individual muscles, at least in expert hands, may be managed with surgery alone (see Table 11.1 and Fig. 11.1) (RYDHOLM et al. 1991). In contrast, evidence strongly suggests that for most other situations surgery which does not achieve wide clearance through normal tissue has a significantly higher rate of local failure. Even in some small lesions adverse outcomes may be observed (FLEMING et al. 1999), although the literature on this subject is controversial concerning the benefit from the addition of RT in small (<5 cm) high-grade lesions (ALEKTIAR et al. 2002). Nevertheless, the benefit of adjuvant RT with conservative surgical resection in a large number of STS cases has been demonstrated in three recent randomized clinical trials (O'SULLIVAN et al. 2002a; PISTERS et al. 1996; YANG et al. 1998).

Table 11.1. Surgery alone for selected STS*

Author (year)	Center	No.	Selection	L Fail	D Fail
GEER et al. (1992)	MSKCC	117	T1, primary	8%	5%
RYDHOLM et al. (1991)	Lund	56	«Contained» clear margin	7%	NR
KARAKOUSIS et al. (1986)**	Roswell	116	2 cm margin	10%	NR
BALDINI et al. (1999)	Harvard	74	Not specified	7%	12%
FABRIZIO et al. (2000)	Mayo	34	Not specified	20%	14%

* Lower metastatic rates than is typical for STS, implying selection of favorable cases

** Additional cases receiving RT had a worse outcome in some series

L Fail: local failure rate; *D Fail:* distant failure rate; *NR:* not reported

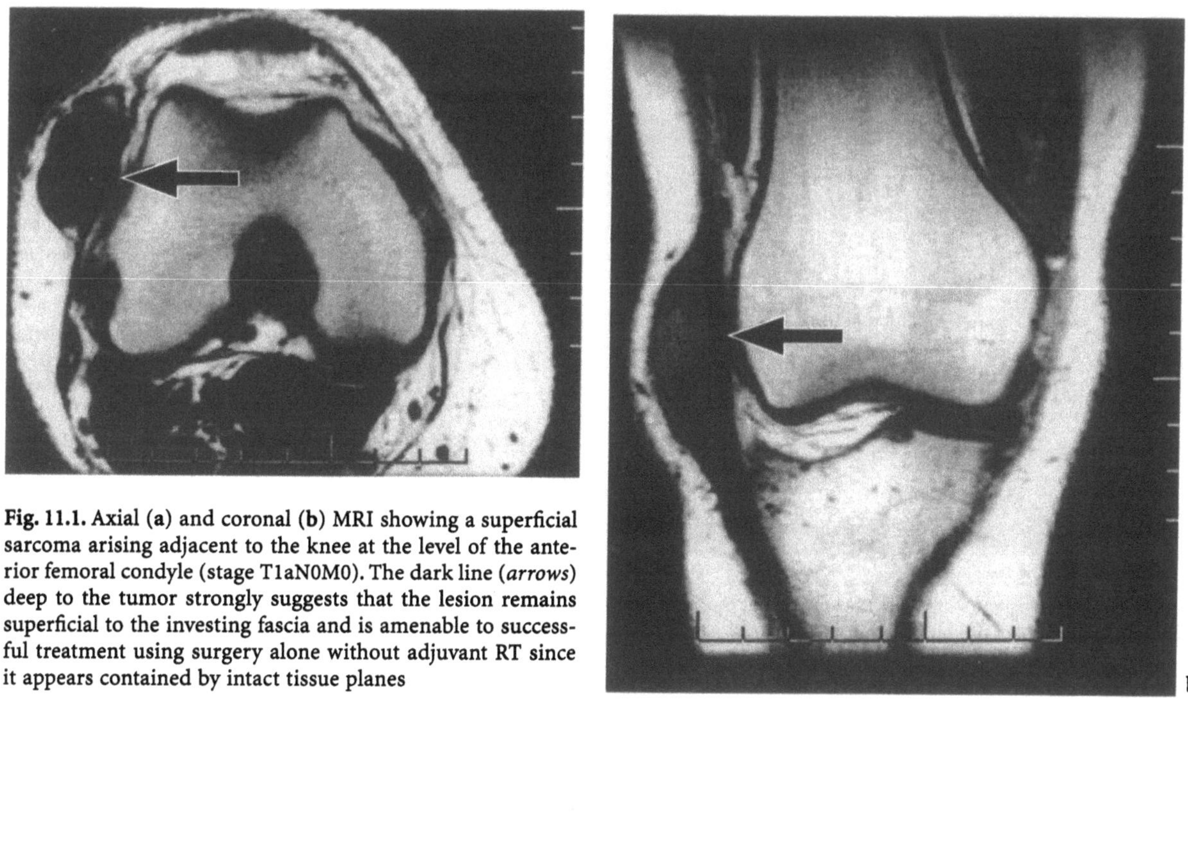

a

b

Fig. 11.1. Axial (**a**) and coronal (**b**) MRI showing a superficial sarcoma arising adjacent to the knee at the level of the anterior femoral condyle (stage T1aN0M0). The dark line (*arrows*) deep to the tumor strongly suggests that the lesion remains superficial to the investing fascia and is amenable to successful treatment using surgery alone without adjuvant RT since it appears contained by intact tissue planes

11.3.2 'Unplanned' Excision

About one-third of new patients referred to a specialized center may well have undergone an 'unplanned' excision with wound contamination by tumor (NORIA et al. 1996). Typically imaging will not have been performed prior to surgery and the sarcoma specialist evaluating the patient will often have difficulty in deciding the exact site of tumor origin, the extent of the original surgical field, or the actual zone of contamination. This differs from the positive microscopic resection margin which may occur along critical structures (e.g. major nerve, vessel, bone) following a planned attempt at complete resection by the sarcoma specialist as part of multidisciplinary care with combined surgery and RT (GERRAND et al. 2001). In the 'unplanned' resection, there is likely to be a substantial amount of residual tumor in the wound, although this is rarely detectable by CT scan or MRI.

Whether or not to recommend postoperative (or preoperative) radiation in this situation is not always certain. If microscopic evidence of sarcoma is identified following re-excision of the initial surgical bed and area of risk, RT is generally recommended unless particularly extensive surgery has been undertaken after specialist assessment. Sarcoma can spread a considerable distance into the surrounding soft tissues following an 'unplanned' resection and it is often difficult to be sure that all contaminated tissue has been excised (see Fig. 11.2). Therefore, patients with this referral pattern usually require RT because of inadvertent seeding in the wound, even if the presenting lesion was small and confined prior to the attempted resection (O'SULLIVAN et al. 2002b). The principles in the choice of RT volumes should be those outlined below for either preoperative or postoperative RT. However the preoperative volumes differ compared to the usual practice for the surgically 'naive' case, and should be extended further in an attempt to include an appropriate margin surrounding all surgically violated tissues in addition to the tumor.

11.3.3 Determinants of Extent of RT Targets

11.3.3.1 RT Planning Principles in STS

The basic premise in RT planning is to initially define a gross tumor volume (GTV) on a series of thin slice

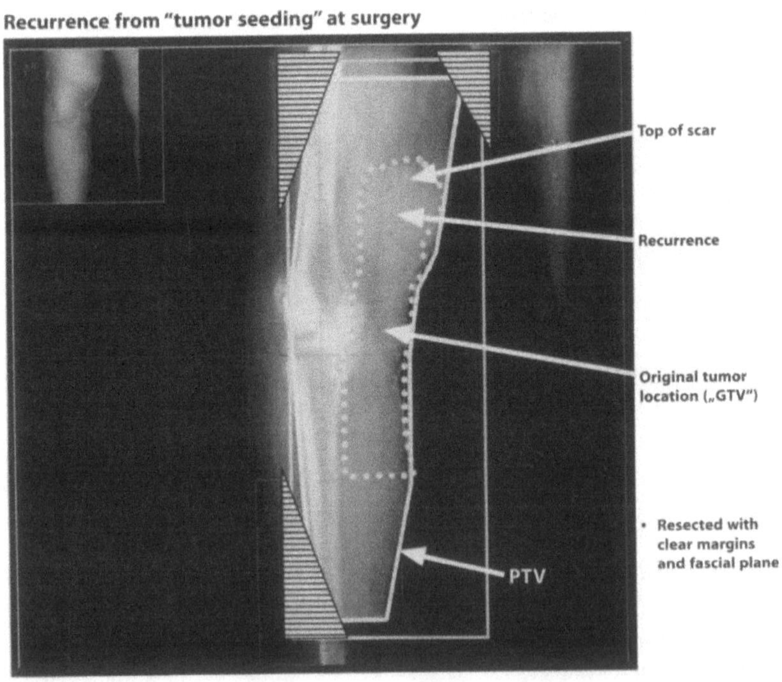

Fig. 11.2. Recurrent high-grade sarcoma presenting at the proximal limit of a previous surgical field. This patient initially underwent an 'unplanned' excision for a tumor limited to the popliteal fossa (see text for details; Sect. 11.3.2). Because of coexisting diabetes and peripheral vascular disease RT was not performed due to concern about unacceptable sequelae including problematic and prolonged wound breakdown. Instead, surgery was performed with preservation of the neurovascular structures and clear surgical resection margins. A subsequent recurrence is located at a considerable distance from the original high-risk area, indicating the degree of contamination possible from an unplanned excision. The location of the recurrence adjacent to the scar can be seen on the 3D surface image (see *insert*). This figure also shows the planned field borders to provide preoperative RT in an attempt to salvage this case. A putative target volume (*dotted line*) is indicated, encompassing the known recurrence as well as the likely risk area of the previous unplanned excision that includes the original GTV location. Although no disease is evident at this site, the area was considered at high risk. The area intended to receive a RT dose capable of eradicating microscopic foci of sarcoma (50 Gy in 25 fractions) is illustrated by the PTV that encompasses a CTV with a margin for additional security. The cross-hatching indicates shielding blocks for beam shaping, although multileaf collimation is frequently used in contemporary treatment delivery

CT scans used for dose volume delineation. An appropriate margin is then placed around the GTV to encompass tissues at risk of harboring microscopic disease (the clinical target volume or CTV) (ICRU Report 1993, 1999). Beyond the CTV, an additional zone is outlined to account for uncertainties in treatment delivery (termed the planning target volume or PTV; see below) (ICRU Report 1993, 1999). Strictly, in the postoperative setting no actual GTV exists. However, the principle of initially contouring the high-risk area (i.e. original site of disease with or without postoperative changes; see Sect. 11.5.1.2) remains sound and facilitates subsequent contouring of the CTV on the RT planning CT slices.

Soft tissue sarcomas tend to spread in a longitudinal direction within the muscle groups of the extremity. They generally respect barriers to tumor spread in the axial plane of the extremity such as bone, interosseous membrane, major fascial planes, etc. Thus the margins of RT must be wide in the cephalo-caudal direction but in the cross section there may be much greater security in defining non-target structures. For non-extremity lesions, the direction of sarcoma growth is also along the involved musculature, but care must be taken to ensure that the fascial planes are appropriately recognized and encompassed in the radiation target volume.

11.3.3.2
Principle of Fascial Containment (e.g. Thigh)

A complete description of all the body's anatomic planes and fascial compartments is not possible in this chapter. This is unfortunate, since they determine to a large extent the principles used to manage these lesions and why there exists such heterogeneity, individualization and complexity in planning STS. However, for discussion of the most common STS case, that normally found in the proximal thigh, attention will be paid to the anatomy of this region. In turn, this will illustrate some of the concepts in treatment planning with broad applicability to other sites.

The fascia of the thigh invests the whole of this region of the limb, although its thickness may vary in different parts. It is particularly dense in the region of the upper and lateral thigh, where it is intimately associated with the insertions of both the gluteus maximus and the tensor fascia lata muscles. Medially and proximally, it is much more attenuated, readily revealing underlying muscle structures. The lateral side coalesces to form the iliotibial tract, stretching from the iliac crest to the lateral tibial plateau. The fascial structures in this region are important because they divide the thigh into three osteofascial compartments, each containing a muscle unit with its nerve (the extensor/quadriceps group anteriorly and the femoral nerve; the flexor/hamstring group posteriorly and the sciatic nerve; the medially located adductor muscles and the obturator nerve) (see Fig. 11.3a, b). The three thigh compartments are created by the passage of three intermuscular septa from the fascia investing the external contour of the muscle to the linea aspera on the posterior aspect of the femur (see Fig. 11.3b). Termed the lateral, medial, and posterior intermuscular septa, they are of varying strength and consistency. The lateral septum is strong and represented by a fibrous partition separating the vastus lateralis and intermedius from the short head of the biceps femoris, one of the posteriorly located hamstring muscles (see Fig. 11.3b). The other two septa are represented only by thin fascial layers on the front and back of the adductor muscles. The medial septum is anterior to the adductor brevis, longus and magnus muscles and the posterior septum is the thin layer between the adductor magnus and the hamstrings.

The importance of the osteofascial compartments of the thigh is that, from an anatomic standpoint, they operate as functional units and are protected from each others' risks of tumor contamination provided inappropriate violation of the septa has not taken place. The latter may occur as a result of misplaced surgical intrusion, including inappropriate placement of drain or biopsy tracts (Mankin et al. 1996). Thus the septa provide sanctuary containment of tumor in the radial direction and uncontaminated compartments may be protected from both high-dose radiation and surgical interventions. It is usual to limit the target to include the adjacent septum to ensure coverage of an involved compartment. Longitudinally, tumor tends to track along within the compartment of origin while respecting adjacent fascial boundaries (Fig. 11.4).

In general, within the compartments of the thigh, individual muscles are intimately related to one another and may share musculoaponeurotic structures as well as neurovascular supply. We would not normally regard these individual muscles as independently free of risk of involvement by infiltrating tumor within adjacent muscles in the same compartment, except in the case of rare small contained lesions without extramuscular extension. Of the latter exceptions, the sartorius muscle, in addition to being the longest muscle in the body, is a narrow ribbon-like muscle crossing the thigh diagonally from the hip laterally to the knee medially. The sartorius possesses it own fascia, thereby

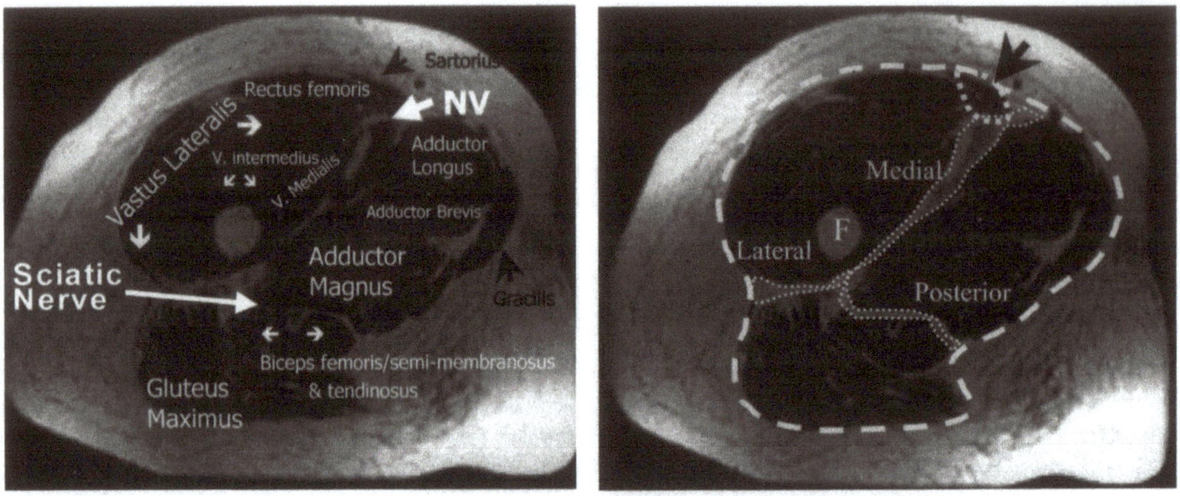

a b

Fig. 11.3. a Cross-sectional anatomy of the proximal thigh in the supine position indicating the principal contents of the region (labels generally indicate names of muscles) including the femoral neurovascular structures (*NV*) anterior to the adductor longus. The sciatic nerve (*long white arrow*) is not seen as readily, but lies between the adductor magnus muscle belly and the hamstring group of muscles posteriorly. The unlabeled obturator nerve is sandwiched between the bodies of the adductor magnus and brevis and is exceptional among the three major nerves of the region in not being contained within one of the intermuscular septa shown in part b of this figure. **b** Axial MRI of the proximal thigh in part a of this figure showing the three osteofascial compartments created by the passage of 'medial', 'lateral', and 'posterior' intermuscular septa (*stippled areas* and *lines*) extending from the fascia investing the external contour of the muscle (*dashed line*) to the linea aspera on the posterior aspect of the femur (*F*). The investing fascia also separates the region into superficial and deep compartments. The importance of the osteofascial compartments of the thigh is that they are protected from each other's risks of tumor contamination provided disruption of the septa has not taken place. Note that the sartorius is protected by its own fascia (*dotted line* and *arrow*)

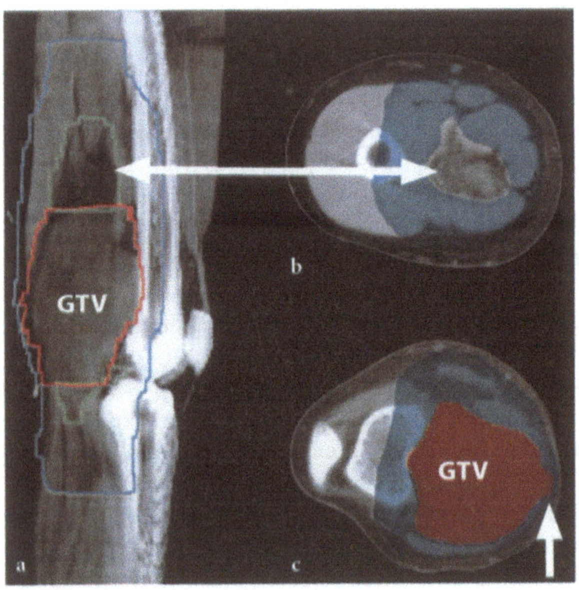

Fig. 11.4. A digitally reconstructed radiograph (**a**) and two axial CT slices (**b, c**) from a virtually 'fluoroscoped' three-dimensional treatment plan for a sarcoma arising in the popliteal fossa. The normal tissue isodense GTV is evident, tracking longitudinally in the compartment of origin (depicted in *red*; **a, c**). In addition, proximal and distal lower isodense peritumoral edema are shown (in *green*; **a**) and have been left colorless (**b**) to exhibit the density difference from normal muscle in the proximal part of the target (*long double-headed arrow*). In this case, the CTV includes a 5-cm margin beyond the limit of the peritumoral edema. Note that the GTV and CTV are extended posteriorly (*arrowhead*; **c**) because of a biopsy located in this region (see Sect. 11.5.2)

facilitating complex action (flexion of the leg on the thigh, the thigh on the pelvis, as well as thigh abduction and lateral rotation). Lesions originating in the sartorius often present relatively early in the disease course, and if small may occasionally be successfully managed with resection of the muscle body and its independent surrounding fascia without need for RT (see Fig. 11.3b). A similar situation may also exist for small tumors confined to the tensor fascia muscle as well as the gluteus maximus.

The fascial structures are also important throughout the body because they create similar compartments to those in the thigh and also separate tumors arising superficially to the fascia investing the muscles of the region (see dashed line; Fig. 11.3b). Such tumors arising in subcutaneous (s.c.) tissues are classified as 'T' subcategory 'a' lesions in the 'TNM' classification (Greene et al. 2002; Sobin and Wittekind 2002) (Fig. 11.1), as opposed to those arising deep to the fascia, the so-called 'T' subcategory 'b' lesions Greene et al. 2002; Sobin and Wittekind 2002). The same treatment principles operate as those for deep lesions involving the muscular compartments. Most specifically, inappropriate violation of the fascia should not take place because tumors can ordinarily be considered to involve either the superficial compartment or the deep compartment, but rarely both. In the event that the fascia overlying the muscle has been disrupted or removed, as is often the case following an 'unplanned' sarcoma resection with positive margins, it may provide a route for deep contamination with tumor. In this case, re-excision, RT, or frequently both may be required, and RT should generously include the deep compartment together with the original s.c. tissue site. For most superficial ('Ta' subtype) sarcomas, the clinician's main preoccupation is with radial margins, since the tumor may liberally extend in these directions. The deep margin can be safely secured by either: (1) resecting the lesion *en bloc* with the investing fascia which acts as a 'wide' deep resection margin; or (2) alternatively, performing RT after a negative but not wide margin excision of the lesion in which the fascia remains intact. In this latter situation, RT coverage only needs to encompass the superficial tumor region widely with the underlying fascia, but not the deeper muscle compartment. We would stress, however, that RT is not ordinarily indicated in the presence of adequate resection margins, irrespective of pathologic features including grade, since the principle of anatomic containment and tissue protection should govern the use of the local treatment modalities.

11.3.3.3
Uncertainties regarding Anatomic Principles

It is important to be aware of the different and numerous variations between the different anatomic locations of the body, any of which could be involved by a primary STS. As mentioned, this is beyond the scope of this text. Nevertheless some specific anatomic issues in STS management merit comment. In small deep tumors, unperturbed involvement of the peripheral limb circumference may permit RT volumes to be concentrated at the central and diseased area of the limb, with tissue sparing at selected peripheral areas. This principle may be particularly useful in rare instances where tumors may arise from a fascial boundary or intermuscular septum. The principle is virtually impossible to observe in the postoperative setting with any confidence, for the reasons discussed below (see Sect. 11.4.2). For lesions arising adjacent to the interosseous membranes that separate the anterior and posterior compartments in the forearm and leg, penetrating vascular structures may provide a route for tumor transgression (or peritumoral edema; see Sect. 11.5.1.2) from one compartment to another, and this needs to be accounted for in planning (see Fig. 11.5). Also, iatrogenic surgical misadventure may also lead to involvement of multiple compartments. In these circumstances it may not be possible to choose an appropriate tissue region to spare from high-dose RT, and more extensive surgery and RT need to be considered with the attendant risk of substantial functional loss (O'Sullivan et al. 1999).

In some situations fascial planes may not exist, and a sufficient margin is required within immediately adjacent normal tissues to encompass the GTV, even though these may not contain gross or

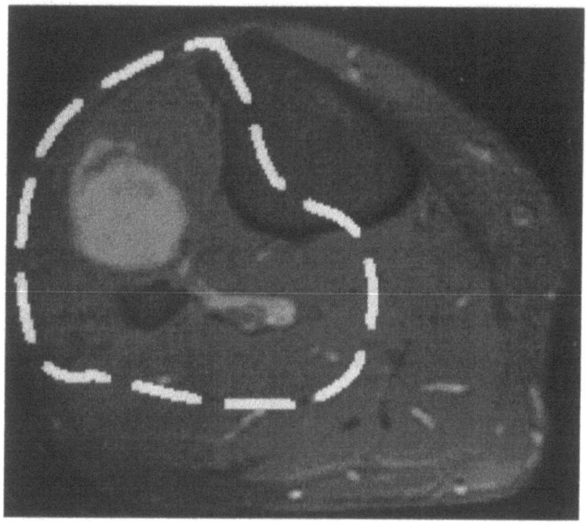

Fig. 11.5. Axial MRI showing a soft tissue sarcoma of the pretibial region. Peritumoral edema can be seen transgressing the interosseous membrane. The CTV is shown for this case treated with preoperative RT (*dashed line*) and takes account of the additional unexpected extension to the posterior leg compartment

microscopic disease. Typically this may be the case in the preoperative RT of tumors which extend into the abdominal or thoracic cavities (e.g. retroperitoneal sarcomas; see Fig. 11.6). Generally for such situations it is useful to exploit any advantage that may be present: for example, inclusion of the non-perturbed peritoneal surface of retroperitoneal tumors within the target volume since the tumor may still be contained by this barrier. This is discussed below under 'Retroperitoneal sarcoma' (see Sect. 11.7.2).

An additional feature in RT target delineation concerns that of allowance for uncertainties in set-up and treatment delivery. The latter may be particularly relevant in anatomical areas affected by respiratory movement (e.g. abdominal and thoracic areas) in contrast to limb and head and neck sites where such movement does not apply to the same extent, and immobilization methods can be readily used to facilitate set-up and treatment delivery. In either case, clinical judgment is needed to determine the extent of additional margin required to account for uncertainties, and this volume should be defined around the CTV as the PTV. In the remainder of the chapter the discussion will generally focus on the GTV and CTV, but the PTV must also be considered in appropriate planning considerations.

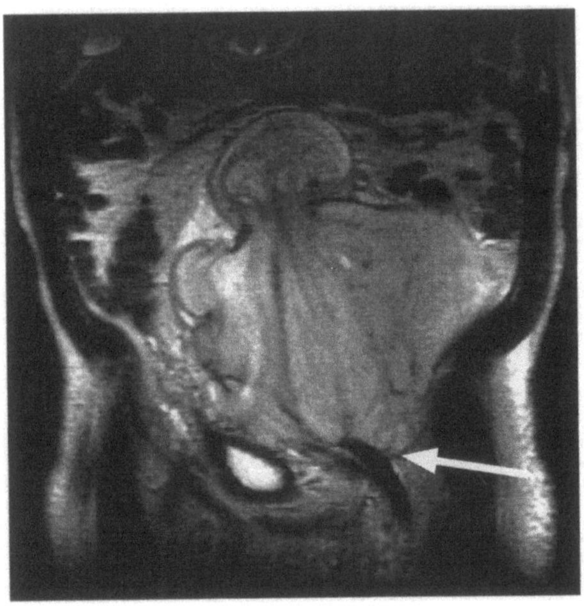

Fig. 11.6. Coronal view MRI of a retroperitoneal sarcoma involving the abdomen and pelvis with extension into the inguinal region. Encasement of the external iliac and femoral artery (*arrow*) needs to be accounted for in the RT planning and surgery of this case. Preoperative RT planning for this case is also shown in Fig. 11.14

11.4 Scheduling RT

11.4.1 'Shrinking Field Technique'

The classical external beam approach consists of delivering at least two phased volumes of treatment, especially when using postoperative RT. Generally an initial Phase 1 volume is chosen for treatment to a dose capable of sterilizing microscopic disease (e.g. equivalent to 50 Gy in 2 Gy per fraction delivered over 5 weeks). Following this, a 'reducing field' strategy may deliver a 'boost' of 10–16 Gy. In most institutions, the total dose from both phases (60–66 Gy, or a biologically equivalent fractionation) is administered in the postoperative setting. In preoperative RT, the most usual dose approximates 50 Gy in 25 fractions to the Phase 1 volume and a postoperative boost (10–16 Gy) is generally restricted to cases with positive resection margins.

In cases where the postoperative boost would exceed the tolerance of regional anatomic structures, the former may not be administered, or may be given using BRT. Our comments will focus on outlining principles in defining the Phase 1 volumes for both preoperative and postoperative RT. Phase 2 'boost' volumes are not described in detail since they are the most variable depending on institutional practice, and our earlier general comments about verification of target volumes are even more relevant in this setting. However, they should comprise reduction of the Phase 1 volume to include the immediate region of the surgical bed and scar that is at greatest risk with a minimum CTV coverage of the high-risk area of least a 1 cm margin. Typically a 2 cm coverage of the surgical bed and the scar is employed. In some protocols, a third phase may be added to a very small 'boost' region for the final two or three fractions to further minimize the risk of late toxicity (Lindberg et al. 1981).

One dilemma concerns the volume to consider when delivering a Phase 2 field reduction in the uncommon case already treated with preoperative RT. This postoperative boost is usually restricted to situations with positive resection margins following preoperative RT, and it is administered after the wound is fully healed. However, whether to administer a large volume sufficient to encompass the entire postoperative surgical field or restrict the volume to the original Phase 1 region used preoperatively has not yet been determined. Our practice is to use a postoperative Phase 2 volume that is similar to the initial preoperative volume and concentrate particularly on the area of the 'positive' margin. The rationale for this is that any tumor cells that may have migrated to other regional areas will have already received a 'microscopic' dose of RT preoperatively, and the goal of the 'boost' is to enhance the local control in the area of greatest risk where the margin was positive, while minimizing the high-dose target volume because of the potential for RT damage to these tissues (O'Sullivan et al. 2002). It is also of interest that the value of the post-operative 'boost' following preoperative radiotherapy itself remains unproven, and there is evidence that patients who electively do not receive this phase may have satisfactory outcome (Tanabe et al. 1994) in addition to cases where it was omitted because of wound healing problems (Sadoski et al. 1993; Wilson et al. 1994). As noted below, this phase of treatment is often intentionally omitted when treating disease in the vicinity of critical organs that may be injured by doses exceeding 50 Gy (e.g. the base of the skull, paraspinal, intrathoracic or intra-abdominal lesions).

Table 11.2. Relative advantages and disadvantages for postoperative and preoperative external beam RT in the management of STS

Postoperative RT

- No potential added problems with impaired wound healing over baseline risk (about 15% risk for postoperative RT in a randomized trial; O'Sullivan et al. 2002a)
- Final margins available to help determine need for RT
- Less requirement for preoperative multidisciplinary assessment (an operational advantage of dubious benefit)
- Increased late tissue morbidity (dose and volume related) evident in a randomized trial (O'Sullivan and Davis 2001)

Preoperative RT

- Well-defined treatment volume – better tissue sparing possible
- Better blood supply – possibly lower dose needed to control disease
- Increased risk to wound healing compared to postoperative phase (risk confined to lower extremity in a randomized trial; O'Sullivan et al. 2002a)
- Potential to reduce micrometastasis, may confer survival advantage (O'Sullivan et al. 2002a)
- Requires preoperative multidisciplinary assessment (major benefit)

11.4.2 Timing of External Beam RT

Preoperative and postoperative RT represent the two usual approaches to external beam delivery for STS. Because there is no clear distinction between cases treated with either schedule, RT treatment planning basically comprises two disease 'scenarios' from the practical point of view of describing targets. Depending on which schedule is preferred, there are differences in RT planning volumes.

Although not a prime focus of this discussion, a number of advantages and disadvantages present themselves in the protocol timing that may influence the choice of schedule (see Table 11.2). These considerations have now been borne out in a randomized controlled Phase 3 trial (O'Sullivan et al. 2002a). In particular from the planning perspective the larger fields and greater doses used in postoperative RT present real consequences for patients including enhanced late toxicity (O'Sullivan and Davis 2001). In comparison, preoperative RT is associated with significant early morbidity related to delayed wound healing (O'Sullivan et al. 2002a). Otherwise, both approaches provide high rates of local control (local control rates of 93% in both groups of the trial) although a dubious and surprising survival advantage has also been noted after 3.3 years of median follow-up in favor of the preoperative group. These observations certainly warrant longer follow-up.

From a RT planning perspective, scheduling for pre- or postoperative RT may have substantially different implications in a given case. The size of the CTV is certainly smaller with preoperative RT (O'Sullivan et al. 2002a) as compared to postoperative RT, and this may provide advantages in certain situations (Table 11.3) (O'Sullivan et al. 2002a). In addition, because the postoperative 'boost' beyond 50 Gy is not normally used, there is a dividend in restricting the dose when treating sensitive areas. Therefore, while there is a greater risk of wound complications with preoperative RT, especially in lower extremity lesions (O'Sullivan et al. 2002a), this should be balanced against the greater risk of late complications with higher dose postoperative RT. These factors need to be considered in the decision algorithm. The influence of the timing of RT may be further apparent when one compares two cases, one managed with preoperative RT and the other managed with postoperative RT with a positive margin in a distal satellite nodule with peritumoral edema and extensive soft tissue reconstruction (see Figs. 11.4 and 11.7).

11.4.3 Treatment After Neoadjuvant Chemotherapy in Responsive Tumors

Some STS are routinely treated with initial systemic chemotherapy prior to local management. Although the

Table 11.3. Relative indications for preoperative RT

Treatment context/sarcoma site	Issues of concern	Comments
Head and neck and paraspinal:		
Paranasal sinus	Proximity to optic apparatus (eye, optic nerves and chiasma)	Major functional deficit (visual) may be avoided or tumor control achieved with lower RT dose. Other 'lesser' morbidities (dental, xerostomia) may also be due to reduced doses and volumes
Skull base	Proximity to spinal cord, brainstem	
Cheek and face		
Paraspinal	Proximity to spinal cord	
Split thickness skin graft reconstruction (especially lower limb):		
	Skin graft breakdown and consequent infection	Significant disability may occur during healing (rare)
Large volume GTV or CTV occupying celomic cavities:		
Retroperitoneal	Proximity to bowel, liver, kidney	Critical organs may be displaced by tumor, or not fixed or adherent as is likely in postoperative setting Entire tumor treated prior to possible contamination of cavity
Some small bowel lesions with side wall adherence	Proximity to critical anatomy especially intestine	Contamination of abdominal cavity renders postoperative RT unsuitable
Thoracic wall/pleura	Proximity to lung or cardiac structures	Lung may be displaced by chest wall or pleural tumor and can be avoided with preoperative, or permits GTV to be treated prior to operative contamination
Abdominal trunk walls pelvic side-wall	Proximity to kidney, bowel, liver, ovaries	Avoid CTV encroachment on vulnerable anatomy
GTV adjacent to dose-limiting critical anatomy:		
Thoracic inlet/upper chest wall low neck	Proximity to brachial plexus	Dose limitation to critical anatomy lends itself to preoperative treatment Additional volume considerations
Medial thigh (young male)	Proximity to testes	Permanent infertility may be avoided
Central limb tumor	Proximity to other compartments	Permit partial circumferential sparing which would not be feasible in postoperative setting

Modified with permission from O'Sullivan et al. (1999)

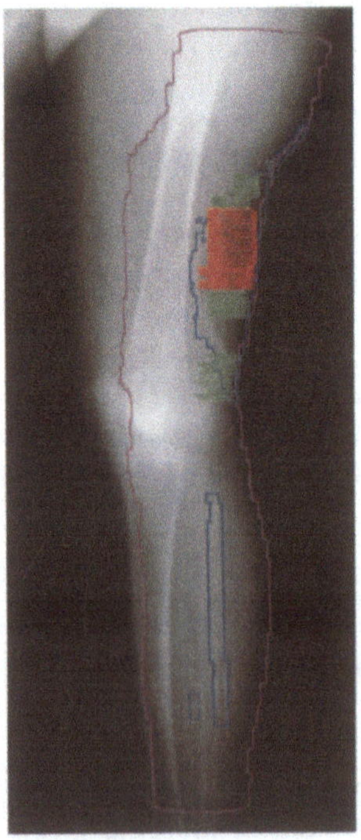

Fig. 11.7. 3D volume display from virtual simulation to indicate the CTV required to encompass the surgical scars for Phase 1 of a postoperative RT plan for a STS originating in the lower hamstring region. The GTV is shown in *red* while the CTV is indicated in *purple*. Additional peritumoral change beyond the overt gross tumor is exhibited in *green*. Note the discontiguous area that was located 5 cm away from the tumor without intervening disease and turned out to be a tumor nodule resected separately with positive margins in the popliteal fossa. This patient also required non-primary wound closure because of skin resection resulting from dermal involvement by tumor. The surgical scars are shown in blue. Proximally the immediate region of the surgical scar and non-primary wound closure at the site of the primary tumor is evident. Distally the donor site for the rotationplasty in the calf is evident as a long scar with an associated drain site. All these areas were included in the Phase 1 CTV because of the involved margins (see Sect. 11.7.3). The MRI for this case is shown in Fig. 11.10, and also illustrates the volume that would have been used for a preoperative plan, provided the isolated tumor nodule distal to the primary tumor was recognized in the planning process

use of systemic chemotherapy remains controversial in STS overall (Bramwell 2001; Sarcoma Meta-analysis Collaboration 1997), embryonal and alveolar rhabdomyosarcoma should initially be managed with systemic approaches (Ruymann and Grovas 2000; Stevens 2002). RT is also essential, since chemotherapy alone is not likely to cure this disease (Stevens 2002), while RT combined with chemotherapy provides high rates of local control. Surgery may not be used, at least in locally advanced parameningeal sites, because of the significant potential detriment from surgical intervention of such lesions which can infiltrate extensively in the base of the skull. The exceptions include small accessible lesions that can be readily resected, especially when lymph node involvement is less likely, as well as extremity lesions.

Frequently such cases also present with regional nodal metastasis in the young adult (see Fig. 11.8) and, even if not manifesting overt clinical lymph node disease, the nodal drainage areas should be considered for inclusion in the treatment volume. Of importance, by the time RT is ordinarily scheduled to commence, vigorous tumor response will likely have manifested and little if any radiologically apparent disease may be present at the time of RT planning (see Figs. 11.8 and 11.9). The initial prechemotherapy volume is the reference for treatment planning, implying that imaging studies must be carefully performed and recorded to facilitate subsequent RT planning.

In the difficult base of the skull locations, rhabdomyosarcoma planning generally attempts to encompass the GTV region with a CTV margin of at least 1 cm wherever possible, recognizing that these margins are significantly more restricted than those ordinarily used in 'regular' STS treatment (see Sect. 11.5.2 below) because of the need to respect adjacent critical structure tolerance. In addition, the neck should be treated together with the primary tumor and a minimum dose of 50 Gy in 2 Gy fractions delivered to the potentially uninvolved nodal chains. Sites originally containing macroscopic disease should generally receive at least 60 Gy, bearing in mind the usually excellent clinical response to chemotherapy. As mentioned earlier, the nodes should be encompassed by the similar types of volume as those recommended by others for head and neck lymph node regions (Gregoire et al. 2000; Nowak et al. 1999; Wijers et al. 1999) and which have been described in detail in the head and neck chapter of this book.

The same RT planning principles hold for other chemosensitive small round cell tumor types when chemotherapy is generally used initially. Examples include primitive neurectodermal tumors and extraosseous Ewing's sarcoma followed by RT with or without surgery, apart from the fact that they are not associated with the same risk of regional lymph node involvement.

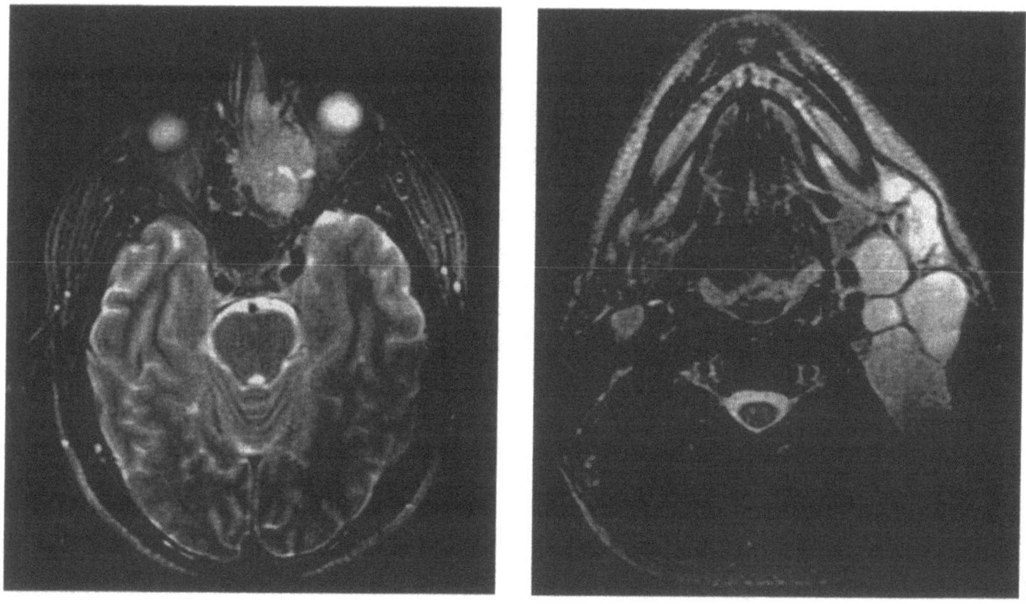

a b

Fig. 11.8a, b. MRI of an alveolar rhabdomyosarcoma of the ethmoid sinus in a young adult. **a** Axial view showing extensive orbital invasion; **b** axial view showing concurrent extensive regional lymphadenopathy. See additional planning details in Fig. 11.9

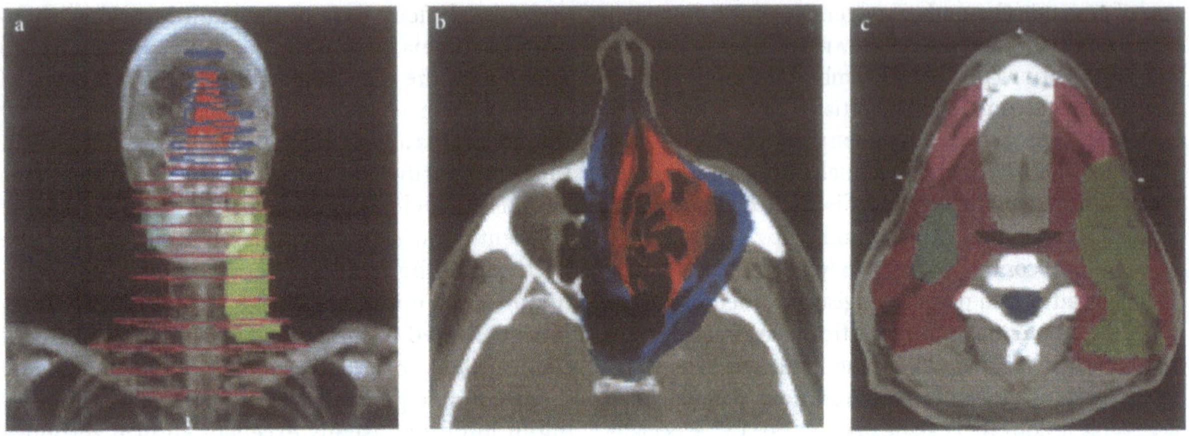

Fig. 11.9. DRR (**a**) and axial CT slices at the plane of the primary tumor (**b**) and through a portion of level 2 of the neck (**c**) for the case shown in Fig. 11.8. **a** The wire frame of the CTV (*dark blue* for the primary; *purple* for the neck node regions) sufficiently spaced to reveal the GTV for the primary tumor (*red*) and prechemotherapy lymph node involvement (*yellow/green* and *pale blue*) in this coronal view. **b, c** Dramatic response at both the primary and the neck is apparent following combination chemotherapy with cyclophosphamide, actinomycin D, vincristine (CAV) and etoposide combined with ifosfamide. In **b**, despite the chemotherapy response, the same *blue* color as in **a** indicates that the CTV is contoured widely to include the primary GTV (again in *red*) from the prechemotherapy imaging (Fig. 11.8). This also pertains to the GTV contours for the lymph nodes in the neck shown in yellow/green surrounded by the purple CTV (**c**)

11.5 Target Coverage

11.5.1 Defining Primary Tissues at Risk

11.5.1.1 Physical Determinants of 'Putative' at Risk Zones

Two attributes underpin the choice of RT target volumes for both adjuvant RT and for the rare occasions where RT is the sole local modality. These are: (1) the distance from the GTV, or alternatively, the distance of potentially contaminated tissues from the GTV following any prior surgery; and (2) the presence of intact anatomic barriers to tumor extension which can permit a smaller margin to be placed around the GTV or surgical volume (whichever is the closest). Thus bone, interosseous membranes and fascial planes are considered barriers to tumor spread in axial directions. Descriptions of radiation target margins employed are principally in the cranio-caudal direction (see Sect. 11.5.2 below).

11.5.1.2 Interpretation of Radiological 'Disease'

A complicating factor in defining the GTV concerns the interpretation of radiologically defined disease and in particular the presence of peritumoral edema. Sarcomas are characterized by the presence of a peripheral surrounding reactive 'pseudocapsule', which itself contains malignant cells that indeed may extend along the compartment beyond the clinically and radiologically detectable tumor. The description of the importance of fascial compartments in controlling sarcoma spread (see Sect. 11.3.3.1) and the concept of the reactive 'pseudocapsule' at the periphery of the lesion are important aspects in the surgical understanding of STS pathoanatomy and for radiation oncology volume determination that have been appreciated for more than two decades (Enneking et al. 1981). More recently, since the advent of MRI for the staging of sarcomas, extensive peritumoral edema that extends along fascial planes and may lie at some distance from the primary tumor has also been taken into account (see Figs. 11.4 and 11.10) (Panicek and Schwartz 1997). It is uncertain to what extent such edema contains viable tumor cells (Manaster 1991), and studies correlating the radiological imaging to the pathological findings are required. The inclusion of edema within the GTV can influence the extent of the treatment field considerably. Our policy is to include this area as part of the GTV in preoperative RT treatment planning (see Fig. 11.4a–c) but we admit that this is not a universally accepted approach. Our concern about this finding is illustrated by the pathologic evaluation of peritumoral edema extending into the popliteal fossa from a lesion originating in the distal hamstring region of the thigh (Fig. 11.10).

a b

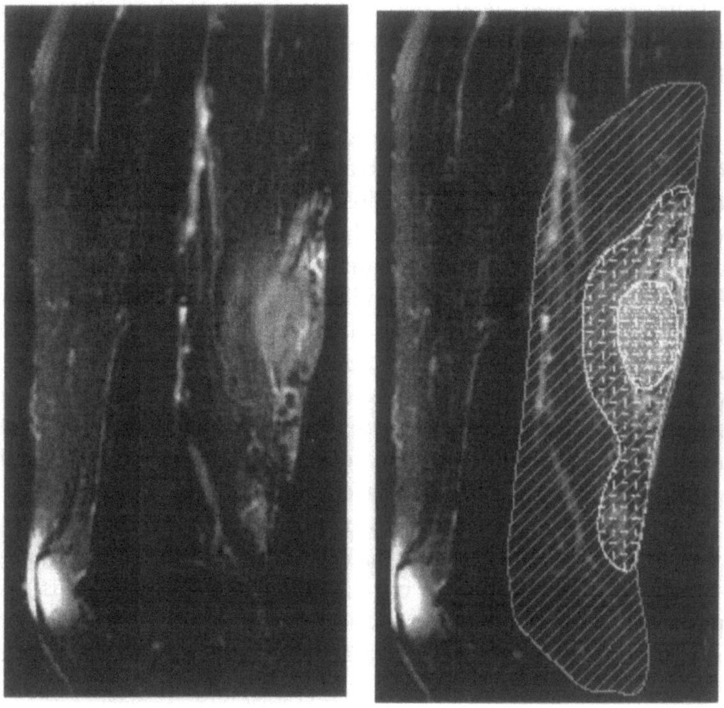

Fig. 11.10. Coronal MRI indicating a STS of the distal hamstring region (**a**). Note the presence of additional separate enhancement remotely in the popliteal fossa and separate from the main tumor mass. Ideally, a preoperative RT plan would identify the GTV as the stippled hatched area encompassed by a larger CTV shown as diagonal cross-hatching in **b**. In fact this case was managed with surgery initially and the separate popliteal nodule was recognized 5 cm distal to the main tumor mass. There were no other nodules. The nodule was resected with a positive resection margin. This case is the same as that shown in Fig. 11.7

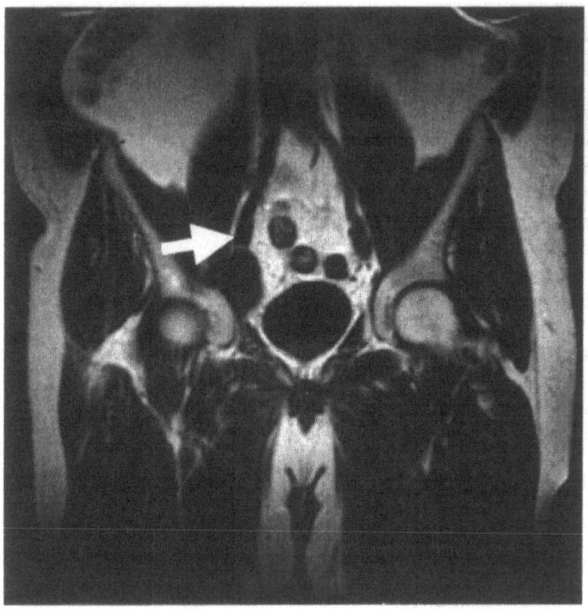

a

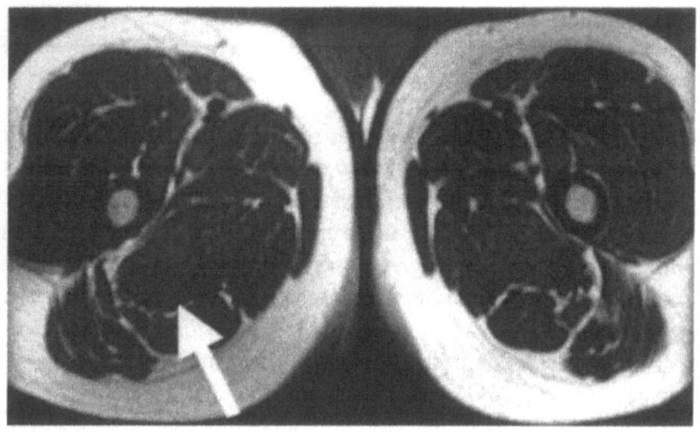

b

Fig. 11.11. a Coronal MRI view revealing an intrapelvic external iliac lymph node located adjacent to the iliac vessel (*arrow*). **b** An axial MRI of the mid-thigh in the same case shows a synchronous primary in the hamstring muscle group (*arrow*). This case is described in detail in Sect. 11.6.3

A further complicating issue concerns the significance of postoperative change visualized on MRI and whether this area, often quite remote from the original GTV and peritumoral edema, also represents an at risk 'target' for RT when this is indicated. For practical purposes, we regard the MRI changes in this setting as the operative 'fingerprint' indicating those tissues that potentially contain microscopic sarcoma because of surgery, and we include such findings in the CTV although this is unlikely to be a universal practice among treating centers.

11.5.2 Extent of Target Coverage

Unfortunately the literature lacks information to address optimal RT margin dimensions in a critical fashion. All available comparative data derive from retrospective observations, although some of the cohorts comprise prospective trial data collected to address other controversies (O'Sullivan et al. 2002a; Pisters et al. 1996; Yang et al. 1998). Our protocols have used consistent margins and therefore do not provide variable field parameters from which to explore whether different outcomes might result (either superior or inferior control rates) and retrospective interpretations, whether within or between cohorts, fall prey to selection bias in identifying cases at different risk of relapse independent of the RT volumes used. This applies to all currently available data concerning field coverage.

Our policy follows the protocol used in the National Cancer Institute of Canada Clinical Trials Group multicenter randomized trial that compared preoperative to postoperative RT (O'Sullivan et al. 2002a). In that protocol, no attempt was made to include the entire length of the compartment in either the preoperative or postoperative approaches. The essential guidelines for primary tumor target coverage are outlined (see Table 11.4). In Phase 1, a longitudinal field margin of 5 cm is included encompassing the GTV or region at risk, including any peritumoral edema, irrespective of grade or size of the tumor. A longitudinal strip of skin and s.c. tissue of a limb is left untreated for at least half of the course or is treated to a dose <40 Gy, unless it reduces the RT margin around the target region to less than 2 cm at any point unconfined by an intact fascial boundary. Joints are handled similarly and are generally excluded from the target region for doses beyond 40 Gy in 2 Gy per fraction, unless there is overt evidence that this would encroach on the high-risk target. As mentioned above (see 'shrinking field technique'), we typically use 2 cm coverage of the surgical bed and the scar for the Phase 2 volume.

In general, the scar is considered part of the target. For this reason, material with radio-isodense qualities similar to normal soft tissue (termed 'bolus') is positioned over the scar during postoperative RT. For preoperative RT, care should be given to determine

Table 11.4. Guidelines for CTV external beam RT treatment planning for the primary tumor site of STS using accepted premises from the literature (O'Sullivan et al. 1999)

CTV definition (Phase 1)

Preoperative:

Minimum 4 cm longitudinal margin from radiological GTV, including peritumoral edema where appropriate
Minimum 2 cm axial margin from the radiological GTV, unless confined by an intact and durable fascial surface
Where the principle of fascial containment is used, the adjacent fascia of the compartment containing tumor should be included in the CTV. This also applies to treatment of superficial vs deep compartments or vice versa
Bolus[§] generally placed over superficial tissues depending on whether skin resection is to be performed (see Sect. 11.5.2)
Include biopsy scar to increase surface dose where needed, using bolus[§]

Postoperative:

Minimum 4 cm longitudinal margin (field margin of 5 cm) from tissues involved by tumor originally or dissected during surgery (manifested by scars and surgical clips); include MRI stigma (postoperative 'fingerprint'; see Sect. 11.5.1.2) within CTV
Minimum 2 cm axial margin from surgically dissected tissues, unless confined by an intact and durable fascial surface
Principle of fascial inclusion in CTV as for preoperative RT
Bolus[§] is generally placed over all surgical scars, drain sites, or other areas of superficial involvement
Include in continuity donor sites if tumor resection margins were positive

CTV definitions (Phase 2)

Preoperative:

Generally only indicated if surgical margins are positive
Generally use CTV identical to Phase 1 (see Sect. 11.4.1)

Postoperative:

Generally indicated in all cases
2 cm CTV margin to include the surgical bed and scar, including original site of GTV
Generally omit donor sites because of prohibitive volumes concerned

Pre- and postoperative (avoidance targeting):

Protect one-third limb circumference (protect for 50% of course or receive <40 Gy)
Protect joint surfaces if possible to <40 Gy
Maintain dose volume constraints for critical anatomy where needed in non-extremity sites or other constraint exists (e.g. head and neck, paraspinal, retroperitoneal, prior RT). Therefore doses and volumes may be less, depending on circumstance
Avoid full thickness bone irradiation if periosteal stripping is to be/has been performed in extremity (limb) irradiation
Use missing tissue compensators, wedging or segmental field techniques as appropriate (including IMRT if preferred) to maintain appropriate dose variation to achieve acceptable normal tissue outcome (minimize s.c. fibrosis, limb edema, neurovascular fibrotic entrapment)

Implies MRI and/or CT staging prior to resection
§Bolus: isodense tissue-like material

whether tumor is present in the superficial or deep compartments and whether the dermis is involved by the disease. This is important, as it must be ascertained whether the surgeon intends resecting overlying skin or will close existing skin flaps primarily. If skin resection is not planned and disease is present superficially in the 'build-up' zone of the RT target volume, tissue-like 'bolus' material should also be considered for the skin to avoid underdosage, since this area must be considered 'target'. In addition the biopsy scar in some situations should also be considered 'target' in the preoperative RT setting and be 'bolussed' with medium of radio-isodense tissue quality to 'bring' the dose to the surface (see Fig. 11.4c).

Of interest, practice varies with respect to the zone at risk of harboring microscopic involvement (CTV). At Massachusetts General Hospital (MGH), the suggested longitudinal target margins are: <5 cm for small grade 1; 5–10 cm for larger grade 1; and small grade 2–3 and 10–15 cm for large grade 2–3 sarcomas (Suit and Spiro 1994). Lindberg at the MD Anderson Cancer Center advocated a 5 cm and 7 cm longitudinal margin for low- and high-grade lesions, respectively (Lindberg et al. 1981). As a general rule however, most centers no longer advocate the use of complete compartmental irradiation, from origin to insertion of the muscle groups, which had been recommended in the early years of conservation management with limb sparing surgery.

11.5.3
Alternative Knowledge About Target Coverage

One small retrospective study suggested a dramatically low 5-year local control of 30% (of 12 patients) when the postoperative RT radiation field margin encompassing the tumor bed/scar was <5 cm, compared to 93% for larger fields (Mundt et al. 1995). In contrast with the latter, and apparently also with the external beam data in general, the BRT protocol at Memorial Sloan Kettering Cancer Center (MSKCC) uses margins of only 2 cm around the surgical bed (Pisters et al. 1996). Despite these marked differences, the local control rates reported are approximately 90% if low-grade lesions are excluded from the BRT data (Pisters et al. 1996). This suggests that the zone of microscopic involvement may be less than previously thought, and studies examining this issue are required. Recent advances in surgical techniques may lessen the need to irradiate all surgically handled tissues, and the issue of scars and drain sites may be overstated today. An additional caveat is that it is not certain if cases treated with BRT are indeed comparable in all ways to those treated with external beam. Evaluation of these issues would require a randomized trial accounting for different selection factors.

11.6
Treatment of Lymph Node Metastasis

11.6.1
Histologic Subtypes at Risk

In STS generally, there is no real link between histologic subtype and biologic behavior or the need for any specific therapeutic interventions such as regional lymph node treatment. Important exceptions to this generalization include epithelioid sarcoma, clear cell sarcoma, angiosarcoma, and embryonal rhabdomyosarcoma (see Table 11.5) (Fong et al. 1993; Mazeron and Suit 1987). Thus, treatment strategies may differ

Table 11.5. Histologic type of sarcomas and lymph node metastasis. Number (*n*) of nodal metastases/all sarcoma patients in 2 studies and proportion (%) of all lesions

Histologic subtype	Mazeron, 1987 series		Fong, 1993 series	
	n	(%)	*n*	(%)
Alveolar soft part	3/24	12.5	0/13	0
Angiosarcoma	–	–	5/37	13.5
Chondrosarcoma	–	–	1/46	2.2
Clear cell sarcoma	11/40	27.5	–	–
Epithelioid sarcoma	14/70	20	2/12	16.7
Fibrosarcoma	54/215	4.4	0/162	0
Hemangiopericytoma	–	–	0/21	0
Leiomyosarcoma	21/524	4.0	9/328	2.7
Liposarcoma	16/504	3.2	3/403	0.7
Lymphangiosarcoma	–	–	1/4	25.0
Malignant fibrous histiocytoma	84/823	10.2	8/316	2.6
Neurofibrosarcoma /MPNT	3/476	0.6	2/96	2.1
Osteosarcoma	–	–	0/11	0
Rhabdomyosarcoma (embryonal)	–	–	12/88	13.6
Rhabdomyosarcoma (other)	201/1354	14.8	1/35	2.9
Synovial Sarcoma	117/851	13.7	2/145	1.4
Undifferentiated spindle cell	–	0	0/42	–
Vascular	43/376	11.4	–	–
Other	–	–	0/27	0
Total	567/5257	10.8	47/1772	2.6

Data from Mazeron and Suit, summarizing literature studies (Mazeron and Suit 1987) and Fong et al. from a single institution (Fong et al. 1993)

for these histologic subtypes, and in particular whether the nodal regions should be investigated (i.e. staged) or treated. Whether the nodal regions should or should not be treated electively will not be discussed in detail. However, in the presence of overt regional lymph node disease they would generally be included, if the patient is being considered for curative management although we recognize that institutional preference may vary in this regard. General guidelines for the use of adjuvant RT following lymph node resection are indicated below (and see Table 11.6).

Table 11.6. Guidelines for external beam RT treatment planning for regional lymph node irradiation of STS using accepted premises from the literature (O'Sullivan et al. 1999)

- Indications for lymph node irradiation
  - Established lymph node involvement (initial presentation or recurrent) with adverse features for complete resection based on pathological or radiological criteria:
    - Matted or fixed multiple lymph nodes or extracapsular extension
    - Positive resection margins at node dissection
    - Lymph nodes >3 cm in maximum dimension
- Specific histological subtype without clinical disease (rhabdomyosarcoma most typically)
  - Absence of distant metastasis
- Targeting lymph node disease
  - Treating lymph node zone based on the existing vascular supply of the region of the primary site. Therefore, contour CTV for lymph nodes to follow arterial supply of the region
  - Treating next echelon of lymph nodes proximal to/beyond established area of macroscopic nodal disease. This is especially important if surgical dissection of lymph node chain will not include these proximal sites of potential nodal disease
- General approaches (scheduling)
  - Treating adjuvant RT of primary and regional node disease in continuity where indicated and if feasible
  - Treating pre- or postoperatively for adjuvant RT
  - Generally treating primary and regional disease in continuity if RT is sole treatment approach (with or without chemotherapy) such as management of rhabdomyosarcoma

11.6.2 Description of Lymph Nodes at Risk

The treatment of regional lymph node metastasis and the areas of potential lymphatic involvement should follow similar principles to those used for other anatomic sites. As noted earlier, in the head and neck the zones at risk mirror those described elsewhere (Gregoire et al. 2000; Nowak et al. 1999; Wijers et al. 1999) and which have also been discussed in the head and neck chapter, and illustrated in the present chapter (see Fig. 11.9). A more comprehensive account of other nodal sites should also be consulted in this book (e.g. the chapter on breast cancer for the description of the supraclavicular nodes, the chapter on gynecological tumors for the pelvic and inguinal nodes). As discussed earlier, it is not possible to present a detailed scheme for all the anatomic sites for the rare occasions when lymph node treatment is needed. Generally, lymph node involvement has an adverse prognosis in STS as evidenced by its assignment to the highest stage in TNM (Greene et al. 2002; Sobin and Wittekind 2002), although the greatest risk is for distant metastasis, which is not likely to be influenced by nodal RT. Nevertheless, features such as the size, multiplicity and the presence of extracapsular extension outside the regional lymph nodes carry a high risk of recurrence and the need for adjuvant RT should be considered.

11.6.3 Targeting the Lymphatics in Limb STS

The target volume should include a zone of potential lymph node bearing tissues along the limb or drainage region of the primary site of the tumor. This may be problematic depending on the anatomic site of involvement, and especially because of the huge range of potential possible routes. In the limbs, but also the head and neck, the lymph node vessels comprise deep and superficial sets. The deep lymphatics are more reliably and easily targeted because they follow the principal vascular and neurovascular bundles of the region. The superficial vessels are much more problematic because they generally follow the superficial veins of the region with variable degrees of consistency. Thus in targeting the lymphatic drainage areas, it is usual to treat the chain along the vascular supply to eventually reach the terminal group of lymph nodes that are at highest risk (Table 11.6). In STS this usually means that the lymph nodes are clinically involved since it is not usual to treat lymph nodes electively. Also, when treating overt lymph node disease, it is advisable to also treat the next echelon of potential lymph node involvement beyond the known area of macroscopic disease, particularly if this is an area not usually included in the surgical resection of the lymph node chains (see case description below). Thus in the pelvis, treatment of the common iliac chain is preferred as well (see Figs. 11.11 and 11.12); similarly, for axillary lymph node involvement, it is our practice to extend the RT target volume to also include the supraclavicular fossa.

Again, the choice between preoperative or postoperative RT needs to be decided, and the rationale

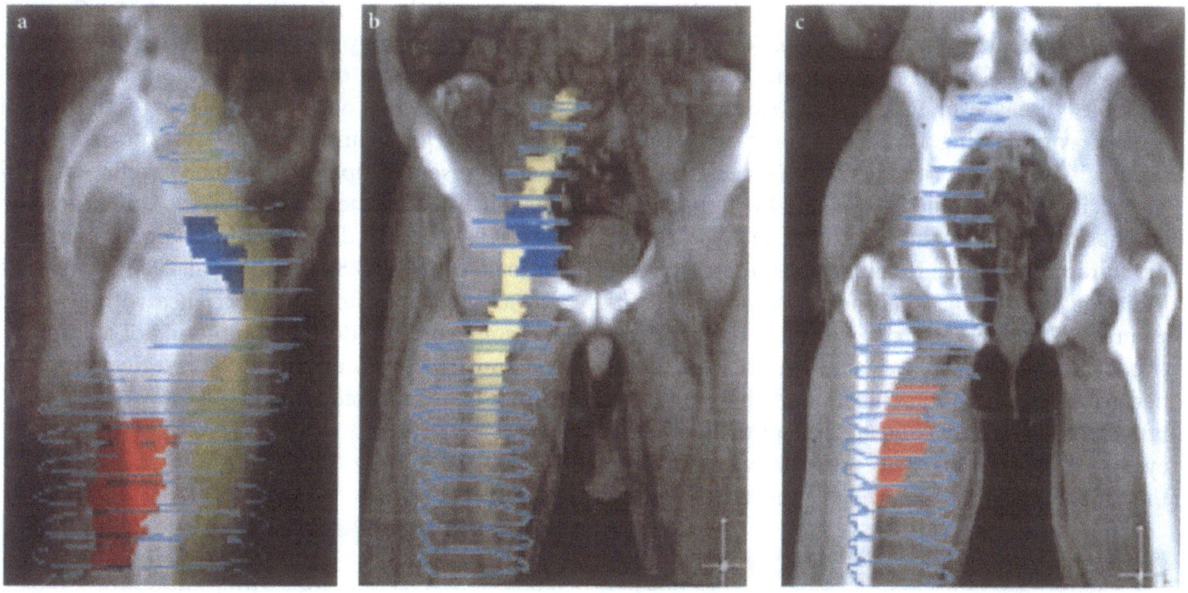

Fig. 11.12a–c. DRR for three representations of the RT planning volumes for the case shown in Fig. 11.11. The sagittal view (**a**) shows the GTV for the primary (*red*), the solitary external iliac lymph node (*dark blue*) and the CTV (*pale blue* wire frame) for concurrent preoperative RT of the primary and the lymphatic areas. Note that the CTV for the nodal region encompasses both the vascular structures (*yellow*) and the GTV for the macroscopic lymph node. The CTV also extends to include the common iliac region in the upper part of the figure. **b, c** The coronal projections with targets marked in the same colors as those used in **a**. Because of differences in their positional planes, only the vascular target (*yellow*) and the lymph node GTV (*dark blue*) are shown in **b** and the primary GTV (*red*) is seen in **c**. This case is described in detail in Sect. 11.6.3.1 (see 'Case example of lymphatic treatment')

for the choice probably should follow the principles mentioned earlier. Frequently, the RT target volumes described will also cover the primary tumor and the target should be designed jointly in this case. As noted, we generally regard the regional nodes at risk as following the vascular drainage for the involved site, and in particular the arterial supply.

11.6.3.1
Case Example of Lymphatic Treatment (Limb STS)

An example is provided to illustrate the principles for an epithelioid thigh sarcoma in a young male. In this case the patient presented with an external iliac lymph node mass located immediately adjacent to the right common iliac artery (Fig. 11.11a). The primary tumor was subclinical and identified in the posterior thigh compartment in adductor magnus and close to the sciatic nerve (Fig. 11.11b). Because of the complexity of the target, preoperative RT was chosen to include both the primary tumor and the femoral, external iliac and common iliac lymph node regions. The CTV was delineated by cross-sectional contouring in the usual manner. However the primary tumor CTV was contoured using the principles noted earlier to encompass the radiologic GTV, and was included with a 'lymph node area' CTV extending beyond the overt lymph node mass and following the femoral and iliac artery into the pelvis (Fig. 11.12a–c). Postoperative RT could have equally been used, but the volume would have been substantially larger and the dose likely greater (i.e. approximately 60–66 Gy by 'shrinking field' technique) with the expectation of greater morbidity.

Of interest, the patient concerned has remained disease-free 2 years following treatment with 50 Gy in 25 fractions administered preoperatively, followed by resection of both the primary tumor and involved lymph nodes. He also received neoadjuvant chemotherapy without apparent response prior to RT.

11.7
Specific Anatomic Issues

11.7.1
Minimizing Dose to Critical Anatomy

In some situations, disease presentations are adjacent to vulnerable anatomy where critical organ function or life-threatening consequences may be at stake. Fortunately such situations are rare, but most commonly occur in the head and neck, especially in the base of the skull, or in paraspinal locations. For example, disease (in this case a leiomyosarcoma) is seen compressing the optic nerve with orbital proptosis in the base of the skull (see Fig. 11.13a). These situations should be evaluated with particular emphasis on maximizing control of the disease with the minimum volume feasible, while also restricting radiation dose to the tolerance of adjacent regional anatomy. The safest strategy may be to use preoperative RT since the structures at risk in the case identified comprise the optic chiasm and the uninvolved but closely situated contralateral optic nerve and eye (see Fig. 11.13b). The potential advantages of this approach are evidenced by the target volume chosen and the restricted dose used (50 Gy in 25 fractions). For this patient, it was recognized that the ipsilateral eye and optic nerve had to be sacrificed to realize the most optimal oncologic result. In addition, the target volume was severely but necessarily compromised compared to usual practice but this was governed by the circumstances. Our experience with this approach demonstrates a good opportunity for local control (O'Sullivan et al. 2000), potentially surpassing our historical experience with resection and compromised dose and targeting of a surgically contaminated volume since the surgical resection cannot be performed *en bloc* (Le Vay et al. 1994).

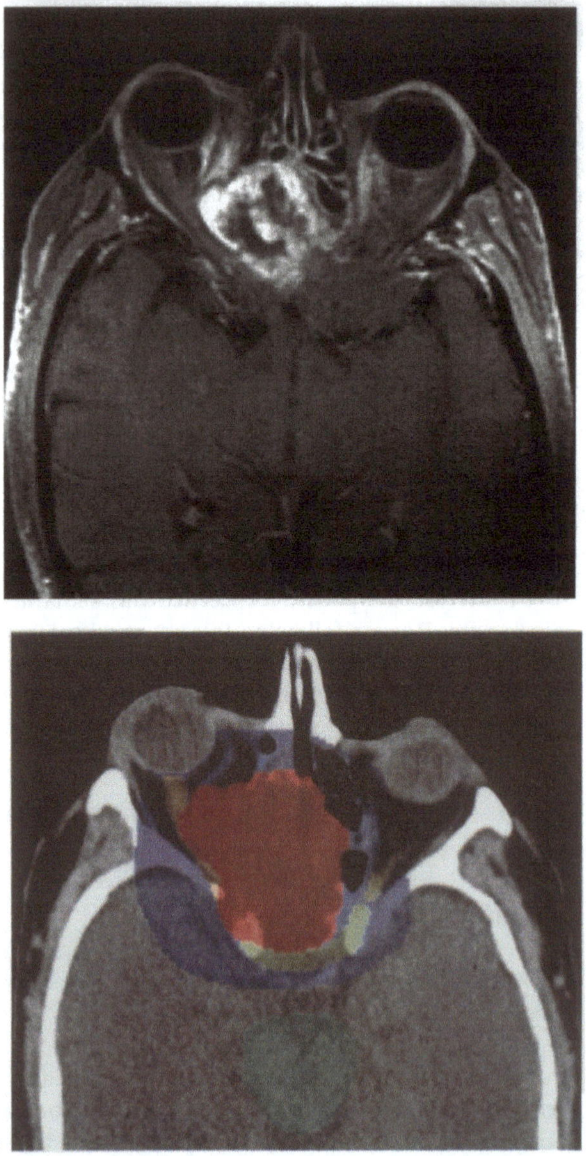

a

b

Fig. 11.13. Axial MRI view (a) and axial RT treatment planning CT slice depicting a leiomyosarcoma arising in the base of the skull. In a the tumor is seen occupying the ethmoid and orbital area with compression of the right optic nerve and proptosis. The GTV (*red*) for preoperative RT is shown in b together with the CTV (*purple*) and the *yellow* contour of the optic nerves and chiasm. The brain stem is shown in *green*. See Sect. 11.7.1. Note also that lymph nodes are not included because of the minimal risk of involvement in this histological subtype

11.7.2 Retroperitoneal Sarcoma

Retroperitoneal sarcoma (RPS) presents a formidable challenge to the oncology team. A variety of approaches have been considered, although the most usual is to employ adjuvant RT with definitive surgical resection. Chemotherapy may also be considered in higher grade lesions, and some centers also provide postoperative or intraoperative boost treatment (Gieschen et al. 2001; Petersen et al. 2002). The more usual approach is with postoperative RT, but evidence of its true value is scant and it is vulnerable to several substantial problems of dose delivery. In the first instance, treatment is already compromised severely by the need to restrict dose because of sensitive normal structures within the proposed target volume, particularly the radiosensitive small bowel. The inherent radiosensitivity of the small bowel, coupled with the fact that the bowel will frequently have to be relocated and become potentially tethered or fixed at the original location of the tumor makes this treatment very problematic to deliver. In addition, based on sarcoma principles in general, it is extremely difficult to determine the potential target areas at risk from operative seeding.

Notwithstanding these problems, an apparent delay in time to recurrence has been observed with postoperative RT (Catton et al. 1994). More recently, we reported a trial using preoperative RT where we have found substantial advantages by virtue of displacement of the small bowel from the target area and almost complete elimination of bowel toxicity from external beam RT. No patient experienced bowel toxicity from preoperative RT exceeding RTOG/EORTC gastrointestinal toxicity of grade 2 in this prospective series (Jones et al. 2002). A further advantage of this approach is that the entire tumor, including peritoneal coverage, can be encompassed in the RT volume prior to potential seeding of tumor cells within the abdomen. The results in this trial, accepting short follow-up, justify additional studies (Brennan 2002).

Target volume delineation in RPS is determined largely by the tolerance of the normal regional anatomy. Ideally we would advise a CTV encompassing the GTV by 2–5 cm in the proximal and distal dimension and accept a more restricted target in the axial dimension (i.e. a 2 cm CTV margin around the GTV). In practice, the longitudinal margins are often determined by the amount of coverage needed to ensure adequate treatment of the diaphragm superiorly and the pelvic floor inferiorly, since these lesions are of such magnitude. Because of their large size, organ sacrifice is often required, most usually the ipsilateral kidney, because of the need to resect it *en bloc* with the tumor. Attempted protection of the kidney from the RT target is futile unless one is attempting the exceptional goal of ipsilateral renal protection in the presence of a single functioning kidney. In all cases bilateral assessment of renal function, potentially by radionucleotide scan, is advisable prior to embarking on surgery and performing RT for this condition.

Another difficult problem, especially in immense lesions of the right abdomen, is liver protection. Not infrequently the primary tumor is 'hooded' by the liver and there is extreme difficulty in delivering adequate radiation doses without exceeding hepatic tolerance. General guidelines for this situation are provided and planning should generally rely on strict examination of dose volume histograms and volumetric tolerance of the liver (O'Sullivan et al. 1999). Again, surgery is part of the overall plan and resection of the liver may be required if parenchymal infiltration of the liver by the tumor is present. If this is needed, it is most important that the multidisciplinary team review all dosimetric volume data jointly at the time of resection, to be certain that adequate unirradiated liver is not also removed at surgery.

In terms of planning, whether the circumstance presented is preoperative or postoperative, every attempt should be made to provide a CTV encompassing the GTV (or the gross tumor prior to resection) with a minimum margin of 2 cm. In this situation, imaging is of paramount importance (see Fig. 11.6 and Fig. 11.14a–c). At times local extension of disease to involve adjacent structures may be present and should be encompassed in the target volume (see Fig. 11.14c). For these plans, reliance on conformal techniques is essential, and in certain instances targets may not be adequately encompassed without resort to IMRT.

11.7.3 Influence of Tissue and Wound Reconstruction on Target Definition

The nature of the reconstruction following STS resection may also influence approaches undertaken in the delivery of external beam treatment. For example when the tumor is resected with vessel or bone and reconstruction performed, all aspects of the treatment should be planned beforehand, including the RT. Generally we plan the RT fields to be as small as possible, and deliver RT preoperatively. If possible, excision of structures and reconstruction can then take place outside the limits of the RT fields to minimize problems related to the radiation dose at the points of reconstruction. Alternatively, postoperative RT can be administered but the reconstructed tissues must receive larger volumes and doses of treatment. For bone reconstruction this seems to be less problematic if radiation is withheld until 3–4 weeks postoperatively to permit union to take place (Spear et al. 1999), but the tolerance of vascular reconstructed tissues may differ.

When planning postoperative RT, another consideration relates to the influence of donor sites of tissues used for reconstruction. Inclusion of the donor site provides a prohibitively large volume and is not ordinarily performed even when the donor site is contiguous to the primary resection site. The exception is when the margins are positive at the resection site and there is concern that the adjacent donor site may have been contaminated. In such situations, we normally extend the Phase 1 volume to include both the contiguous donor site and the primary target area within the same volume (see Fig. 11.7). If preoperative RT was given and a positive surgical margin ensued, we would only treat the preoperative volume for phase 2. The rationale for this approach has been discussed earlier (see Sect. 11.4.1).

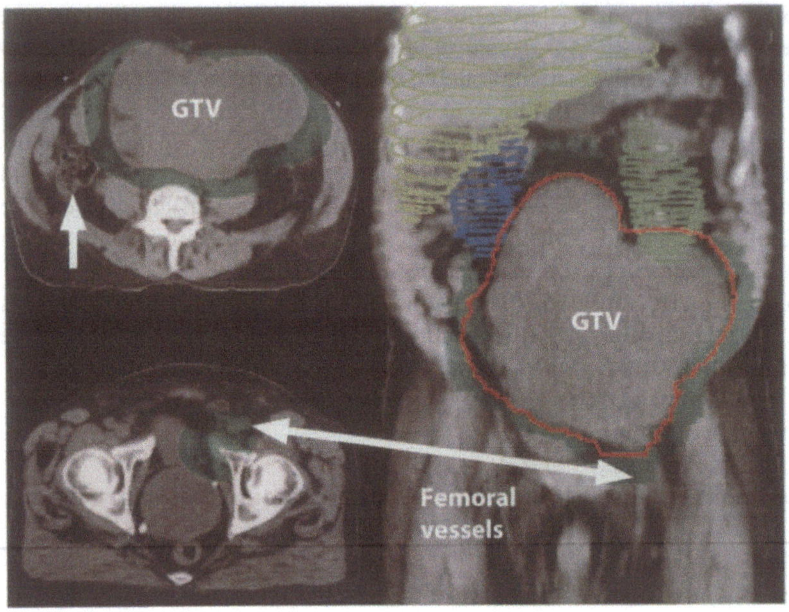

Fig. 11.14a–c. Preoperative RT planning for the retroperitoneal sarcoma shown in Fig. 11.6. **a** An axial cut indicating the GTV and CTV through the equator of the lesion below the kidneys. The CTV is shown in *green* and extends at least 2 cm beyond the peritoneum covering the tumor or where the abdominal wall confines the tumor extension. The CTV extension along the femoral vessels is also shown (**b**). **c** A digitally reconstructed radiograph showing soft tissues in addition to contours for normal tissues to be protected (liver and both kidneys) with the GTV surrounded in *red*, and the *green* CTV extension to include the vessels is again seen. Note also that the preoperative RT delivered in this fashion permits the small bowel to be displaced by tumor from the immediate GTV region and remains mobile. An additional advantage is the preservation of the peritoneal covering around the GTV while treating the entire tumor before potential seeding takes place within the abdominal cavity at surgery

11.7.4 'Uncontained' Anatomic Situations

Certain anatomic situations present additional difficulties because they have poorly developed fascial coverage compared to the proximal thigh, for example. Some are potential spaces without good definition from the standpoint of tumor containment, and in such situations it is usual to design the RT target volume to encompass the extreme limits of the structure or region in question (generally determined by where the fascial reflections eventually merge). Areas such as the axilla, popliteal fossa, femoral triangle, and the entire s.c. compartment present problems of target volume coverage that must be determined on an individual basis. As previously discussed, evaluation of the region in terms of potential tissues involved or tissues that have already been violated is paramount in deciding the most appropriate volume to treat. Again, the principles are determined by the proximity of the most reliable barrier to tumor invasion (hopefully an intact durable fascial boundary) or failing that, an effective distance from the highest risk area most typically manifested by the present GTV or the preoperative GTV, bearing in mind the surgical–pathologic findings at the time of resection. Usually the 'distance guideline' calls for target coverage of at least 2–5 cm surrounding the high-risk area, recognizing that this is impossible in some anatomic sites (see Fig. 11.13).

11.7.5 Treatment of Previously Irradiated Sites

This problem arises for irradiation-induced sarcoma or locally recurrent disease following previous combined management. Appropriate treatment for either of these situations is often curative, and the approach to management would be similar to that adopted with a primary tumor. However, effective management is often complex and influenced by tumor location and extent, and the nature of prior local therapies. An approach to the overall evaluation and management of locally recurrent soft tissue sarcoma is also available (Catton et al. 1999). In addition, in STS the potential also exists for adjuvant chemotherapy to enhance local control (Bramwell et al. 1994), although its effects in this regard are typically minimal when added to the ability of contemporary approaches to achieve high local control rates even in recurrent cases.

Normally RT is considered, but individualization is needed in previously irradiated areas. Tumor bed implantation with BRT catheters in conjunction with wide local excision is usually preferred. If resection margins are closer than 1 cm, BRT is administered 5–7 days postoperatively (Catton et al. 1999). Alternatively, small dose per fraction (altered fractionation) external beam RT may provide tissues with some protection from late damage. Target coverage tends to be individualized, employing smaller volumes than with previously unirradiated tissues, and the total dose is also less. We prefer to administer preoperative RT if external beam is judged a necessity, since it appears more suited to the volume and dose constraints of this setting (Catton et al. 1999).

11.8 Future RT Targeting

To date, treatment planning has focused on conformal methods but without strict modification and shaping of complex targets in STS. A potential question is whether wound complication risk following preoperative RT can be ameliorated with techniques such as IMRT that are capable of conforming doses more closely to the target and protecting more normal tissue from acute injury. In addition, the ability of IMRT to achieve concave volume planning may be of further benefit given the knowledge that an increased risk of irradiation induced bone fracture is evident with doses of 60 Gy or greater (Holt et al. 2002). Lesions in proximity to vital structures may need specific volume modifications in order to encompass disease while sparing normal tissue. This may be particularly attractive for disease sites such as the retroperitoneum where liver protection may be of paramount importance, yet undertreatment of the target poses additional risks. This approach may have the added benefit of potentially achieving kidney protection, as well as spinal cord or lung avoidance in different situations (see Fig. 11.15).

11.9 Conclusions

The use of RT in STS should follow similar principles to those for the surgical approaches to this disease. Individualization is an important principle coupled with a strong commitment to understanding the anatomic areas at risk of involvement. The latter vary substantially depending on the local anatomy of the site of involvement, and will be further influenced by whether native anatomic boundaries to tumor spread are present and not physically disrupted. In principle, for the majority of STS, RT for local tumor is applied

a

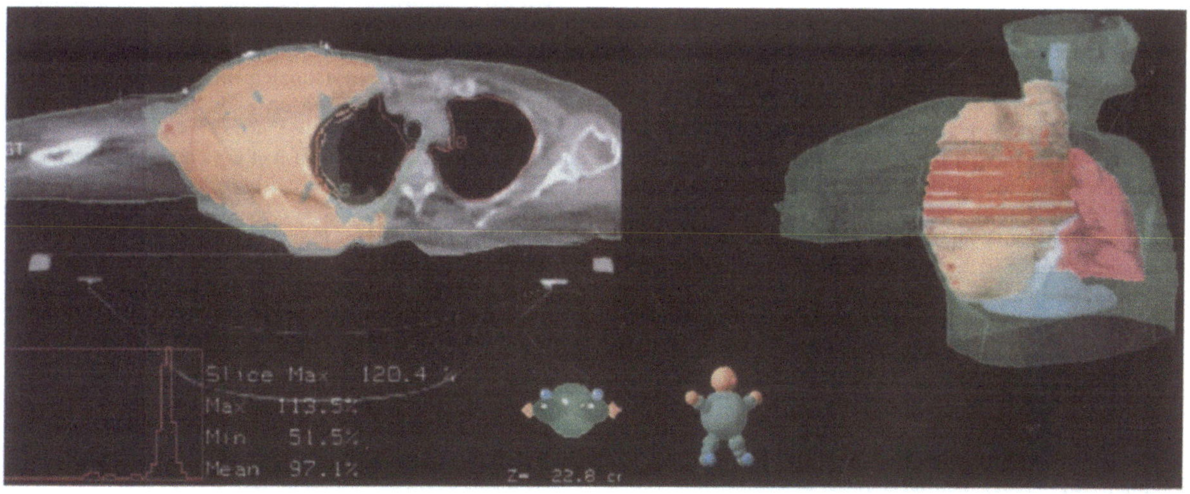

b

Fig. 11.15. a Axial CT slice of treatment of an extensive tumor of the right deltoid. Note the sculpting of dose around the lung achieved with an IMRT plan delivered with the arm abducted from the body. Of note, this was planned with a wide-bore CT scanner for virtual simulation in this position where the arm is abducted from the torso to maximize access and skin preservation. **b** A three-dimensional representation of the GTV and CTV, and normal anatomy for dose optimization including the lungs and spinal cord

to areas of potential microscopic involvement by STS (either as part of the process of local invasion in preoperative RT or including additional areas of potential contamination in postoperative RT), while surgery is used to treat macroscopic disease. RT is not ordinarily indicated in the presence of adequate resection margins, irrespective of pathologic features including grade, since the principle of anatomic containment and tissue protection should govern the use of local treatment modalities.

In regional lymph node treatment, the most usual approach is again a combination of surgery and RT except for very radioresponsive tumors (e.g. rhabdomyosarcomas). Regional lymph node treatment of STS with RT ordinarily follows the zones containing lymphatics and nodes along the arterial supply to the area of interest. In addition, regional node zone treatments should cover lymph node echelons proximal to the defined areas of macroscopic involvement, particularly if surgical dissection is not intended for these areas, since these stations are at high risk of harboring microscopic disease. The indications for using RT in the treatment of STS lymph node areas is a complex issue, and based on the histologic subtype of the primary or recurrent tumor, whether the tumor is primary or recurrent, and whether there are adverse features for recurrence detected either directly at pathologic assessment or indirectly based on the imaging studies.

References

Alektiar KM, Leung D, Zelefsky MJ et al (2002) Adjuvant radiation for stage II-B soft tissue sarcoma of the extremity. J Clin Oncol 20:1643–1650

Baldini EH, Goldberg J, Jenner C et al (1999) Long-term outcomes after function-sparing surgery without radiotherapy for soft tissue sarcoma of the extremities and trunk. J Clin Oncol 17:3252–3259

Bramwell VH (2001) Adjuvant chemotherapy for adult soft tissue sarcoma: is there a standard of care? J Clin Oncol 19:1235–1237

Bramwell VH, Rouesse J, Steward W et al (1994) Adjuvant CYVADIC chemotherapy for adult soft tissue sarcoma – reduced local recurrence but no improvement in survival: a study of the European Organization for Research and Treatment of Cancer Soft Tissue and Bone Sarcoma Group. J Clin Oncol 12:1137–1149

Brennan MF (2002) Retroperitoneal sarcoma: time for a national trial? Ann Surg Oncol 9:324–325

Catton CN, O'Sullivan B, Kotwall C et al (1994) Outcome and prognosis in retroperitoneal soft tissue sarcoma. Int J Radiat Oncol Biol Phys;29:1005–1010

Catton C, Swallow CJ, O'Sullivan B (1999) Approaches to local salvage of soft tissue sarcoma after primary site failure. Semin Radiat Oncol 9:378–388

Enneking WF, Spanier SS, Malawer MM (1981) The effect of the anatomic setting on the results of surgical procedures for soft parts sarcoma of the thigh. Cancer 47:1005–1022

Fabrizio PL, Stafford SL, Pritchard DJ (2000) Extremity soft-tissue sarcomas selectively treated with surgery alone. Int J Radiat Oncol Biol Phys 48:227–232

Fleming JB, Berman RS, Cheng SC et al (1999) Long-term outcome of patients with American Joint Committee on Cancer stage IIB extremity soft tissue sarcomas. J Clin Oncol 17:2772–2780

Fong Y, Coit DG, Woodruff JM et al (1993) Lymph node metastasis from soft tissue sarcoma in adults. Analysis of data from a prospective database of 1772 sarcoma patients. Ann Surg 217:72–77

Geer RJ, Woodruff J, Casper ES et al (1992) Management of small soft-tissue sarcoma of the extremity in adults. Arch Surg 127:1285–1289

Gerrand CH, Wunder JS, Kandel RA et al (2001) Classification of positive margins after resection of soft-tissue sarcoma of the limb predicts the risk of local recurrence. J Bone Jt Surg [Br] 83B:1149–1155

Gieschen HL, Spiro IJ, Suit HD et al (2001) Long-term results of intraoperative electron beam radiotherapy for primary and recurrent retroperitoneal soft tissue sarcoma. Int J Radiat Oncol Biol Phys 50:127–131

Greene FL, Page D, Fleming ID et al (2002) AJCC cancer staging manual, 6th edn. Springer, Berlin Heidelberg New York

Gregoire V, Coche E, Cosnard G et al (2000) Selection and delineation of lymph node target volumes in head and neck conformal radiotherapy. Proposal for standardizing terminology and procedure based on the surgical experience. Radiother Oncol 56:135–150

Holt GE, Wunder JS, Griffin AM et al (2002) Fractures following radiation therapy and limb salvage surgery for soft tissue sarcomas: high versus low dose radiotherapy. Proc Muskuloskelet Tumor Soc p 41

ICRU Report 50 (1993) Prescribing, recording, and reporting photon beam therapy. International Commission on Radiation Units and Measurement, Bethesda

ICRU Report 62 (1999) Prescribing, recording, and reporting photon beam therapy (supplement to ICRU Report 50). International Commission on Radiation Units and Measurement, Bethesda

Jones JJ, Catton CN, O'Sullivan B et al (2002) Initial results of a trial of preoperative external-beam radiation therapy and postoperative brachytherapy for retroperitoneal sarcoma. Ann Surg Oncol 9:346–354

Karakousis CP, Emrich LJ, Rao U et al (1986) Feasibility of limb salvage and survival in soft tissue sarcomas. Cancer 57:484–491

Le Vay J, O'Sullivan B, Catton C et al (1994) An assessment of prognostic factors in soft-tissue sarcoma of the head and neck. Arch Otolaryngol Head Neck Surg 120:981–986

Lindberg RD, Martin RG, Romsdahl MM et al (1981) Conservative surgery and postoperative radiotherapy in 300 adults with soft-tissue sarcomas. Cancer 47:2391–2397

Manaster BJ (1991) Musculoskeletal oncologic imaging. Int J Radiat Oncol Biol Phys 21:1643–1651

Mankin HJ, Mankin CJ, Simon MA (1996) The hazards of the biopsy, revisited. Members of the Musculoskeletal Tumor Society (see comments). J Bone Jt Surg Am 78:656–663

Mazeron JJ, Suit HD (1987) Lymph nodes as sites of metastases from sarcomas of soft tissue. Cancer 60:1800–1808
Mundt AJ, Awan A, Sibley GS et al (1995) Conservative surgery and adjuvant radiation therapy in the management of adult soft tissue sarcoma of the extremities: clinical and radiobiological results. Int J Radiat Oncol Biol Phys 32:977–985
Noria S, Davis A, Kandel R et al (1996) Residual disease following unplanned excision of soft tissue sarcoma of an extremity. J Bone Jt Surg 78:650–655
Nowak PJ, Wijers OB, Lagerwaard FJ et al (1999) A three-dimensional CT-based target definition for elective irradiation of the neck. Int J Radiat Oncol Biol Phys 45:33–39
O'Sullivan B, Davis A (2001) A randomized phase III trial of pre-operative compared to post-operative radiotherapy in extremity soft tissue sarcoma. Proceedings of the 43rd annual meeting of the American Society of Therapeutic Radiology and Oncology. Int J Radiat Oncol Biol Phys 51 [3 Suppl 1]:151
O'Sullivan B, Wylie J, Catton C et al (1999) The local management of soft tissue sarcoma. Semin Radiat Oncol 9:328–48
O'Sullivan B, Gullane P, Irish J et al (2000) Preoperative radiotherapy for adult head and neck soft tissue sarcoma (STS): assessment of wound complication rates and cancer outcome in a prospective series. Proceedings of the 5th international conference on head and neck cancer. Abstract #215, p 120
O'Sullivan B, Davis A, Turcotte R et al (2002a) Pre-operative versus post-operative radiotherapy in soft issue sarcoma of the limbs: a randomized trial. Lancet 359:2235–2241
O'Sullivan B, Bell RS, Bramwell VHC (2002b) Sarcomas of the soft tissues. In: Souhami RL, Tannock I, Hohenberger P, Horiot J-C (eds) Oxford textbook of oncology, 2nd edn. Oxford University Press, Oxford, pp 2495–2523
Panicek DM, Schwartz LH (1997) Soft tissue edema around musculoskeletal sarcomas at magnetic resonance imaging. Sarcoma 1:189–191
Petersen IA, Haddock MG, Donohue JH et al (2002) Use of intraoperative electron beam radiotherapy in the management of retroperitoneal soft tissue sarcomas. Int J Radiat Oncol Biol Phys 52:469–475
Pisters PW, Harrison LB, Leung DH et al (1996) Long-term results of a prospective randomized trial of adjuvant brachytherapy in soft tissue sarcoma. J Clin Oncol 14:859–868
Ruymann FB, Grovas AC (2000) Progress in the diagnosis and treatment of rhabdomyosarcoma and related soft tissue sarcomas. Cancer Invest 18:223–241
Rydholm A, Gustafson P, Rooser B et al (1991) Limb-sparing surgery without radiotherapy based on anatomic location of soft tissue sarcoma. J Clin Oncol 9:1757–1765
Sadoski C, Suit HD, Rosenberg A et al (1993) Preoperative radiation, surgical margins, and local control of extremity sarcomas of soft tissues. J Surg Oncol 52:223–230
Sarcoma Meta-analysis Collaboration (1997) Adjuvant chemotherapy for localised resectable soft-tissue sarcoma of adults: meta-analysis of individual data. Lancet 350: 1647–1654
Sobin L, Wittekind C (2002) TNM classification of malignant tumours, 6th edn. Wiley-Liss, New York
Spear MA, Dupuy DE, Park JJ et al (1999) Tolerance of autologous and allogeneic bone grafts to therapeutic radiation in humans. Int J Radiat Oncol Biol Phys 45: 1275–1280
Stevens MCG (2002) Malignant mesenchymal tumours of childhood. In: Souhami RL, Tannock I, Hohenberger P, Horiot J-C (eds) Oxford textbook of oncology, 2nd edn. Oxford University Press, Oxford, pp 2525–2538
Stotter A, Fallowfield M, Mott A et al (1990) Role of compartmental resection for soft tissue sarcoma of the limb and limb girdle. Br J Surg 77:88–92
Suit HD, Spiro I (1994) Role of radiation in the management of adult patients with sarcoma of soft tissue. Semin Surg Oncol 10:347–356
Tanabe KK, Pollock RE, Ellis LM et al (1994) Influence of surgical margins on outcome in patients with preoperatively irradiated extremity soft tissue sarcomas. Cancer 73: 1652–1659
Tepper J, Rosenberg SA, Glatstein E (1982) Radiation therapy technique in soft tissue sarcomas of the extremity - policies of treatment at the National Cancer Institute. Int J Radiat Oncol Biol Phys 8:263–273
Wijers OB, Levendag PC, Tan T et al (1999) A simplified CT-based definition of the lymph node levels in the node negative neck. Radiother Oncol 52:35–42
Wilson AN, Davis A, Bell RS et al (1994) Local control of soft tissue sarcoma of the extremity: the experience of a multidisciplinary sarcoma group with definitive surgery and radiotherapy. Eur J Cancer 30A:746–751
Yang JC, Chang AE, Baker AR et al (1998) Randomized prospective study of the benefit of adjuvant radiation therapy in the treatment of soft tissue sarcomas of the extremity. J Clin Oncol 16:197–203

12 Role of Radiotherapy in Lymphomas

A. Bosly

CONTENTS

12.1 Hodgkin's Disease

The indications for radiotherapy (RT) in Hodgkin's disease (HD) are very distinct in two different situations: early stages (I, II, several IIIA) or advanced stages (the majority of III, IV), as defined by the Ann Arbor Staging System (Carbone et al. 1971). The clinical stages (CS) are based on physical and X-ray examinations. The pathological stages (PS) take into account the results of staging laparotomy.

A. Bosly, MD, PhD
Department of Hematology, University Hospital of Mont-Godinne, Catholic University of Louvain, Avenue Therasse 1, 5530 Yvoir, Belgium

12.1.1 Radiotherapeutic Fields

The functional field definition is that used by Mendenhall et al. (1999). The reader will find a comprehensive description of the three-dimensional delineation of the different nodal areas in the other chapters of this book, i.e. chapter 3 for head and neck nodes, chapters 4–6 for mediastinal, axillary and supraclavicular nodes, and chapters 7–10 for pelvic and abdominal lymph nodes.

- *Involved field* (IF) is the minimum radiation field size used for HD. It includes not only the individual clinically enlarged nodes but also the other lymph nodes within the same lymph node region. For example, for patients with disease involving the right cranial jugular node, the target volume includes the cranial, medial and caudal jugular nodes, the submandibular nodes, and the supraclavicular nodes. For patients with disease involving the left inguinal and pelvic lymph nodes, the target volume includes the ipsilateral pelvic and paraaortic lymph nodes. Some examples of target volume projections for cervical or mediastinal localizations are shown in Fig. 12.1.
- *Extended field* (EF).The strict definition includes the involved field as well as all the adjacent lymph node regions. In cases of supraclavicular lesions, the EF would include the mantle field and the upper abdominal nodes and spleen.
- *Mantle field* includes all the supradiaphragmatic lymph nodes: cervical, supraclavicular, axillary, infraclavicular, superior mediastinal, hilar and subcarinal nodes. Minimantle field excludes the mediastinum entirely.
- *Paraaortic/spleen fields* include the paraaortic lymph nodes with a superior border matching the mantle field and the lower border of the field at the aortic bifurcation (L4). Spleen hilar region (in the case of splenectomy) or spleen irradiation is classically associated with the paraaortic field with minimized kidney irradiation.

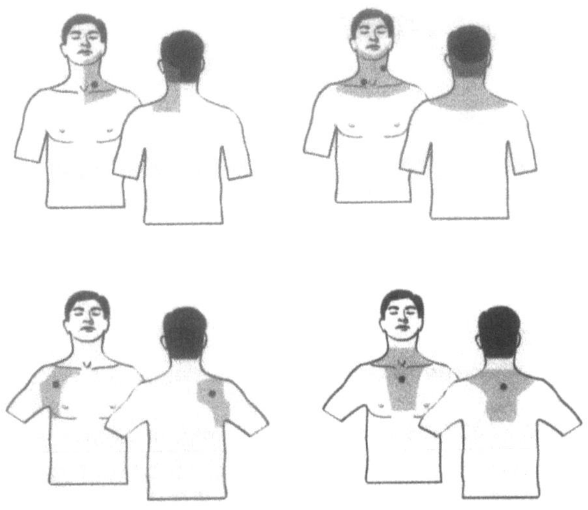

Fig. 12.1. Examples of involved field irradiation adopted from HOPPE (1996)

- *Pelvic field* includes the pelvic and inguinal nodes.
- *Inverted Y field* is the combination of the para-aortic pelvic and inguinal–femoral fields. It may or may not comprise the spleen, and is used for infradiaphragmatic HD.
- *Total lymphoid or total nodal irradiation* (TLI or TNI) is the combination of mantle and inverted Y fields. Certain lymph nodes, rarely affected by HD, are not included: the brachial, epitrochlear, popliteal, sacral, and mesenteric lymph nodes.
- *Subtotal lymphoid or subtotal nodal irradiation* (STLI or STNI) is the combination of mantle and paraaortic/spleen fields and is preferred to TLI in supradiaphragmatic diseases.

12.1.2 Early Stages

12.1.2.1 Radiotherapy Alone

RT alone may be curative in the early stages of HD. The studies of GILBERT (1925) advocated irradiation of involved as well as uninvolved adjacent lymph node chains. Moreover, the data of Vera PETERS (1950) demonstrated that limited HD could be cured by RT given at high dosage and covered involved nodal sites as well as adjacent sites (reviewed in MAUCH 1996). High dosage (40 Gy and over) and large field are essential to obtain these good results.

TNI or STNI (mantle + upper abdominal nodes and spleen) have become the standard treatment for early stages (I, II).

The Stanford Group (ROSENBERG and KAPLAN 1985) showed that STNI was superior to IF for relapse-free survival (RFS; 83% vs 32%). However, overall survival was not modified by the field size.

A recent meta-analysis (SPECHT et al. 1998) grouping eight trials on 1,974 patients and comparing more RT (TNI or STNI) to less RT (IF or EF) showed that more RT was associated with a reduction of events (36.6% ± 6.4) in comparison with less RT (*P*<0.00001). At 10 years, the relapse rate was 43.4% for less RT and 31.3% for more RT: the difference of 12.1% (±2.4) was highly significant (*P*<0.00001).

This reduction of the rate of relapse in the group of more RT was present independently of stage (I or II), age (<20, 20–39, 40+ years), sex, or whether laparotomy was performed or not.

However, no difference in survival was observed between the two groups according to field size. At 10 years, survival rate was 77% in both arms. There was a tendency (not statistically significant) toward less mortality due to HD and more to other causes in the more RT arm. These studies have permitted the description of prognostic factors for HD at a limited stage (Table 12.1). The German Hodgkin Study Group (GHSG; SIEBER et al. 2000) and the European Organization for Research and Treatment of Cancer (EORTC; NOORDIJK et al. 1997) have defined three groups as follows: very favorable, favorable and unfavorable.

Table 12.1. Prognostic factors for Hodgkin's lymphoma: limited stages

	GHSG	EORTC
Very favorable (must meet all criteria)	CS IA Female, age <40 years LP/NS MMR <0.35	
Favorable	All others	All others
Unfavorable (if any criteria)	MMR ≥0.35 High ESR ≥4 sites Age ≥40 years	MMR ≥0.35 High ESR ≥3 sites Extranodal sites Massive splenic disease

From Horwitz and Horning (2000)

CS, Clinical staging; LP/NS, lymphocyte predominance/nodular sclerosis histologies; MMR, mediastinal mass ratio; ESR, erythrocyte sedimentation rate, GHSG, German Hodgkin Study Group, EORTC, European Organization for Research and Treatment of Cancer

For favorable patients, less extensive RT could be safely proposed to patients. In the EORTC favorable group (H5-F), mantle irradiation was as effective as STNI. With a follow-up of 9 years, the event-free survival (EFS) was 69% vs 70%, and the overall survival was 94% and 91% respectively. These results were confirmed after a longer follow-up (Cosset et al. 1997).

Very recently, a prospective American trial on mantle irradiation alone without laparotomy in 87 selected patients with stage IA disease showed very good results at 5 years, with 86% of freedom from treatment failure and a 100% survival rate obtained (Backstrand et al. 2001).

However, the results are not as good as expected, especially for disease control and recent EORTC trials on very favorable HD (H7-VF) showed a 6-year EFS, RFS and overall survival of 66%, 73% and 96% respectively, which is an unacceptably high relapse rate due to which the trial was closed. The EORTC distinction between very favorable and favorable was also abandoned.

12.1.2.2
Combination Chemotherapy–Radiotherapy

Due to these results, combination chemotherapy–RT (CMT) was proposed even for favorable early stages of HD, thereby avoiding laparotomy and splenectomy, which was the standard approach in Europe. In the United States, laparotomy remains the standard treatment before the use of RT alone. For the early stages of HD, CMT was compared to RT alone.

A meta-analysis (Specht et al. 1998) comparing 12 trials on 1,688 patients showed that CMT reduced the relapse rate by 53% (±7.2) in comparison with RT alone ($P<0.00001$). The reduction in relapse rate in the combination arm was present either if radiotherapeutic fields were the same in the combination arm and in the RT alone arm [54% (±12); $P<0.00001$] or even if RT fields were limited in the combination arm [52% (±9); $P<0.00001$].

At 10 years, the failure rate was 32.7% for the RT arm vs 15.8% for the combination arm; the difference 16.8% (± 2.2) was highly significant ($P<0.00001$).

The advantage for CMT was present independently of stage (I, II) age (<20, 20–39, 40+ years), sex, or whether laparotomy was performed or not.

However, the reduction in mortality rate in the CMT arm of 7.6% (±9.1) was not statistically significant.

At 10 years, the overall survival was 79.4% for the CMT and 76.5% for the RT group (NS). There was a tendency for better survival (considering only mortality from HD) in the CMT arm: 87.7% vs 84.6% in the RT arm alone ($P=0.07$).

Very recently, multicentric prospective randomized trials in the USA and Europe have confirmed the superiority of CMT compared to RT alone. The SWOG–CALGB trial on 329 patients (Press et al. 2000) showed that the combination of three courses of chemotherapy (doxorubicin + vinblastine) and STLI was superior to STLI alone (RFS: 93% vs 81%, $P=0.001$). The preliminary results of the EORTC–GELA trial on 543 favorable early-stage HD (Hagenbeek et al. 2000) showed that combination chemotherapy (three courses of MOPP–ABV hybrid) plus IF RT was superior to STNI RT not only for EFS (99% vs 77%; $P<0.001$) but also for overall survival (99% vs 95%; $P=0.019$).

In the GHSG for patients with early HD without adverse prognostic factors, patients were randomized to receive either two cycles of ABVD+EF irradiation or EF alone. complete remission (CR) rates were the same, but EFS was better for CMT, i.e. 96% vs 87% for RT alone (Horwitz and Horning 2000). There was no difference in survival.

Thus, the standard regimen for early-stage HD is the combination of chemotherapy (three courses) and IF RT. For patients with unfavorable prognostic factors, four courses of chemotherapy associated with RT are probably necessary (Fermé et al. 2000b). Ongoing trials are now testing the ideal dosage of RT in favorable patients after chemotherapy.

12.1.3
Advanced Stages

Very recently, a prognostic index was defined for advanced-stage HD (Table 12.2) (Hasenclever and Diehl 1998). Patients with 0–2 adverse prognostic factors have a better survival than patients with 3 adverse prognostic factors (81% to 90% vs 56% to 78%).

In advanced-stages HD, CT is the first-line treatment and IF RT is regularly given after CT (Sieber et al. 2000).

Table 12.2. Prognostic factors for HD: advanced stages (international collaborative study)

Age ≥50 years
Stage IV
Male sex
Leukocyte count ≥15,000/μl
Lymphocyte count <800 cells/μl or <6%
Albumin <4 g/dl
Hb <10.5 g/dl

Hasenclever and Diehl (1998)

A meta-analysis of 16 trials on 1,740 patients compared CT versus CMT in HD has recently been published (LOEFFLER et al. 1998). Two different situations were analyzed. In the first group of eight trials on 918 patients, additive RT was compared versus no treatment after CT. In this situation, there was a benefit of 11% (95% CI: 4% to 18%; $P<0.001$) for additive RT in the rate of continuous complete remission. This advantage was more pronounced in patients with mediastinal involvement, less pronounced in patients with mixed cellularity or lymphocyte depletion histology and virtually absent in stage IV disease and in bulky disease. However, no beneficial effect on overall survival could be identified by additional RT.

The second group of eight trials on 837 patients compared additional RT versus additional CT. In this situation no difference in CR rate was observed between the two arms. Only a moderate but non-significant ($P=0.14$) trend toward improvement of CR rate in the case of mediastinal involvement was observed in the RT arm. Remarkably, the overall survival was improved in the CT alone arm ($P=0.045$). Ten years after the start of treatment, overall survival rates were 8% better (95% CT: 1% to 15%) if only CT was given.

The improvement of survival for CT alone was due to a lower incidence of leukemia-related mortality and also to improved survival after relapse. The latter two situations where CT alone is superior to CMT were not only encountered in the trials where additive CT was administered, but also in the first situation where no additive CT was given.

After the publication of this meta-analysis, the prospective randomized GELA trial (FERMÉ et al. 2000a) compared additive RT (STNI) versus additive CT (two courses) after six courses of CT (MOPP–ABV or ABVPP) in advanced HD. A total of 559 patients were randomized with a median follow-up of 48 months. The 5-year disease-free survival (DFS) and overall survival did not differ between CT and RT (74% and 79%, 85% and 88% respectively).

A prospective randomized trial in Germany (HD12) is ongoing to test the role of additive RT in cases of advanced-stage bulky tumor (30 Gy) versus no radiotherapy (SIEBER et al. 2000).

12.1.4 Other Indications

Localized infradiaphragmatic HD is rare (7% of all early stages). Presentation combination of chemotherapy (ABVD) and Y inverted field without spleen irradiation in stage I but with spleen irradiation in other inguinal situations is the standard therapy (BARTON and O'BRIEN 1999).

Other indications for RT could be first its use in cases of relapse as a salvage regimen because the majority of relapses occur in the primary sites (HOPPE 1996). A last indication is TBI as part of the conditioning regimen before hematopoietic stem cell transplantation. This subject will be treated later in this paper.

12.1.5 Conclusion

RT alone is only advocated for very localized stages without any adverse prognostic factors. Even in this regard, no prospective randomized trial has supported this recommendation and by contrast EORTC studies have shown a too high relapse rate. Thus, in the early stages a combination of three or four courses of CT followed by IF or EF RT has now become the standard regimen either in favorable or unfavorable early stages. Prospective randomized trials are now underway to test the ideal RT dosage.

For advanced stages, despite its efficacy in obtaining more CR in certain situations, additive RT is not indicated in comparison with additive CT because prospective trials have shown no advantage in CR rate and even an adverse effect on overall survival.

A summary of therapeutic options is reported in Table 12.3.

Table 12.3. Therapeutic options in HD

	First choice	Alternative
Early stages		
Supradiaphragmatic		
Very favorable	Cfr favorable	Mantle field irradiation
Favorable	Chemotherapy + IF (3 courses)	STNI
Unfavorable	Chemotherapy + IF (4 courses at least)	-
Infradiaphragmatic	Chemotherapy + Y inverted	Chemotherapy + IF
Advanced stages	Chemotherapy (8 courses)	Chemotherapy (6 courses) + consolidation radiotherapy (STNI or IF)

12.2 Non-Hodgkin's Lymphoma

Recent classifications of non-Hodgkin's lymphoma: i.e. REAL (HARRIS et al. 1994) and that made by the WHO (HARRIS et al. 1999) are now largely used and permit the differentiation of two major subclasses of lymphoma: indolent and aggressive. Follicular lymphoma is the most frequently observed indolent lymphoma and diffuse large B cell lymphoma constitutes the majority of aggressive lymphomas.

These two categories will be discussed separately in localized or in advanced stages. Thereafter, some special situations possibly requiring RT will be examined: primary gastric, mediastinal B cell, central nervous system (CNS) and cutaneous (T cell or B cell) lymphomas.

Finally, the role of TBI as a conditioning regimen before stem cell transplantation will be examined.

12.2.1 Indolent Lymphoma

12.2.1.1 Localized Early Stages (I and II)

This situation occurs in 15% to 20% of follicular lymphomas. For patients treated with RT alone, EFS at 10 years varies from 43% to 85% (CARDE et al. 1984; CHEN et al. 1979; GOSPORODOWICZ et al. 1994; HUDSON et al. 1994; KAMATH et al. 1999; PARYANI et al. 1983;PENDLEBURY et al. 1996; REDDY et al. 1989) (Table 12.4).

For these patients, the generally admitted dose is 35 Gy (at least more than 25 Gy) with a weekly dose of 5×2 Gy. With this dosage, local relapse rate may be as low as 10% (BUSH et al. 1997). An important prospective multicentric trial on 117 patients has shown that the in-field relapse rate was 17% for stage I, 40% for stage II and 35% for stage IIIa. The major factor for recurrence was a decrease of more than 20% from the assigned total radiation dose (STUSCHKE et al. 1997). Field size was not standardized in this case, because no superiority of STNI over EF or IF was demonstrated.

Adverse prognostic factors for EFS are: age >60 years, stage II, B symptoms and tumor size >5 cm (GOSPORODOWICZ et al. 1994). The majority of relapses occur in non-irradiated lymph nodes. For patients with stage I, a plateau around 50% with no relapse after seven years was observed in the disease-free survival curve. Thus RT alone can cure stage I low-grade lymphoma (MAC MANUS and HOPPE 1996) and stage II disease without adverse prognostic factors. RT can even induce a molecular response in patients with a localized stage and a low International Prognostic Index (IPI) score (HA et al. 2001).

The role of CMT in treating localized indolent lymphoma remains controversial. CMT therapy results in a 63% freedom from relapse rate in comparison with 35% for RT alone, but this long-term assessment (15 years) was performed retrospectively at the MD Anderson Cancer Center (BESA et al. 1995). In a British prospective trial (KELSEY et al. 1999), where RT alone was compared to RT followed by chlorambucil, the difference was not statistically significant (RFS: 33% versus 41%, respectively).

12.2.1.2 Advanced Stages

Despite the fact that some stage III treated by RT alone have a median EFS of 5.1 years (MURTHA et al. 2001), RT alone in stage III or IV indolent lymphoma is not currently recommended because of a high

Table 12.4. RT alone in limited-stage (I–II) low-grade lymphoma

Authors	*n* Patients	Relapse at irradiated site (%)	Relapse-free survival (%)
CHEN et al. (1979)	26	0	83%
PARYANI ET AL. (1983)	124	2	I 52 II 42
GOSPORODOWICZ et al. (1994)	248	10	53
REDDY et al. (1989)	24	N.D.	I 83 II 43
CARDE et al. (1984)	45	2	47
HUDSON et al. (1994)	208	NP	49
PENDLEBURY et al. (1996)	58	9	43
KAMATH et al. (1999)	67	6	47

adapted from SOLAL-CELIGNY et al. (1997)
N.D.: Not done

relapse rate even in irradiated sites (Solal-Celigny et al. 1997) due to the characteristics of disseminated disease. Chemotherapy alone with or without anthracyclines is the standard regimen (Kimby et al. 1994). However a prospective randomized trial comparing chemotherapy associated with interferon versus chemotherapy alone showed a superiority in EFS and in survival for the chemotherapy + interferon arm, and this regimen is considered standard by the GELA group (Solal-Celigny et al. 1993).

High-dose therapy and autologous stem cell transplantation are probably the best treatment options for relapsing patients (Apostolidis et al. 2000; Freedman et al. 1999) and are very effective as first-line treatment (Freedman et al. 1996), although until now no randomized trial has been able to demonstrate the superiority of this approach over conventional treatment.

The availability of chimeric monoclonal anti-CD20 antibody (Rituximab) has completely modified the approach in advanced stages of indolent lymphoma. Rituximab is effective as unique agent in cases of relapse (McLaughlin et al. 1998) or in first-line treatment (Colombat et al. 2001). Moreover, the association of Rituximab and chemotherapy is even more effective (Czuczman et al. 1999), and is now being compared to chemotherapy and interferon in a prospective trial.

A non-classical RT procedure for advanced stages of indolent lymphoma is low-dose TBI (0.1 to 0.25 Gy) administered several times a week at a total dose of 1.5–2 Gy. Its efficacy may be explained by three mechanisms: immunomodulation, induction of apoptosis and hypersensitivity to low radiation doses. This technique was used in the 1970s (Safwat 2000a) and was compared to chemotherapy with a comparable CR rate and 5-year overall survival (reviewed in Safwat 2000b). However, the increased risk of secondary leukemia following low-dose TBI, and an even greater risk when TBI is combined with chemotherapy is a limiting factor for its use in patients with long-term survival expectation and so this technique has now been largely abandoned.

The association of radioisotopes ^{131}iodine or ^{90}yttrium and anti-CD20 antibodies is also an effective treatment for indolent lymphoma either in conventional (Vose et al. 2000; Witzig et al. 1999b) or in myeloablative dosage (Press et al. 2000). Comparison of radioimmunotherapy (anti-CD20 ^{90}Y) versus immunotherapy (anti-CD20) in 90 patients showed a higher response rate for radioimmunotherapy, with an objective response of 80% vs 44%, and a CR of 21% vs 7% (P<0.001) (Witzig et al. 1999a). However, the duration of the response was not increased, and a comparison between radioimmunotherapy and chemoimmunotherapy is necessary to assess the precise role of the former.

12.2.2 Aggressive Lymphoma

12.2.2.1 *Early Stages*

RT alone can obtain up to 90% CR rate. The RT dose for local control is at least 40 Gy with 1.8 to 2 Gy per session, five times a week. However, relapse is frequent and only 55% of patients are relapse-free at 5 years (Ganem and Thirion 1999; Sutcliffe et al. 1985).

Due to the curative potential of chemotherapy for aggressive lymphoma, the association of chemotherapy and RT is superior to RT alone (Nissen et al. 1983) and the issue is now to compare chemotherapy alone versus CMT.

Stage is not the only prognostic factor in aggressive lymphoma (Shipp et al. 1993). The IPI adapted to age, includes performance status and LDH level in addition to stage, and must be taken into account in the therapeutic decision.

The South West Oncology Group (SWOG) (Miller et al. 1998) conducted a prospective randomized trial comparing chemotherapy alone (eight courses of CHOP) with the association of chemotherapy (three courses of CHOP) and RT (40–55 Gy involved field) in localized aggressive lymphoma, stage I and II without bulky tumors. In this trial, 70% of the patients were graded as low-risk by the IPI scoring system. At 5 years, EFS was 64% for CHOP and 77% for CHOP+RT (P=0.03) and overall survival was 72% for CHOP and 82% for CHOP+RT (P=0.02), demonstrating the superiority of CMT over chemotherapy alone.

A very recent study by the GELA (Reyes et al. 2000) compared three courses of CHOP+IF RT to three courses of ACVBP + sequential consolidation chemotherapy in young patients with low-risk IPI score. By contrast, results were very different from those of the SWOG study. EFS was 75% for three CHOP+RT versus 82% for ACVBP + consolidation chemotherapy (P=0.03). Overall survival was 80% for three CHOP+RT versus 88% for ACVBP + consolidation chemotherapy (P=0.08). Of interest, results of the arm three CHOP+RT was very similar in the two studies, but in the SWOG study the CMT arm was superior to eight CHOP, and in the GELA study CMT was inferior to three ACVBP + consolidation chemotherapy. It is important to note that the chemotherapy alone arms were very different in the SWOG and in the GELA study.

The advantage of chemotherapy alone in the GELA study was present for the whole population and for bulky tumors. More follow-up is necessary to determine if a statistically significant difference in overall survival will appear in the GELA study. Thus, at the present time, even if CMT is the standard treatment in localized stages of aggressive lymphoma (Van der Maazen et al. 1998), high-dose induction chemotherapy plus sequential consolidation offers even better results.

12.2.2.2 Advanced Stages

Advanced-stage aggressive lymphomas are treated by chemotherapy such as CHOP (Fisher et al. 1993) or sequential ACVBP + consolidation (Coiffier 1995). No large prospective randomized trial has demonstrated the role of RT in consolidation compared to chemotherapy in bulky disease. However, retrospective analysis (Ferreri et al. 2000) has supported the beneficial effect of RT (IF or EF at a dose of 30–46 Gy) after chemotherapy for bulky stage III–IV diffuse large B cell lymphomas. By multivariate analysis consolidation RT was found to be a favorable prognostic factor for RFS. However, the duration of chemotherapy was variable and the median was not optimal (six courses of CHOP instead of eight). A randomized trial on a limited number of patients was also in favor of consolidation therapy by radiation (Aviles et al. 1994).

But the very recent progress made in the treatment of advanced-stage aggressive lymphoma is the association of anti-CD20 monoclonal antibody (Rituximab) with chemotherapy. This association (immunochemotherapy) is superior to chemotherapy alone, with very impressive results (Coiffier et al. 2000) and has become a new standard of therapy.

Due to these positive results, it is not logical to set up a large prospective randomized trial to test the impact of RT as consolidation treatment in advanced-stage aggressive lymphomas versus chemotherapy alone.

12.2.3 Particular Situations

12.2.3.1 Primary Gastric Lymphoma

The gastric mucosa are the most frequent localization of mucosa-associated lymphoid tissue (MALT) lymphoma. In this disease, the implication of *Helicobacter pylori* (HP) infection has modified the therapeutic approach. Eradication of HP infection by antibiotics is now the first-line treatment for patients with this disease.

For patients in whom no regression of lymphoma has occurred after HP eradication, a conservative approach using RT and/or chemotherapy is advocated, and offers the same EFS and overall survival as the operative approach (Schlechter and Yahalom 2000). RT for MALT gastric lymphoma is not only safe and effective but presents low morbidity and preserves gastric function (Schlechter and Yahalom 2000). Other localizations of low-grade MALT lymphoma such as the larynx can be successfully treated by RT alone (de Bree et al. 1998). There is no real consensus regarding target volumes for localized non-Hodgkin's lymphoma, but IF treatment is most often advocated. For example, for gastric lymphoma, the entire stomach, the perigastric and celiac lymph nodes are included in the target volume. For thyroid lymphoma, the target volume includes the thyroid, the cranial, medial and caudal jugular nodes, the prelaryngeal, recurrent and paratracheal lymph nodes, and the upper mediastinal lymph nodes. A comprehensive description of these various lymph node groups can be found in the other chapters of this book.

For high-grade gastric lymphoma, polychemotherapy is effective and no advantage is obtained by the surgical approach (Salles et al. 1991).

Recently, two large retrospective studies, the first on all histologies and stages of primary gastric lymphoma (Willich et al. 2000) and the second on limited stage (I–II) high-grade primary gastric lymphoma (Ferreri et al. 1999) showed that CMT is at least as efficient as surgery. In the Italian study (Ferreri et al. 1999), the addition of chemotherapy was necessary for improved survival: the results of chemotherapy alone, CMT, and surgery–CMT are superior to surgery–RT or RT alone.

Thus, the treatment approach for high-grade primary gastric lymphoma is not different from that for the nodal localization of high-grade lymphoma (Salles et al. 1991).

12.2.3.2 Cutaneous Lymphoma

Mycosis fungoides (MF) and Sezary syndrome are the most frequently occurring primary cutaneous lymphomas.

This T-cell lymphoma primarily involves the skin, manifesting as plaques; after which it progresses with the development of cutaneous tumors and spreads to visceral sites and nodes. Sezary syndrome is an erythrodermic variant of MF associated with the presence of tumor cells circulating in the blood. Many treatments have been proposed for MF including topical chemotherapy, PUVA therapy, photopheresis, chemotherapy, interferon and immunoconjugates (Diamandidou et al. 1996).

RT in the form of total skin electron beam radiation (TSEBT) has been proposed because of its ability to treat the entire skin. The response rate was between 80% and 100% with 36% to 98% of CR. Duration of response was quite prolonged (2–10 years) and higher CR rates and longer duration of response were observed in limited-stage disease (Bekkend et al. 2000; Diamandidou et al. 1996; Ha et al. 2001; Kirova et al. 1999; Maingon et al. 2000; Zackheim et al. 1999) . For very localized lesions, local RT is preferred to TSEBT (Micaily et al. 1998).

Other types of primary cutaneous lymphoma (Kirova et al. 1999) are less common; $CD30^+$ (anaplastic) large T cell lymphoma can be localized in the skin and be primary or secondary. For secondary cutaneous localizations, $CD30^+$ T cell lymphoma should be treated as a nodal $CD30^+$ T cell lymphoma. Only primary cutaneous $CD30^{++}$ T cell lymphoma has a particularly good prognosis. If lesions are solitary or localized, the treatment of choice is RT (± methotrexate). For multifocal lesions (lymphomatoid papillosis), various approaches – no treatment, methotrexate or PUVA therapy – may be proposed depending on the clinical evolution (Bekkend et al. 2000).

B cell lymphomas can involve the skin either as a manifestation of nodal lymphomas or even as the only localization (primary cutaneous B cell lymphoma). RT is also required for these cases even if the prognosis is poor (Bekkend et al. 1999) when the localization involves the lower limbs.

However, the prognosis for cutaneous B cell lymphoma is poor and only cases of limited disease have shown prolonged EFS (Kirova et al. 1999).

12.2.4 Primary Mediastinal Large B-cell Lymphoma

This condition has been recognized in the REAL classification as a distinct clinico-pathological entity. It occurs preferentially in young women with symptoms including a rapidly enlarging mass in the upper anterior mediastinum, and is commonly localized at diagnosis. CMT is highly effective, and in a retrospective comparison was found to be even superior to chemotherapy alone (Martelli et al. 1998).

However, larger studies consider a specific prognosis for this disease in comparison with other large B cell lymphomas very debatable, and there is no reason for special treatment to be administered for this condition (Cazals-Hatem et al. 1996).

12.2.5 Primary CNS Lymphoma

Primary CNS lymphoma is a rare disease with a poor prognosis. Median overall survival is only 12 to 48 months when treated by RT alone, which is the standard treatment for these patients (Abrey et al. 2000). Improvements have been obtained with combination chemotherapy. Effective drugs are those which have a sufficient concentration in the CNS. High-dose methotrexate and Ara-C have been shown in retrospective studies to be associated with a better prognosis (Blay et al. 2000).

In a recent study, 52 patients were treated with high-dose methotrexate, procarbazine and vincristine followed by whole-brain RT (45 Gy) in 30 patients. Twenty-two older patients received deferred RT to lessen the risk of delayed neurotoxicity. Most patients (n=35) received high-dose Ara-C post-RT.

Young patients receiving the whole-brain treatment did not reach median overall or EFS after a 50-month follow-up. The 5-year overall survival was 80%. In older patients, the neurotoxicity associated with RT was high. Survival at 5 years was less than 40%, and was not different for patients receiving RT or not (Abrey et al. 2000).

In conclusion, in young patients, maximal therapy (high doses of chemotherapy and RT) was associated with much better survival than previously reported. The situation was not the same for older patients because of the treatment-associated toxicity, which meant that effective doses could not be delivered.

12.2.6 Total-body Irradiation Transplantation

(Reviewed in Aristei and Tabilio 1990)

The rationale for using TBI in the conditioning regimen before marrow or stem-cell transplantation is the sensitivity of lymphoma cells to radiation.

The addition of TBI to chemotherapy offers several advantages:

Table 12.5. Therapeutic options in non-Hodgkin's lymphoma

	First choice	Alternative
Indolent lymphoma		
Localized	IF RT	Wait and watch
Generalized: low-burden	Wait and watch	Rituximab
Generalized: high-burden	Chemotherapy + IFN	Chemotherapy + Rituximab + IFN
Aggressive lymphoma		
Localized	CHOP + IF[a]	Chemotherapy
Generalized	CHOP + Rituximab	Chemotherapy
MALT gastric lymphoma resistant to HP eradication	IF radiotherapy	Surgery
Non-gastric MALT lymphoma (larynx, thyroid)		
Localized	IF radiotherapy	Alkylant chemotherapy
Generalized	Alkylant chemotherapy	-
T cell cutaneous lymphoma		
Generalized	PUVA + IFN	Electron beam irradiation
Localized	Electron beam irradiation	Methotrexate
B cell cutaneous lymphoma	Radiotherapy + chemotherapy	-
Primary mediastinal B cell lymphoma	Chemotherapy	Chemotherapy + IF
CNS lymphoma	Chemotherapy + whole-brain irradiation	Chemotherapy

[a]Possible modification for near future; see text

1) there is no cross-resistance with chemotherapy
2) irradiation of the body is performed homogeneously
3) some organs (e.g., the lungs) can receive a reduction of the dose by the use of shields
4) there is no sanctuary site sparing.

Different techniques can be used: single dose (8 to 10 Gy), fractionated dose (one fraction a day for several days), or hyperfractionated dose (two or three fractions a day for several days).

The most frequently used technique is hyperfractionated TBI: two fractions a day for three days at a total of 12 Gy. The best schedule still remains to be defined for maximum efficacy and also for the least toxicity.

For low-grade NHL, TBI is frequently used in association with cyclophosphamide and etoposide in the conditioning regimen. Despite a very good rate of response, the relapse rate is quite frequent (21% to 55%) when HDT + ASCT is performed as second-line treatment. Some retrospective analyses have shown a better EFS when the conditioning regimen comprises TBI (Darrington et al. 1994). Acute toxicity is acceptable (4% to 12% of treatment-related mortality) but late complications include minor toxicity (hypothyroidism, cataract) and major toxicity (myelodysplasia, MDS) (Van der Maazen et al. 1998). The actual risk for MDS is as high as 19.8% at 10 years (Friedberg et al. 1999). However, this incidence is probably overestimated and other series suggest an incidence of 4% at 7 years (Mounier and Gisselbrecht 2000).

For aggressive NHL, no advantage was observed in retrospective analysis for the TBI conditioning regimens versus chemotherapy alone (Mounier and Gisselbrecht 1998).

An alternative to TBI is the use of IF before or after transplantation.

In HD, TBI is frequently avoided because of the pulmonary toxicity in previously irradiated patients. In this situation, IF irradiation pre- or post-ASCT is preferred to TBI.

References

Abrey LE, Yahalom J, DeAngelis LM (2000) Treatment for primary CNS lymphoma: the next step. J Clin Oncol 18: 3144–3150

Apostolidis J, Gupta RK, Grenzelias D et al (2000) High-dose therapy with autologous marrow support as consolidation of remission in follicular lymphoma: long-term clinical and molecular follow-up. J Clin Oncol 18:527–536

Aristei C, Tabilio A (1990) Total-body irradiation in the conditioning regimens for autologous stem cell transplantation in lymphoproliferative diseases. Oncologist 4:386–397

Aviles A, Delgado S, Nambo MJ et al (1994) Adjuvant radiotherapy to sites of previous bulky disease in patients with stage IV diffuse large cell lymphoma. Int J Radiat Oncol Biol Phys 30:799–803

Backstrand KH, Ng AK, Takvorian RW et al (2001) Results of a prospective trial of mantle irradiation alone for selected patients with early-stage Hodgkin's disease. J Clin Oncol 19:736–741

Barton M, O'Brien P (1999) Hodgkin's disease presenting below the diaphragm. In: Mauch PM, Armitage JO, Diehl

V et al (eds) Hodgkin's disease. Lippincott/Williams and Wilkins, Philadelphia, pp 727–739

Bekkend MW, Vermeer MH, Geerts ML et al (1999) Therapy of multifocal primary cutaneous B-cell lymphoma: a clinical follow-up study of 29 patients. J Clin Oncol 17:2471–2478

Bekkend MW, Geelen FAM, van Voorst Vader PC et al (2000) Primary and secondary cutaneous $CD30^{+}$ lymphoproliferative disorders: a report from the Dutch Cutaneous Lymphoma Group on the long-term follow-up data of 219 patients and guidelines for diagnosis and treatment. Blood 95:3653–3661

Besa PC, McLaughlin PW, Cox JD (1995) Long-term assessment of patterns of failure and survival in patients with stage I and II follicular lymphoma. Cancer 75:2361–2367

Blay JY, Ongolo-Zogo P, Sebban C et al for the FNCLCC (2000) Primary cerebral lymphomas: unsolved issues regarding first-line treatment, follow-up, late neurological toxicity and treatment of relapses. Ann Oncol 11 [Suppl 1]:S39–S44

Bush RS, Gospodorowicz M, Sturgeon J et al (1997) Radiation therapy of localized non-Hodgkin's lymphoma. Cancer Treat Rep 61:1129–1136

Carbone PP, Kaplan HS, Musshoff K et al (1971) Report of the committee on Hodgkin's disease staging classification. Cancer Res 31:1860–1861

Carde P, Burgers JMV, Van Glabbeke M et al (1984) Combined radiotherapy–chemotherapy for early stages of non-Hodgkin's lymphoma: the 1975–1980 EORTC controlled lymphoma trial. Radiother Oncol 2:301–312

Cazals-Hatem D, Lepage E, Brice P et al (1996) Primary mediastinal large B-cell lymphoma. A clinicopathologic study of 141 cases compared with 916 nonmediastinal large B-cell lymphomas, a GELA ("Groupe d'Etudes des Lymphomes de l'Adulte") study. Am J Surg Pathol 20:877–888

Chen MG, Prosnitz LR, Gonzales-Serva A et al (1979) Results of radiotherapy in control of stage I and II non-Hodgkin's lymphoma. Cancer 43:1245–1254

Coiffier B (1995) Fourteen years of high-dose CHOP (ACVB regimen): preliminary conclusions about the treatment of aggressive-lymphoma patients. Ann Oncol 6:211–217

Coiffier B, Lepage E, Herbrecht R et al (2000) Mabthera (Rituximab) plus CHOP is superior to CHOP alone in elderly patients with diffuse large B-cell lymphoma (DLCL): interim results of a randomized GELA trial [abstract 950]. Blood 96:223a

Colombat P, Salles G, Brousse N et al (2001) Rituximab (anti-CD20 monoclonal antibody) as single first-line therapy for patients with follicular lymphoma with a low tumor burden: clinical and molecular evaluation. Blood 97:101–106

Cosset JM, Henry-Amar M, Noordijk E et al (1997) The EORTC trials for adult patients with early-stage Hodgkin's disease: a 1997 update. American Society for Therapeutic Radiology and Oncology Syllabus

Czuczman MS, Grillo-Lopez AJ, White CA et al (1999) Treatment of patients with low-grade B-cell lymphoma with the combination of chimeric anti-CD20 monoclonal antibody and CHOP chemotherapy. J Clin Oncol 17:268–276

Darrington DL, Vose JM, Anderson JR et al (1994) Incidence and characterization of secondary myelodysplastic syndrome and acute myelogenous leukemia following high-dose chemoradiotherapy and autologous stem-cell transplantation for lymphoid malignancies. J Clin Oncol 12:2527–2534

de Bree R, Mahieu HF, Ossenkoppele GP et al (1998) Malignant lymphoma of mucosa-associated lymphoid tissue in the larynx. Eur Arch Otorhinolaryngol 255:368–370

Diamandidou E, Cohen PR, Karzrock P (1996) Mycosis fungoides and Sezary syndrome. Blood 88:2385–2409

Fermé C, Sebban C, Hennequin C et al (2000a) Comparison of chemotherapy to radiotherapy as consolidation of complete or good partial response after six cycles of chemotherapy for patients with advanced Hodgkin's disease: results of the Groupe d'Etudes des Lymphomes de l'Adulte H89 trial. Blood 95:2246–2252

Fermé C, Eghbali H, Hagenbeek A et al for the EORTC Lymphoma Group and the Groupe d'Etudes des Lymphomes de l'Adulte (2000b) MOPP/AVB (M/A) hybrid and irradiation in unfavourable supradiaphragmatic clinical stages (CS) I–II Hodgkin's disease (HD): comparison of three treatments modalities. Preliminary results of the EORTC–GELA H8-V randomized trial in 995 patients [abstract 2473]. Blood 96:575a

Ferreri AJM, Cordio S, Paro S et al (1999) Therapeutic management of stage I–II high-grade primary gastric lymphomas. Oncology 56:274–282

Ferreri AJM, Dell'Oro S, Reni M et al (2000) Consolidation radiotherapy to bulky or semibulky lesions in the management of stage III–IV diffuse large B-cell lymphomas. Oncology 58:219–226

Fisher RI, Gaynor ER, Dahlberg S et al (1993) Comparison of a standard regimen (CHOP) with three intensive chemotherapy regimens for advanced non-Hodgkin's lymphoma. N Engl J Med 328:1002–1006

Freedman A, Gribben J, Neuberg D et al (1996) High-dose therapy and autologous bone marrow transplantation in patients with follicular lymphoma during first remission. Blood 88:2780–2786

Freedman AS, Neuberg D, Mauch P et al (1999) Long-term follow-up of autologous bone marrow transplantation in patients with relapsed follicular lymphoma. Blood 94: 3325–3333

Friedberg JW, Neuberg D, Stone RM et al (1999) Outcome in patients with myelodysplastic syndrome after autologous bone marrow transplantation for non-Hodgkin's lymphoma. J Clin Oncol 17:3128–3135

Ganem G, Thirion P (1999) Place de la radiothérapie dans le traitement des formes ganglionnaires des lymphomes non Hodgkiniens de l'adulte. Cancer Radiother 3:129–140

Gilbert R (1925) La roentgenthérapie de la granulomatose maligne. J Radiol Electrol 9:509

Gosporodowicz MK, Bush RS, Brown TC et al (1994) Prognostic factors in nodular lymphomas: a multivariate analysis based on the Princess Margaret Hospital experience. Int J Radiat Oncol Biol Phys 10:489–492

Ha CS, Tucker SL, Lee MS et al (2001) The significance of molecular response of follicular lymphoma to central lymphatic irradiation as measured by polymerase chain reaction for (t 14; 18) (q 32; q 21). Int J Radiat Oncol Biol Phys 49:727–732

Hagenbeek A, Eghbali H, Fermé C et al for the EORTC Lymphoma Group and the Groupe d'Etudes des Lymphomes de l'Adulte (2000) Three cycles of MOPP–ABV (M–A) hybrid and involved-field irradiation is more effective than subtotal nodal irradiation (STNI) in favorable supradiaphragmatic clinical stages (CS) I–II Hodgkin's disease (HD): preliminary results of the EORTC–GELA H8-F randomized trial in 543 patients [abstract 2472]. Blood 96:575a

Harris NL, Jaffe ES, Stein H et al (1994) A revised European-American classification of lymphoid neoplasms: a proposal from the International Lymphoma Study Group. Blood 84:1361–1392

Harris NL, Jaffe ES, Diebold J et al (1999) World Health Organization classification of neoplastic diseases of the hematopoietic and lymphoid tissues: report of the Clinical Advisory Committee meeting, Airlie House, Virginia, November 1997. J Clin Oncol 17:3835–3849

Hasenclever D, Diehl V (1998) A prognostic score for advanced Hodgkin's disease. International prognostic factors project on advanced Hodgkin's disease. N Engl J Med 339: 1505–1514

Hoppe RT (1996) Hodgkin's disease. The role of radiation therapy in advanced disease. Ann Oncol 7 [Suppl 4]:S99–S103

Horwitz SM, Horning SJ (2000) Advances in the treatment of Hodgkin's lymphoma. Curr Opin Hematol 7:235–240

Hudson BV, Hudson GV, McLennan KA et al (1994) Clinical stage I non-Hodgkin's lymphoma: long-term follow-up of patients treated by the British National Lymphoma Investigation with radiotherapy alone as initial therapy. Br J Cancer 69:1088–1093

Kamath SS, Marcus RB, Lynch JW et al (1999) The impact of radiotherapy dose and other treatment-related and clinical factors on in-field control in stage I and II non-Hodgkin's lymphoma. Int J Rad Oncol Biol Phys 44:563–568

Kelsey SM, Newland AC, Vaughan-Hudson G et al (1999) A British National Lymphoma Investigation randomised trial of single-agent chlorambucil plus radiotherapy versus radiotherapy alone in low-grade localized non Hodgkin's lymphoma. Med Oncol 11:19–25

Kimby E, Bjorkholm M, Garhrton G et al (1994) Chlorambucil/prednisone vs CHOP in symptomatic low-grade non-Hodgkin's lymphomas: a randomized trial from the Lymphoma Group of Central Sweden. Ann Oncol 5:S67–S77

Kirova YM, Piedbois Y, Haddad E et al (1999) Radiotherapy in the management of mycosis fungoides: indications, results, prognosis. Twenty years experience. Radiother Oncol 51: 147–151

Kirova YM, Piedbois Y, Pan Q et al (1999) Radiothérapie des lymphomes cutanés. Cancer/Radioth 3:105–111

Loeffler M, Brosteanu O, Hasenclever D et al (1998) Meta-analysis of chemotherapy versus combined modality treatment trials in Hodgkin's disease. J Clin Oncol 16:818–829

Mac Manus MP, Hoppe RT (1996) Is radiotherapy curative for stage I and II low-grade follicular lymphoma? Results of a long-term follow-up study of patients treated at Stanford University. J Clin Oncol 14:1282–1290

Maingon P, Truc G, Dalac S et al (2000) Radiotherapy of advanced mycosis fungoides: indications and results of total skin electron beam and photon beam irradiation. Radiother Oncol 54:73–78

Martelli MP, Martelli M, Pescarmona E et al (1998) MACOP-B and involved field radiation therapy is an effective therapy for primary mediastinal large B-cell lymphoma with sclerosis. Ann Oncol 9:1027–1029

Mauch PM (1996) Management of early stage Hodgkin's disease: the role of radiation therapy and/or chemotherapy. Baillière's Clin Haematol 9:531–541

Mc Laughlin P, Grillo-Lopez AJ, Link BK et al (1998) Rituximab chimeric anti-CD20 monoclonal antibody therapy for relapsed indolent lymphoma: half of patients respond to a four-dose treatment program. J Clin Oncol 16:2825–2832

Mendenhall NP, Hoppe RT, Prosnitz LR et al (1999) Principles of radiation therapy in Hodgkin's disease. In: Mauch PM, Armitage JO, Diehl V et al (eds) Hodgkin's disease. Lippincott/Williams and Wilkins, Philadelphia, pp 337–376

Micaily B, Miyamoto C, Kantor G et al (1998) Radiotherapy for unlesional mycosis fungoides. Int J Radiat Oncol Biol Phys 42:361–364

Miller TP, Dahlberg S, Cassady JR et al (1998) Chemotherapy alone compared with chemotherapy plus radiotherapy for localized intermediate and high-grade non-Hodgkin's lymphoma. N Engl J Med 339:21–26

Mounier N, Gisselbrecht C (1998) Conditioning regimens before transplantation in patients with aggressive non-Hodgkin's lymphoma. Ann Oncol 9 [Suppl 1]:S15–S21

Mounier N, Gisselbrecht C (2000) Myelodysplasia after autotransplantation. J Clin Oncol 18:3446–3447

Murtha AD, Know SJ, Hoppe RT et al (2001) Long-term follow-up of patients with stage III follicular lymphoma treated with primary radiotherapy at Stanford University. Int J Radiat Oncol Biol Phys 49:3–15

Nissen NI, Ersboll J, Hansen MM et al (1983) A randomized study of radiotherapy versus radiotherapy plus chemotherapy in stage I–II non-Hodgkin's lymphomas. Cancer 52:1–7

Noordijk E, Carde P, Hagenbeek A et al (1997) Combination of radiotherapy and chemotherapy is advisable in all patients with clinical stage I–II Hodgkin's disease. Six-year results of the EORTC-GPMC controlled clinical trials H7-VF, H7-F and H7 V. Proc Am Soc Ther Radiol Oncol 39:173

Paryani SB, Hoppe RT, Cox RS et al (1983) Analysis of non-Hodgkin's lymphomas with nodular and favourable histologic stage I and II. Cancer 52:2300–2307

Pendelbury S, El Awadi M, Ashley S et al (1996) Radiotherapy results in early low-grade nodal non-Hodgkin's lymphoma. Radiother Oncol 36:167–171

Peters MV, Middlemiss KCH (1958) A study of Hodgkin's disease treated by irradiation. Am J Roentgenol 79:114

Press OW, Eary JF, Gooley T, Gopal AK, Liu S, Bush SA, Durack LD, Martin PJ, Fisher DR, Wood B, Borrow JW, Porter B, Smith JP, Matthews DC, Appelbaum FR, Bernstein ID (2000) A phase I/II trial of iodine-131 tositumomab (anti-CD20), etoposide, cyclophosphamide, and autologous stem cell transplantation for relapsed B-cell lymphomas. Blood 96(9):2934–2942

Press OW, LeBlanc M, Lichter A et al (2000) A phase III randomized intergroup trial of subtotal lymphoid irradiation (STLI) versus doxorubicin, vinblastine, and STLI for stage IA–IIA Hodgkin's disease (SWOG 9133, CALGB 9391) [abstract 2471]. Blood 96:575a

Reddy S, Saxema VS, Pelletiere EV et al (1989) Stage I and II non-Hodgkin's lymphomas: long-term results of radiation therapy. Int J Radiat Oncol Biol Phys 16:687–692

Reyes F, Lepage E, Munck JN et al for the GELA (2000) Superiority of the ACVBP regimen over a combined treatment with three cycles of CHOP followed by involved field radiotherapy in patients (pts) with low risk localized agressive non Hodgkin's lymphoma: results of the LNH93-1 study. Blood 96:575a (abstract 3595)

Rosenberg S, Kaplan H (1985) The evolution and summary results of the Stanford of the management of Hodgkin's disease/1962–1984. Int J Radiat Oncol Biol Phys 11:5–22

Safwat A (2000a) The immunobiology of low-dose total body irradiation: more questions than answers. Radiat Res 153: 599–604

Safwat A (2000b) The role of low-dose total body irradiation in the treatment of non-Hodgkin's lymphoma: a new look at an old method. Radiother Oncol 56:1–8

Salles G, Herbrecht R, Tilly H et al (1991) Aggressive primary gastrointestinal lymphomas, review of 91 patients treated with the LNH-84 regimen, a study of the Groupe d'Etudes des Lymphomes de l'Adulte. Am J Med 90:77–84

Schechter NR, Yahalom J (2000) Low-grade MALT lymphoma of the stomach: a review of treatment options. Int J Radiat Oncol Biol Phys 46:1093–1103

Shipp MA, Harrington DP for the International Non-Hodgkin's Lymphoma Prognostic Factors Project (1993) A predictive model for aggressive non-Hodgkin's lymphoma. N Engl J Med 329:987–994

Sieber M, Engert A, Diehl V et al (2000) Treatment of Hodgkin's disease: results and current concepts of the German Hodgkin's lymphoma study group. Ann Oncol 11:581–585

Solal-Celigny P, Lepage E, Brousse N et al (1993) Recombinant interferon-alfa 2b combined with a regimen containing doxorubicin in patients with advanced follicular lymphomas. N Engl J Med 329:1608–1613

Solal-Celigny P, Brousse N, Tilly H et al (1997) Lymphomes folliculaires. In: Solal-Celigny P et al (eds) Lymphomes. Frison-Roche, Paris, pp 171–203

Specht L, Gray RG, Clarke MJ et al for the International Hodgkin's Disease Collaborative Group (1998) Influence of more extensive radiotherapy and adjuvant chemotherapy on long-term outcome of early-stage Hodgkin's disease: a meta-analysis of 23 randomized trials involving 3,888 patients. J Clin Oncol 16:830–843

Stuschke M, Hoederath A, Sack H et al (1997) Extended field and total central lymphatic radiotherapy in the treatment of early stage lymph node centroblastic – centrocytic lymphomas. Cancer 80:2273–2284

Sutcliffe SB, Gospodorowicz MK, Bush RS et al (1985) Role of radiation therapy in localized non-Hodgkin's lymphoma. Radiother Oncol 4:211–223

Van der Maazen RWM, Noordijk EM, Thomas J et al (1998) Combined modality treatment is the treatment of choice for stage I–IE intermediate and high grade non-Hodgkin's lymphomas. Radiother Oncol 49:1–7

Vose JM, Wahl RL, Saleh M et al (2000) Multicenter phase II study of iodine-131 tositumomab for chemotherapy-relapsed/refractory low-grade and transformed low-grade B-cell non-Hodgkin's lymphomas. J Clin Oncol 18:1316–1323

Willich NA, Reinartz G, Horst EJ et al (2000) Operative and conservative management of primary gastric lymphoma: interim results of a German multicenter study. Int J Rad Oncol Biol Phys 46:895–901

Witzig TE, White CA, Gordon LI et al (1999a) Prospective randomized controlled study of Zevalin (IDEC Y_2B_8) radioimmunotherapy compared to Rituximab immunotherapy for B-cell NHL: report of interim results [abstract 2805]. Blood 94:631a

Witzig TE, White CA, Wiseman GA et al (1999b) Phase I–II trial of IDEC-Y2B8 radioimmunotherapy for treatment of relapsed or refractory CD20(+) B-cell non-Hodgkin's lymphoma. J Clin Oncol 17:3793–3803

Zackheim HS (1999) Cutaneous T cell lymphoma: update of treatment. Dermatology 199:102–105

Subject Index

List of Contributors

K. Kian Ang, MD, PhD
Department of Radiation Oncology
UT MD Anderson Cancer Center
Houston, TX 77030
USA

André Bosly, MD, PhD
Department of Hematology
Cliniques Universitaires de Mont Godinne
5530 Yvoir
Belgium

Robert Bristow, MD
Department of Radiation Oncology
University of Toronto
Princess Margaret Hopsital
Toronto M5G 2M9
Canada

Mustafa Cengiz, MD
Radyasyon Onkolojisi
Hacettepe Universitesi
Ankara
Turkey

K. S. Clifford Chao, MD
Radiation Oncology Center
Washington University School of Medicine
4939 Children's Place, Suite 5500
St. Louis, MO 63110
USA

Emmanuel E. Coche, MD
Department of Radiology
Université Catholique de Louvain
St-Luc University Hospital
10 Avenue Hippocrate
1200 Brussels
Belgium

Guy Cosnard, MD
Professor, Department of Radiology
Université Catholique de Louvain
St-Luc University Hospital
10 Avenue Hippocrate
1200 Bruxelles
Belgium

Thierry Duprez, MD
Department of Radiology
Université Catholique de Louvain
St-Luc University Hospital
10 Avenue Hippocrate
1200 Brussels
Belgium

Pascal A. Gervaz, MD
Fellow in Colorectal Surgery
Mayo Clinic and Mayo Medical School
Rochester, MN 55905
USA

Mary Gospodarowicz, MD
Princess Margaret Hospital
Department of Radiation Oncology
Toronto M5G 2M9
Canada

Vincent Grégoire, MD, PhD
Department of Radiation Oncology
Université Catholique de Louvain
Cliniques Universitaires Saint-Luc
10 Avenue Hippocrate
1200 Bruxelles
Belgium

Leonard L. Gunderson, MD, MS
Professor and Chair of Oncology
Consultant in Radiation Oncology
Department of Radiation Oncology
Mayo Clinic and Mayo Medical School
Desk SR Charlton Building
Rochester, MN 55905
USA

Michael G. Haddock, MD
Assistant Professor of Oncology
Consultant in Radiation Oncology
Department of Radiation Oncology
Mayo Clinic and Mayo Medical School
Desk SR Charlton Building
Rochester, MN 55905
USA

Marc Hamoir, MD
Professsor, Department of Otorhinolaryngology
and Head & Neck Surgery
Université Catholique de Louvain
St-Luc University Hospital
10 Avenue Hippocrate
1200 Brussels
Belgium

Karin Haustermans, MD, PhD
Department of Radiation Oncology
University Hospital, K.U. Leuven
3000 Leuven
Belgium

T. Haycocks, MD
Department of Radiation Oncology
University of Toronto
Princess Margaret Hopsital
Toronto M5G 2M9
Canada

Thomas Herzog, MD
Division of Gynecologic Oncology
Department of Obstetrics and Gynecology
Washington University School of Medicine
4939 Children's Place, Suite 5500
St. Louis, MO 63110
USA

Ion-Christian Kiricuta, MD, PhD
Associate Professor, Institute for Radiation Oncology
St. Vincenz-Hospital Limburg/Lahn
Auf dem Schafsberg
65649 Limburg/Lahn
Germany

Benoit Lengelé, MD, PhD, FCCP
Department of Plastic Surgery
Cliniques Universitaires St-Luc
1200 Brussels
Belgium

Atoon Lerut, MD
Thoracic Surgery
UZ Gasthuisberg
3000 Leuven
Belgium

Max Lonneux, MD, PhD
Department of Radiology
Cliniques Universitaires St-Luc
Université Catholique de Louvain
Avenue Hippocrate, 10
1200 Brussels
Belgium

Pierre Loubeyre, MD
Service de Radiologie
Hopital Cantonal Universitaire de Geneve
CH-1211 Geneve
Switzerland

Michael Milosevic, MD
Department of Radiation Oncology
University of Toronto
Princess Margaret Hopsital
Toronto M5G 2M9
Canada

Françoise Mornex, MD
Department of Radiotherapy
Centre Hospitalier Lyon Sud
69495 Pierre Bénite
France

Heidi Nelson, MD
Professor and Chair of Colorectal Surgery
Mayo Clinic and Mayo Medical School
Rochester, MN 55905
USA

Brian O'Sullivan, MD
Princess Margaret Hospital
Department of Radiation Oncology
Toronto M5G 2M9
Canada

Peter W. T. Pisters, MD, FACS
Department of Surgery
University of Texas M.D. Anderson Cancer Center
Houston, TX 77030
USA

Laurette Renard, MD
Department of Radiation Oncology
Université Catholique de Louvain
Cliniques Universitaires St-Luc
1200 Brussels
Belgium

Hervé Reychler, MD, DMD
Professor, Department of Oral and Maxillo-Facial Surgery
Université Catholique de Louvain
St-Luc University Hospital
10 Avenue Hippocrate
1200 Brussels
Belgium

Pierre Rocmans, MD
Department of Thoracic Surgery
Hôpital Erasme
1070 Brussels
Belgium

Pierre Scalliet, MD, PhD
Department of Radiation Oncology
Université Catholique de Louvain
Cliniques Universitaires Saint-Luc
Avenue Hippocrate 10, UCL 10/4752
1200 Bruxelles
Belgium

Bertrand Tombal, MD
Department of Urology
Cliniques Universitaires St-Luc
1200 Brussels
Belgium

Paul van Houtte, MD, PhD
Department of Radiation Oncology
Institut Jules Bordet
rue Héger-Bordet 1
1000 Bruxelles
Belgium

François Vaylet, MD
Department of Respiratory Diseases
Hôpital d 'Instruction des Armées Percy
92141 Clamart
France

J. Wunder, MD, FRCSC
Department of Surgical Oncology
Princess Margaret Hospital
and University Musculoskeletal Oncology Unit
Mount Sinai Hospital
University of Toronto
Toronto M5G 2M9
Canada

MEDICAL RADIOLOGY Diagnostic Imaging and Radiation Oncology

Titles in the series already published

RADIATION ONCOLOGY

Lung Cancer
Edited by C.W. Scarantino

Innovations in Radiation Oncology
Edited by H. R. Withers and L. J. Peters

Radiation Therapy of Head and Neck Cancer
Edited by G. E. Laramore

Gastrointestinal Cancer – Radiation Therapy
Edited by R.R. Dobelbower, Jr.

Radiation Exposure and Occupational Risks
Edited by E. Scherer, C. Streffer, and K.-R. Trott

Radiation Therapy of Benign Diseases
A Clinical Guide
S.E. Order and S. S. Donaldson

Interventional Radiation Therapy Techniques – Brachytherapy
Edited by R. Sauer

Radiopathology of Organs and Tissues
Edited by E. Scherer, C. Streffer, and K.-R. Trott

Concomitant Continuous Infusion Chemotherapy and Radiation
Edited by M. Rotman and C. J. Rosenthal

Intraoperative Radiotherapy – Clinical Experiences and Results
Edited by F. A. Calvo, M. Santos, and L.W. Brady

Radiotherapy of Intraocular and Orbital Tumors
Edited by W. E. Alberti and R. H. Sagerman

Interstitial and Intracavitary Thermoradiotherapy
Edited by M. H. Seegenschmiedt and R. Sauer

Non-Disseminated Breast Cancer
Controversial Issues in Management
Edited by G. H. Fletcher and S.H. Levitt

Current Topics in Clinical Radiobiology of Tumors
Edited by H.-P. Beck-Bornholdt

Practical Approaches to Cancer Invasion and Metastases
A Compendium of Radiation Oncologists' Responses to 40 Histories
Edited by A. R. Kagan with the Assistance of R. J. Steckel

Radiation Therapy in Pediatric Oncology
Edited by J. R. Cassady

Radiation Therapy Physics
Edited by A. R. Smith

Late Sequelae in Oncology
Edited by J. Dunst and R. Sauer

Mediastinal Tumors. Update 1995
Edited by D. E. Wood and C. R. Thomas, Jr.

Thermoradiotherapy and Thermochemotherapy

Volume 1:
Biology, Physiology, and Physics

Volume 2:
Clinical Applications
Edited by M.H. Seegenschmiedt, P. Fessenden, and C.C. Vernon

Carcinoma of the Prostate
Innovations in Management
Edited by Z. Petrovich, L. Baert, and L.W. Brady

Radiation Oncology of Gynecological Cancers
Edited by H.W. Vahrson

Carcinoma of the Bladder
Innovations in Management
Edited by Z. Petrovich, L. Baert, and L.W. Brady

Blood Perfusion and Microenvironment of Human Tumors
Implications for Clinical Radiooncology
Edited by M. Molls and P. Vaupel

Radiation Therapy of Benign Diseases
A Clinical Guide
2nd Revised Edition
S. E. Order and S. S. Donaldson

Carcinoma of the Kidney and Testis, and Rare Urologic Malignancies
Innovations in Management
Edited by Z. Petrovich, L. Baert, and L.W. Brady

Progress and Perspectives in the Treatment of Lung Cancer
Edited by P. Van Houtte, J. Klastersky, and P. Rocmans

Combined Modality Therapy of Central Nervous System Tumors
Edited by Z. Petrovich, L. W. Brady, M. L. Apuzzo, and M. Bamberg

Age-Related Macular Degeneration
Current Treatment Concepts
Edited by W. A. Alberti, G. Richard, and R. H. Sagerman

Radiotherapy of Intraocular and Orbital Tumors
2nd Revised Edition
Edited by R. H. Sagerman, and W. E. Alberti

Biological Modification of Radiation Response
Edited by C. Nieder, L. Milas, and K. K. Ang

Radiation Oncology for Cure and Palliation
R. G. Parker, N. A. Janjan, and M. T. Selch

Clinical Target Volumes in Conformal and Intensity Modulated Radiation Therapy
A Clinical Guide to Cancer Treatment
Edited by V. Grégoire, P. Scalliet, and K. K. Ang

Springer

Medical Radiology Diagnostic Imaging and Radiation Oncology

Titles in the series already published

Diagnostic Imaging

Innovations in Diagnostic Imaging
Edited by J. H. Anderson

Radiology of the Upper Urinary Tract
Edited by E. K. Lang

The Thymus - Diagnostic Imaging, Functions, and Pathologic Anatomy
Edited by E. Walter, E. Willich, and W. R. Webb

Interventional Neuroradiology
Edited by A. Valavanis

Radiology of the Pancreas
Edited by A. L. Baert, co-edited by G. Delorme

Radiology of the Lower Urinary Tract
Edited by E. K. Lang

Magnetic Resonance Angiography
Edited by I. P. Arlart, G. M. Bongartz, and G. Marchal

Contrast-Enhanced MRI of the Breast
S. Heywang-Köbrunner and R. Beck

Spiral CT of the Chest
Edited by M. Rémy-Jardin and J. Rémy

Radiological Diagnosis of Breast Diseases
Edited by M. Friedrich and E.A. Sickles

Radiology of the Trauma
Edited by M. Heller and A. Fink

Biliary Tract Radiology
Edited by P. Rossi

Radiological Imaging of Sports Injuries
Edited by C. Masciocchi

Modern Imaging of the Alimentary Tube
Edited by A. R. Margulis

Diagnosis and Therapy of Spinal Tumors
Edited by P. R. Algra, J. Valk, and J. J. Heimans

Interventional Magnetic Resonance Imaging
Edited by J. F. Debatin and G. Adam

Abdominal and Pelvic MRI
Edited by A. Heuck and M. Reiser

Orthopedic Imaging
Techniques and Applications
Edited by A. M. Davies and H. Pettersson

Radiology of the Female Pelvic Organs
Edited by E. K.Lang

Magnetic Resonance of the Heart and Great Vessels
Clinical Applications
Edited by J. Bogaert, A. J. Duerinckx, and F. E. Rademakers

Modern Head and Neck Imaging
Edited by S. K. Mukherji and J. A. Castelijns

Radiological Imaging of Endocrine Diseases
Edited by J. N. Bruneton in collaboration with B. Padovani and M.-Y. Mourou

Trends in Contrast Media
Edited by H. S. Thomsen, R. N. Muller, and R. F. Mattrey

Functional MRI
Edited by C. T. W. Moonen and P. A. Bandettini

Radiology of the Pancreas
2nd Revised Edition
Edited by A. L. Baert
Co-edited by G. Delorme and L. Van Hoe

Emergency Pediatric Radiology
Edited by H. Carty

Spiral CT of the Abdomen
Edited by F. Terrier, M. Grossholz, and C. D. Becker

Liver Malignancies
Diagnostic and Interventional Radiology
Edited by C. Bartolozzi and R. Lencioni

Medical Imaging of the Spleen
Edited by A. M. De Schepper and F. Vanhoenacker

Radiology of Peripheral Vascular Diseases
Edited by E. Zeitler

Diagnostic Nuclear Medicine
Edited by C. Schiepers

Radiology of Blunt Trauma of the Chest
P. Schnyder and M. Wintermark

Portal Hypertension
Diagnostic Imaging-Guided Therapy
Edited by P. Rossi
Co-edited by P. Ricci and L. Broglia

Recent Advances in Diagnostic Neuroradiology
Edited by Ph. Demaerel

Virtual Endoscopy and Related 3D Techniques
Edited by P. Rogalla, J. Terwisscha Van Scheltinga, and B. Hamm

Multislice CT
Edited by M. F. Reiser, M. Takahashi, M. Modic, and R. Bruening

Pediatric Uroradiology
Edited by R. Fotter

Transfontanellar Doppler Imaging in Neonates
A. Couture and C. Veyrac

Radiology of AIDS
A Practical Approach
Edited by J.W.A.J. Reeders and P.C. Goodman

CT of the Peritoneum
Armando Rossi and Giorgio Rossi

Magnetic Resonance Angiography
2nd Revised Edition
Edited by I. P. Arlart, G. M. Bongratz, and G. Marchal

Pediatric Chest Imaging
Edited by Javier Lucaya and Janet L. Strife

Applications of Sonography in Head and Neck Pathology
Edited by J. N. Bruneton in collaboration with C. Raffaelli and O. Dassonville

Imaging of the Larynx
Edited by R. Hermans

3D Image Processing
Techniques and Clinical Applications
Edited by D. Caramella and C. Bartolozzi

Imaging of Orbital and Visual Pathway Pathology
Edited by W. S. Müller-Forell

Pediatric ENT Radiology
Edited by S. J. King and A. E. Boothroyd

Radiological Imaging of the Small Intestine
Edited by N. C. Gourtsoyiannis

Imaging of the Knee
Techniques and Applications
Edited by A. M. Davies and V. N. Cassar-Pullicino

Perinatal Imaging
From Ultrasound to MR Imaging
Edited by Fred E. Avni

Radiological Imaging of the Neonatal Chest
Edited by V. Donoghue

Diagnostic and Interventional Radiology in Liver Transplantation
Edited by E. Bücheler, V. Nicolas, C. E. Broelsch, X. Rogiers, and G. Krupski

Radiology of Osteoporosis
Edited by S. Grampp

Imaging of the Foot and Ankle
Techniques and Applications
Edited by A. M. Davies, R. W. Whitehouse, and J. P. R. Jenkins

Imaging of the Pancreas
Cystic and Rare Tumors
Edited by C. Procacci and A. J. Megibow

Imaging Pelvic Floor Disorders
Edited by C. I. Bartram and J. O. L. DeLancey
Associate Editors: S. Halligan, F. M. Kelvin, and J. Stoker

High Resolution Sonography of the Peripheral Nervous System
Edited by S. Peer and G. Bodner

Radiology Imaging of the Ureter
Edited by F. Joffre, Ph. Otal, and M. Soulie

Interventional Radiology in Cancer
Edited by A. Adam, R. F. Dondelinger, and P. R. Mueller

Imaging and Intervention in Abdominal Trauma
Edited by R. F. Dondelinger

Intracranial Vascular Malformations and Aneurysms
From Diagnostic Work-Up to Endovascular Therapy
Edited by M. Forsting

Springer

MIX
Papier aus verantwortungsvollen Quellen
Paper from responsible sources
FSC® C105338

If you have any concerns about our products,
you can contact us on
ProductSafety@springernature.com

In case Publisher is established outside the EU,
the EU authorized representative is:
Springer Nature Customer Service Center GmbH
Europaplatz 3, 69115 Heidelberg, Germany

Printed by Libri Plureos GmbH
in Hamburg, Germany